Geriatric Medicine and Gerontology: Current Perspectives

Geriatric Medicine and Gerontology: Current Perspectives

Editor: Riley Carter

AMERICAN
MEDICAL PUBLISHERS
www.americanmedicalpublishers.com

AMERICAN
MEDICAL PUBLISHERS
www.americanmedicalpublishers.com

Cataloging-in-Publication Data

Geriatric medicine and gerontology : current perspectives / edited by Riley Carter.
p. cm.
Includes bibliographical references and index.
ISBN 978-1-63927-003-3
1. Geriatrics. 2. Gerontology. 3. Older people--Health and hygiene.
4. Older people--Diseases. I. Carter, Riley.
RC952 .G47 2022
618.97--dc23

American Medical Publishers,
41 Flatbush Avenue,
1st Floor, New York,
NY 11217, USA

ISBN 978-1-63927-003-3 (Hardback)

Contents

Preface IX

Chapter 1 **Exploring Innovative Solutions for Quality of Life and Care of Bed-Ridden Nursing Home Residents through Codesign Sessions** 1
J. van Hoof, M. H. Wetzels, A. M. C. Dooremalen, R. A. Overdiep, M. E. Nieboer, A. M. E. Eyck, P. J. L. M. van Gorkom, E. L. M. Zwerts-Verhelst, S. Aarts, C. Vissers-Luijcks, C. S. van der Voort, M. J. G. A. Moonen, H. A. van de Vrande, C. J. M. L. van Dijck-Heinen and E. J. M. Wouters

Chapter 2 **Clinical Correlates of Awareness for Balance, Function, and Memory: Evidence for the Modality Specificity of Awareness** 15
Megan E. O'Connell, Vanina Dal Bello-Haas, Margaret Crossley and Debra Morgan

Chapter 3 **Learning from "Knocks in Life": Food Insecurity among Low-Income Lone Senior Women** 27
Rebecca J. Green-LaPierre, Patricia L. Williams, N. Theresa Glanville, Deborah Norris, Heather C. Hunter and Cynthia G. Watt

Chapter 4 **Factors affecting Mortality in Elderly Patients Hospitalized for Nonmalignant Reasons** 38
Teslime Ayaz, Serap Baydur Sahin, Osman Zikrullah Sahin, Ozlem Bilir and Halil RakJcJ

Chapter 5 **Differential Item Functioning Related to Age in the Reading Subtest of the Test of Functional Health Literacy in Adults** 45
Raymond L. Ownby and Drenna Waldrop-Valverde

Chapter 6 **Universal Design: A Step toward Successful Aging** 51
Kelly Carr, Patricia L. Weir, Dory Azar and Nadia R. Azar

Chapter 7 **Home-Living Elderly People's Views on Food and Meals** 59
Ellinor Edfors and Albert Westergren

Chapter 8 **The Relationship between Health and Community across Aging Cohorts** 68
Julie Norstrand and Keith T. Chan

Chapter 9 **A Brief Report on the Factor Structure of the Cognitive Measures in the HRS/AHEAD Studies** 78
A. Nayena Blankson and John J. McArdle

Chapter 10 **Robotics to Enable Older Adults to Remain Living at Home** 83
Alan J. Pearce, Brooke Adair, Kimberly Miller, Elizabeth Ozanne, Catherine Said, Nick Santamaria and Meg E. Morris

Chapter 11 **The use of Multiple Correspondence Analysis to Explore Associations between Categories of Qualitative Variables in Healthy Ageing** 93
Patrício Soares Costa, Nadine Correia Santos, Pedro Cunha, Jorge Cotter and Nuno Sousa

Chapter 12 **Cumulative Weight Exposure is Associated with Different Weight Loss Strategies and Weight Loss Success in Adults Age 50 or Above** 105
Martin Sénéchal, Jana Slaght and Danielle R. Bouchard

Chapter 13 **Homeless Aging Veterans in Transition: A Life-Span Perspective** 113
Carla J. Thompson and Nancy L. Bridier

Chapter 14 **Variations in Community Prevalence and Determinants of Recreational and Utilitarian Walking in Older Age** 123
Elizabeth Procter-Gray, Suzanne G. Leveille, Marian T. Hannan, Jie Cheng, Kevin Kane and Wenjun Li

Chapter 15 **The Combined effects of Tai Chi, Resistance Training, and Diet on Physical Function and Body Composition in Obese Older Women** 133
S. A. Maris, D. Quintanilla, A. Taetzsch, A. Picard, J. Letendre, L. Mahler, I. Lofgren, F. Xu and M. J. Delmonico

Chapter 16 **Neighborhood Influences on Late Life Cognition in the ACTIVE Study** 141
Shannon M. Sisco and Michael Marsiske

Chapter 17 **Investment Trait, Activity Engagement, and Age: Independent effects on Cognitive Ability** 152
Sophie von Stumm

Chapter 18 **Active Ageing Level of Older Persons: Regional Comparison** 159
Md. Nuruzzaman Haque

Chapter 19 **Everyday Health among Older People: A Comparison between Two Countries with Variant Life Conditions** 168
Cecilia Fagerström, Lena Sandin Wranker, Zarina Nahar Kabir and Ola Sternäng

Chapter 20 **Risk Factors for Six Types of Disability among the Older People in Thailand in 2002, 2007, and 2011** 176
Pattaraporn Khongboon, Sathirakorn Pongpanich and Robert S. Chapman

Chapter 21 **Novel Combined Training Approach Improves Sleep Quality but does not Change Body Composition in Healthy Elderly Women** 189
Thiago Matheus da Silva Sousa, Bruno Rodrigues, Marco Carlos Uchida, Olivia de Moraes Ruberti, Paulo Adriano Schwingel, Tânia Maria Gaspar Novais, Paula de Lourdes Lauande Oliveira, Fabiano de Jesus Furtado Almeida, Janaína Oliveira Bentivi Pulcherio and Bruno Bavaresco Gambassi

Chapter 22 **Matrix Metalloproteinase-1 Gene Polymorphism Associated with Ultrasound-Assessed Carotid Thickness among Older Adults** 195
Gilberto Santos Morais Junior, Nathalia Oliveira Rodrigues, Adriane Dallanora Henriques, Audrey Cecília Tonet-Furioso, Ciro José Brito, Lucy Oliveira Gomes, Clayton Franco Moraes and Otàvio Toledo Nóbrega

Chapter 23 **The Influence of Video Game Training with and without Subpatelar Bandage in Mobility and Gait Speed on Elderly Female Fallers** 201
Isabela Feitosa de Carvalho, Gianluca Loyolla Montanari Leme and Marcos Eduardo Scheicher

Chapter 24 **Can Driving-Simulator Training Enhance Visual Attention, Cognition, and Physical Functioning in Older Adults?** 207
Mathias Haeger, Otmar Bock, Daniel Memmert and Stefanie Hüttermann

Chapter 25 **Implementation of an Evidence-Based Exercise Program for Older Adults** 216
Richard C. Palmer, Anamica Batra, Chelsie Anderson, Timothy Page, Edgar Vieira and Laura Seff

Chapter 26 **Health Status and Social Networks as Predictors of Resilience in Older Adults Residing in Rural and Remote Environments** 223
Christine McKibbin, Aaron Lee, Bernard A. Steinman, Catherine Carrico, Katelynn Bourassa and Andrea Slosser

Permissions

List of Contributors

Index

Preface

Geriatric medicine is a field of medicine that is concerned with the health care of elderly people. It focuses on maintaining and promoting health by treating diseases and disabilities in older people. There are various subspecialties within geriatric medicine. These include cardiogeriatrics, geriatric dermatology, geriatric neurology, orthogeriatrics, geriatric ophthalmology, geriatric audiology, geriatric pharmacy, etc. Gerontology refers to the study of psychological, cultural and biological aspects of ageing. Gerontological nursing aims to meet the health needs of elderly people. The mental and physical health of an aging population is studied under the domain of geriatric psychology. It focuses on the deteriorating memory, coordination and learning capabilities of individuals in the later stages of life. Such selected concepts that redefine geriatric medicine and gerontology have been presented in this book. The topics covered herein offer the readers new insights in this field. The aim of this book is to present researches that have transformed this discipline and aided its advancement.

This book is a result of research of several months to collate the most relevant data in the field.

When I was approached with the idea of this book and the proposal to edit it, I was overwhelmed. It gave me an opportunity to reach out to all those who share a common interest with me in this field. I had 3 main parameters for editing this text:

1. Accuracy - The data and information provided in this book should be up-to-date and valuable to the readers.

2. Structure - The data must be presented in a structured format for easy understanding and better grasping of the readers

3. Universal Approach - This book not only targets students but also experts and innovators in the field, thus my aim was to present topics which are of use to all

Thus, it took me a couple of months to finish the editing of this book.

I would like to make a special mention of my publisher who considered me worthy of this opportunity and also supported me throughout the editing process. I would also like to thank the editing team at the back-end who extended their help whenever required.

Editor

1

Exploring Innovative Solutions for Quality of Life and Care of Bed-Ridden Nursing Home Residents through Codesign Sessions

J. van Hoof,[1,2] M. H. Wetzels,[3] A. M. C. Dooremalen,[1,4] R. A. Overdiep,[1,2] M. E. Nieboer,[1,2] A. M. E. Eyck,[1,5] P. J. L. M. van Gorkom,[1,4] E. L. M. Zwerts-Verhelst,[1,6] S. Aarts,[2] C. Vissers-Luijcks,[2] C. S. van der Voort,[2] M. J. G. A. Moonen,[2] H. A. van de Vrande,[7] C. J. M. L. van Dijck-Heinen,[1,4] and E. J. M. Wouters[2]

[1]*Fontys University of Applied Sciences, Fontys EGT-Centre for Healthcare and Technology, Dominee Theodor Fliednerstraat 2, 5631 BN Eindhoven, Netherlands*
[2]*Fontys University of Applied Sciences, Institute of Allied Health Professions, Dominee Theodor Fliednerstraat 2, 5631 BN Eindhoven, Netherlands*
[3]*Department of Industrial Design, Eindhoven University of Technology, Den Dolech 2, 5612 AZ Eindhoven, Netherlands*
[4]*Fontys School of People and Health Studies, Fontys University of Applied Sciences, Dominee Theodor Fliednerstraat 2, 5631 BN Eindhoven, Netherlands*
[5]*Fontys University of Applied Sciences, Institute of Information and Communication Technology, Rachelsmolen 1, 5612 MA Eindhoven, Netherlands*
[6]*Fontys University of Applied Sciences, Institute of Human Resource Management and Psychology, Emmasingel 28, 5611 AZ Eindhoven, Netherlands*
[7]*Fontys University of Applied Sciences, Institute of Engineering, Rachelsmolen 1, 5612 MA Eindhoven, Netherlands*

Correspondence should be addressed to J. van Hoof; joost.vanhoof@fontys.nl

Academic Editor: F. R. Ferraro

Bed-ridden nursing home residents are in need of environments which are homelike and facilitate the provision of care. Design guidance for this group of older people is limited. This study concerned the exploration and generation of innovative environmental enrichment scenarios for bed-ridden residents. This exploration was conducted through a combination of participatory action research with user-centred design involving 56 professional stakeholders in interactive work sessions. This study identified numerous design solutions, both concepts and products that are available on the marketplace and that on a higher level relate to improvements in resident autonomy and the supply of technological items and architectural features. The methodology chosen can be used to explore the creative potential of stakeholders from the domain of healthcare in product innovation.

1. Introduction

There are approximately 165,000 persons residing in Dutch long-term care institutions [1]. This is equivalent to around 6% of the Dutch population aged over 65. Nursing homes are often the final place of residence for the occupants. It is, therefore, important that the nursing home is not only a place where care is delivered, but also a place where one lives and feels truly at home making use of a wide array of architectural and technological solutions [1, 2]. This also applies to nursing home residents who are bed-ridden due to their declining health and physical fitness. Bed-ridden residents are confined to bed because of illness or infirmity, especially for a long or indefinite period. This group faces many difficulties in terms of activities of daily living and mobility. The percentage of nursing home residents who are permanently or sometimes bed-ridden was estimated by the Netherlands Institute for Social Research to be about 25%, with the highest percentages found in psychogeriatric wards [3].

To date, not much research has been done on people who are bed-ridden or staying in bed for prolonged periods of time, both in long-term care and hospitals, and how they perceive the space around them. Annemans et al. [4] cited the work by van der Geest and Mommersteeg [5], who concluded that the role of the bed in the general hospital experience is largely under researched: van der Geest and Mommersteeg [5, pages 11-12], *"[t]he importance of the bed for health is obvious [, and] beds in hospitals and other medical settings have a special relation to health. They are tools to organise and realise health recovery. [... Hospital] beds are not meant to provide privacy but rather to allow for optimal access to the patient by clinical staff. Hospital beds are surrounded by medical care providers and medical equipment, facilitating permanent surveillance and the possibility of intervention."* In addition, Annemans et al. [4] showed that persons who are bed-ridden, including patients in hospitals, have a different experience and perception of the space around them. For instance, while being transported through the hospital, the bed is an important mediator between the patient and his or her environment. Annemans et al. [4] concluded that most research on beds and transport seems often restricted to functional matters such as organisation and ergonomics.

The situation in well-facilitated nursing homes, in terms of design and technology, is assumed to be similar to that of hospitals. There are, however, significant differences. As mentioned before, a nursing home is a place of residence, and many residents deal with the consequences of dementia syndrome affecting one's perception and abilities, resulting in further limitations to one's resilience and autonomy [6]. Given the transitions in Dutch long-term care, it is expected that the number of bed-ridden nursing home residents, both with a somatic and a psychogeriatric background will increase. This is a direct consequence of the increased threshold for admission, which is related to one's health status and the ability to carry out activities of daily living independently or with the help of home care services [1]. The way long-term care settings are designed for bed-ridden nursing home residents is different from that for residents who have a degree of mobility. This is because the space bed-ridden residents are able to access and use independently is so limited. This should have implications to the character and appearance of buildings. Apart from guidance concerning fire safety that exists on a national level [7], there is practically no design guidance for this group of residents.

The design and construction of nursing homes are a complex and dynamic process, as the very design of these buildings forces us to consider the technology-human interface directly in terms of living-space, ethics, and social priorities [8]. Moreover, the design process includes a large variety of stakeholders, who further add to the complexity. Technology and architectural solutions can support the well-being, activities of daily living, and quality of life of older residents and support and optimize the work processes of healthcare professionals and professionals in the domain of maintenance [9–11]. In order to meet the needs of future nursing home residents, in particular those who are bed-ridden, new creative and inclusive approaches are needed to come up with new and innovative design solutions. In addition, Annemans et al. [4] mentioned that spatial aspects, for instance, that of the direct environment of a bed-ridden resident, cannot be studied isolated from the activities going on in the spaces considered. Depending on what is happening and who is involved, each experience is shaped differently.

The aim of this study was to explore and generate design concepts for the direct environment of bed-ridden residents of nursing homes through interdisciplinary participatory design sessions. These design concepts should consist of innovative environmental enrichment scenarios, which, in this study, concern the enhancement of a person's physical or social environment.

2. Methodology

2.1. Type of Research Methodology: Participatory Action Research and User-Centred Design. Delhoofen [12] stated that, in the concept phase of a design process, also called the creative phase, creativity is allowed. Creativity, on the one hand, is an important source of inspiration for any dynamic organization, and, on the other hand, it is a capricious and uncontrollable phenomenon which defies any formalization and set of rules. Creativity is hard to manage, even though this is often necessary to find new solutions for complex problems. According to Delhoofen [12], creativity is the ability to ignore restrictive frameworks of thinking and to find original solutions for both everyday and new problems. Creativity is not the same as innovation, but creativity is necessary to come to new innovations. We define innovation as the creation of new products and the improvement and differentiation of products.

A qualitative methodology called participatory action research was used for this study and it provides a tool to deal with the complexity of the design challenge and stakeholder-related needs [13–18]. According to Madden et al. [15], participative frameworks have been shown to be useful in design of environments, and participatory action research has a long history of use with disadvantaged groups in order to assist them to improve their living conditions, with researchers and the research subjects working collaboratively to develop solutions for community issues. Moreover, participatory action research "*involves practitioners as both subjects and co-researchers*" [13, page 613]. According to Howard and Somerville [17], participatory action research is a common methodology among designers but is not often framed as a codesign practice. In this study, participatory action research is integrated with activities of making [19], such as scenario writing and storyboarding, performance ethnography, and collaborative design and prototyping [20–22]. According to Sanders and Stappers [19], "making" is an important activity for designers, as one can bring insights to the surface. Prototypes can play a number of roles, such as evoking a focused discussion in a team, the testing of a hypothesis, and confronting others as the theory is not hidden in abstraction. Other types of visualisation such as scenarios and storyboards can be made to allow designers to experience, test, transform, develop, and complete early ideas [19]. Sanders and Stappers [19, page 6] stated that "*in the very earliest phase of the design process, the focus*

TABLE 1: List of sessions and the characteristics of the participants.

Group/scenario	Group facilitators and assistants	Room	Characteristics of participants	Background
1	CVL	3.416 (single-resident room)	$n = 4$ (1 female, 3 males)	Healthcare real estate, construction and architecture, and environmental health
2	SA, TW	3.417 (single-resident room)	$n = 4$ (3 females, 1 male)	Healthcare, interior design/architecture, and medical beds
3	LZV, LV	3.418 (single-resident room)	$n = 5$ (2 females, 3 males)	Interior design, healthcare, mobility aids, and electrical engineering
4	PG, CH	3.419 (single-resident room)	$n = 5$ (2 females, 3 male)	Healthcare technology, electrical engineering, ICT, and interactive technology
5	EW, JW	3.406 (group room)	$n = 6$ (4 females, 2 males)	Architecture, building physics, healthcare, and medical devices
6	MM, BP	3.406 (group room)	$n = 6$ (3 females, 3 males)	Healthcare, electrical engineering, healthcare technologies, and construction
7	MN, NP, LOW, and CDH	3.403 (group room)	$n = 4$ (1 female, 3 males)	Healthcare, electrical engineering
8			$n = 5$ (1 female, 4 males)	ICT, real estate, healthcare, and electrical engineering
9			$n = 4$ (1 female, 3 males)	Acoustics, assistive technologies, and healthcare
10	CV, AE, TR, and MW	3.408 (group room)	$n = 4$ (3 females, 1 male)	ICT, cleaning, healthcare, and municipality
11			$n = 4$ (2 females, 2 males)	Social innovation, assistive technologies, and technology innovation services
12			$n = 5$ (3 females, 2 males)	Building services, healthcare, electrical engineering, and acoustics
	Total: 10 facilitators, 9 assistants		$n = 56$ (26 females, 30 males)	

is on using making activities for making sense of the future. Here, making activities are used as vehicles for collectively (e.g. designers and codesigners together) exploring, expressing and testing hypotheses about future ways of living." This is why the current study focuses on scenarios and prototyping as a way to think about the future of nursing home care for bed-ridden residents. According to the map of design research by Sanders and Stappers [19, 23], the current research can be classified as user-centred design, more than participatory design research, as end users (bed-ridden nursing home residents) are not included in the study but seen as the subject. At the same time, care professionals, who are end-users of the solutions identified in this study, are also stakeholders who benefit from these solutions. Therefore, we do qualify this study as participatory design research.

2.2. Location, Researchers, and Participants. Work sessions were held in the evening of 18 June 2013 at the educational hospital wards of the Fontys School of People and Health Studies, Eindhoven, the Netherlands (Figure 1). The large nursing rooms (containing 4 beds) were about 50 m^2 and the small rooms (containing 1 bed) 16 m^2 in size. Each session lasted for 120–150 minutes. A total of 12 scenarios were made by 56 participants (Table 1, Figure 2) during the design improvisation sessions that were guided by creative facilitators (10 professional group facilitators and 9 assistant with a background in industrial design and creative techniques). All session facilitators and assistants had been briefed about the procedures and were provided with a manual and an instruction guide prior to the start of the sessions. The role for the session facilitator was to stimulate creativity, supporting the creative process, and to obtain a maximum of variety in responses and input. In the group rooms, session facilitators and assistants supported the various groups of participants. Apart from these facilitators and assistants, JVH, RO, and AD managed the overall processes of the sessions, supported the supply of materials, and collected written documentation. The participants of this study had a mixed background in healthcare, design, housing, and technology (Table 1).

2.3. Procedure and Assignment. At the start of each collaborative design session, a session facilitator welcomed the participants and explained the procedure. Informed consent, covering the permission to use of all written, videographic, and photographic materials, was obtained from the participants at the start of the session. The participants were invited to consider the beds in the rooms as actual nursing home beds and to enhance the environment with materials presented to them in a shared "material library," including paper and card board, sticky tape and ropes, balloons, plastic covers, and various other do-it-yourself materials. These materials allowed the participants with a high degree of freedom to shape the modifications to the bed and use their imagination. The participants were told that the new scenarios and concepts mattered, not the level of perfection of the results or the execution of the modifications. The 12 scenarios

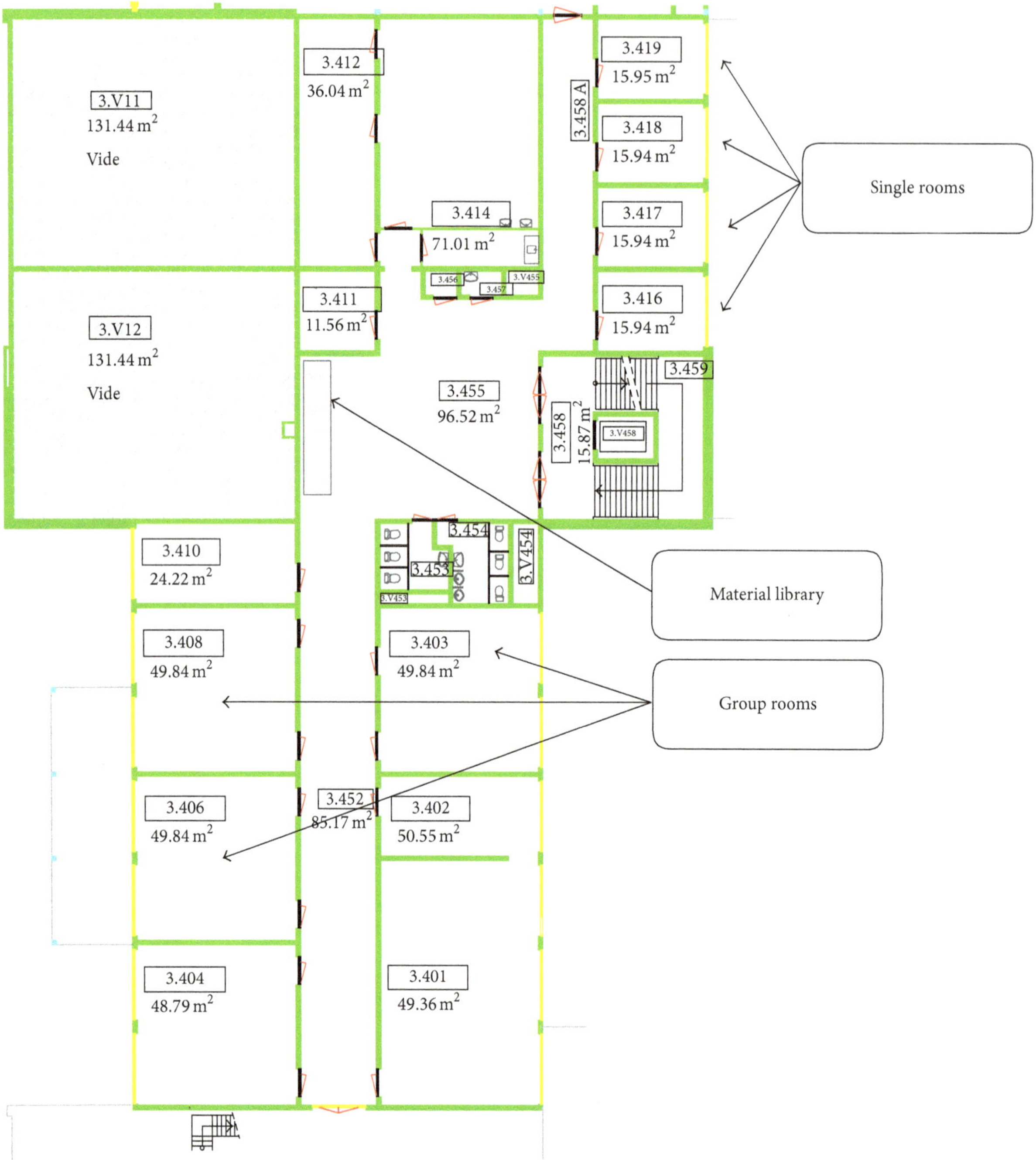

FIGURE 1: Layout of the rooms at the Fontys School of People and Health Studies, Eindhoven, in which the sessions took place.

that the participants developed were based on a persona (a fictional character) of a nursing home resident [21, 22, 24, 25]. Triantafyllakos et al. [21] stated that fictional characters have been used as user representatives, either substituting actual users or supporting idea generation. Their foremost objective is to facilitate the identification of user needs and goals and to support the development of detailed and comprehensive scenarios [21]. The interdisciplinary approach to the sessions was used to minimize stereotypical thinking [26]. Context scenarios were defined as a short story, which represented the use of the bed environment by the resident. The scenarios were represented by making actual changes and adaptations to the beds and the direct surroundings using a wide range of materials, which symbolized actual environmental modifications (Figure 2). At the end of the session, the personas were enacted by participants from each group who served as proxy residents (Figure 2). As creativity cannot be forced upon participants, it was important to create optimal conditions in which new ideas can come to the fore. For creativity to thrive, participants had to be comfortable, motivated, and stimulated through challenging goals [12]. Triantafyllakos et al. [21] found that design alter

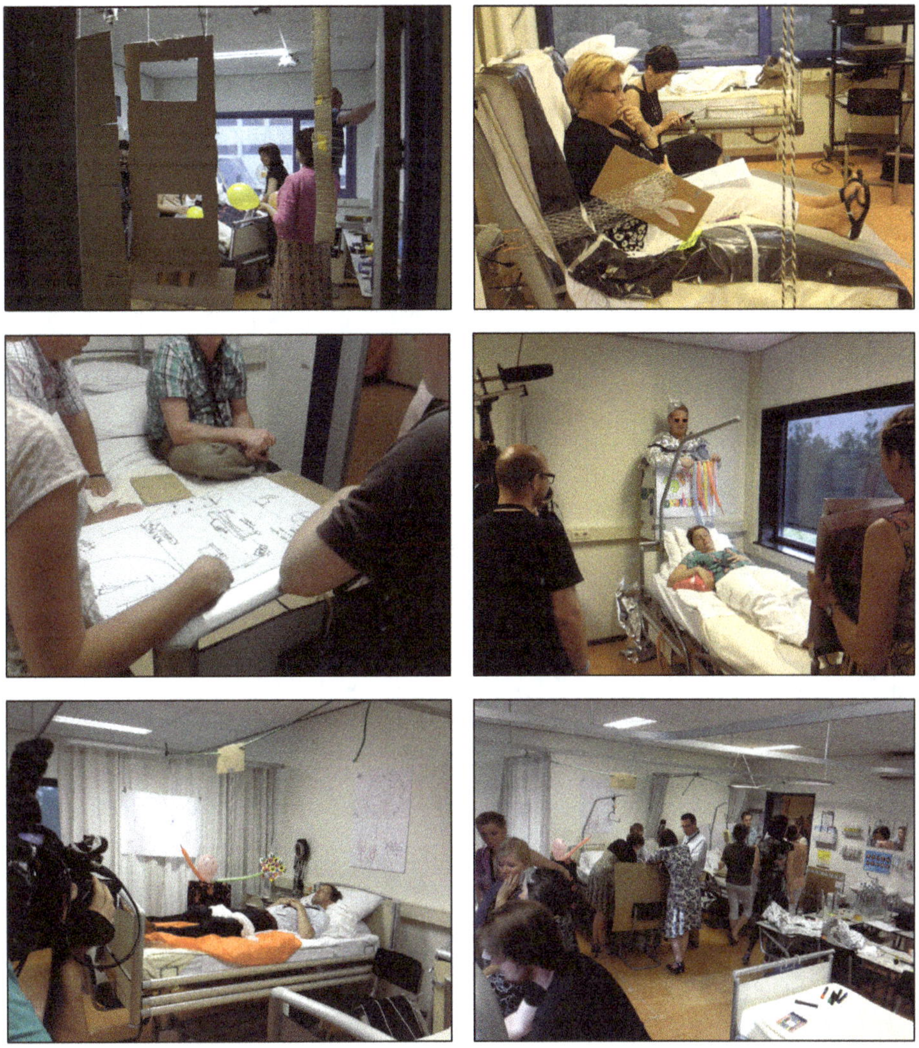

Figure 2: Working together to generate ideas, followed by the enactment and filming of the scenarios.

egos technique liberated the majority of participants from the fear of straightforwardly exposing themselves, supported and enhanced their introspection, stimulated their creativity, and helped to establish an informal and constructive atmosphere throughout the design sessions.

2.4. Data Analysis. The scenarios of the sessions were each documented on paper by the participants and filmed by a professional camera crew for further analysis. This is in line with the narrative videotaping approach to "storytelling laboratory" described by Bate and Robert [22]. The results of all 12 scenarios and the rationale behind each one of them (combination of a context scenario and requirements analysis) are presented as case studies containing potential design innovations that can be thought-through and developed in more detail for implementation in the nursing home setting. The transcripts of the scenarios were analysed in conjunction with the videos, in order to also include visual data. The data were analysed based on the six phases by Braun and Clarke [27] and in conjunction with the steps of content analysis by Krippendorff [28].

First, the transcripts were each read in their entirety. Then, they were read a second time to develop open codes identifying design solutions. Open coding concerns the process of unravelling all of the collected data into fragments or codes. Thereafter, codes were added to the transcripts. Similar codes and quotes were clustered and labelled, and themes emerged from this process. Together, the research team organised the codes and clustered them into smaller thematic groups. The final themes were grouped in amalgamation with graphical material from the films that reflected aspects of these themes, which is a form of axial coding. Thereafter, these themes were reviewed and then defined and named. These themes are made up of design concepts and solutions, which in turn could also be clustered in major themes, that is, to which level of human functioning they relate. Researcher triangulation was applied during the entire process; for example, separate analyses of the scenarios were conducted by two of the authors (J. van Hoof, A. M. C. Dooremalen).

This guarantees that the data are interpreted independently and from different perspectives. A method triangulation was applied due to the use of both written scenarios and video images.

3. Results

The 12 scenarios contained suggestions that can be used for improving the living situation of bed-ridden nursing home residents or for changing product design and are given in the Appendix. Figure 3 shows a composition of the enactments of each of these scenarios. The main themes which emerged from the analysis of the written and video materials are shown in Table 2. A high degree of convergence and data saturation has been found. The interdisciplinary character of the groups (and the interaction between participants) and the mixed location in both single-person and group rooms contributed to the richness of the scenarios and the data. Some of the themes found in this study are overarching (such as the use of tablet computers), whereas smaller themes are an elaboration of the functionalities one should use the tablet computer for (for instance, opening curtains).

The most frequently mentioned theme (11 out of 12) is the use of virtual and interactive walls for displaying pictures, television programs, videos, and materials from the past. This theme is followed by the possibility to have online contacts and to chat with relatives, friends, and fellow residents (8 out of 12). Seven out of twelve scenarios deal with the use of touch screens and tablet computers for the control of the space around them or to place orders for meals and plan the care tasks throughout the day and to control the environment such as curtains. Lights and luminaires, sounds, and music are mentioned (7 out of 12) as important areas for development when designing nursing home environments, for creating a proper atmosphere, for functionality, in order to stimulate day and night rhythms, and in order to make people feel more at ease through music and sounds of nature. The so-called transformer beds, beds that can change their shape into a chair, wheelchair, or bathtub are mentioned by 7 out of 12 scenarios and reflect new products on the market place: beds which can bend and turn and become like real chairs in which residents/patients can sit upright. These developments go together with the desire for smart mattress and smart beds measuring vital signs (6 out of 12) and special mattresses that improve comfort and prevent decubitus (6 out of 12). Seven out of twelve scenarios give attention to the free choice of food and drinks and the need for minibars and coffee corners where visitors can get something to drink. This should contribute to a sense of home and coziness.

Autonomy is an overarching or major theme, which encompasses the freedom and being in control of residents, which is reflected in the choice for meals, planning care activities, being in control of people entering the room, and so on. The smaller themes constituting this overarching theme are numerous. Robotics is a theme mentioned by 3 out of 12 scenarios, mainly in relation to transfers and delivering meals. Homelikeness and atmosphere are another overarching theme, of which smaller themes as flowers, furniture for relatives, and picture frames could be an elaboration.

4. Discussion and Conclusions

4.1. Reflection on Identified Design Solutions. The twelve scenarios resulting from this study contained numerous design ideas and solutions that can be used for improving the quality of life for bed-ridden nursing home residents. In this round of workshops, there was a lot of focus on technologies improving the autonomy of residents and for improving communication capabilities. Overall, the minor and major themes can be on different levels. For instance, tablet computers are things or items and are named as design solutions, whereas the autonomy relates to a personal experience or a human state. The computer tablets, however, can be used for achieving autonomy. The definition of environmental enrichment used in this study, which is the enhancement of a person's physical or social environment, allows for themes that relate to different levels. Various technological solutions were identified, which, apart from the aforementioned tablet computers and touchscreens, include assistive and medical technology such as special beds containing sensors, architectural modifications as windows, and building services solutions including heating, ventilation, and air-conditioning systems and smart home technologies. Although some of the design solutions proposed are futuristic, the vast majority is already available on the marketplace. These innovations are not yet implemented on a large scale in practice, and, therefore, they are still innovative.

Concept generation was at the centre of the study. The goal was to come up with innovative and conceptual design concepts which can be developed into implementable solutions. This study welcomed five types of innovation as distinguished by Delhoofen [12], namely, new products, product improvements, product differentiation, service innovations, and process innovations. The most important aspects of improvement to be achieved with innovations are savings, improvements of functionalities, and extensions of functionalities [12]. Whether the identified solutions can in fact contribute to improvements to healthcare is beyond the scope of the current work.

4.2. Applicability of the Methodology. The chosen approach to this study, participatory action research, has been used within the domain of public health care before. Its combination with user-centred design approaches, however, is relatively new within the domain of healthcare. A small number of scientific publications applying these methodologies within the domain of healthcare and technology are being published (for instance, [29, 30]). The current method had been shown successful in identifying aspects of healthcare facilities which are necessary for the quality of care and life of bed-ridden nursing home residents and for obtaining convergence in design solutions. The creative methodology is very suitable for bringing together people with different backgrounds and quality of knowledge. Cooperation in healthcare innovation is not uncommon in practice. Participatory action research aims to obtain "*knowledge and action directly useful to people, and also to empower people through the process of constructing and using their own knowledge*" [31, p. 225]. The methodology could, therefore, also be applied within healthcare settings

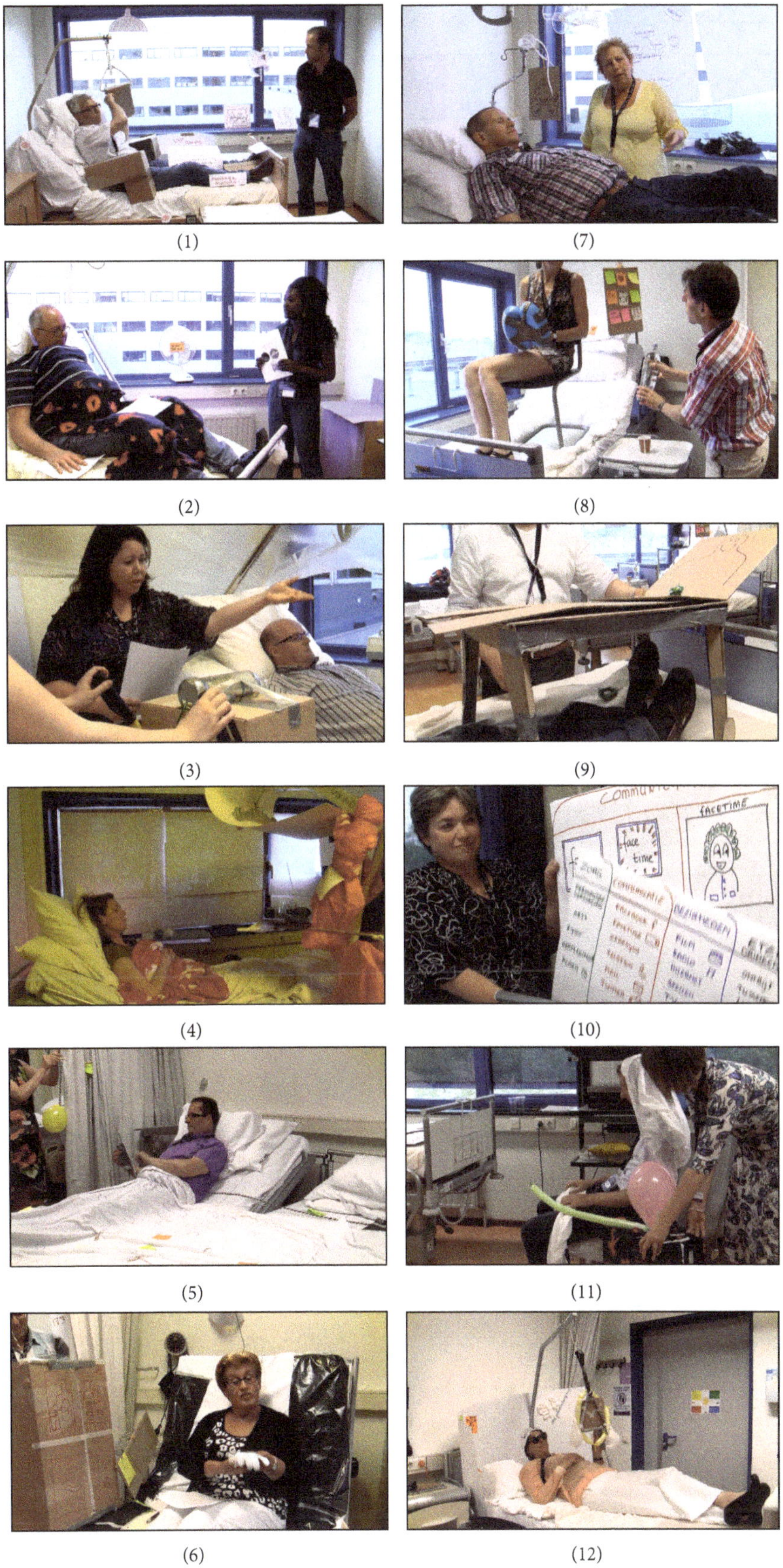

FIGURE 3: A composition of the twelve scenarios written and enacted by the participants.

TABLE 2: Themes or design concepts emerging from the scenarios.

Themes	Scenario
Touchscreens, control panels, and tablet computers	1, 2, 5, 6, 8, 11, and 12
Transformer beds (into chairs and baths)	1, 3, 4, 6, 8, 9, and 12
Sensors in bed for measuring vital functions and analysis	1, 2, 3, 7, and 9
Massage mattress of modified mattress (decubitus)	1, 2, 3, 5, and 9
Arm rests	1
Virtual, interactive walls (displaying pictures, films), and picture frames	1, 2, 3, 4, 5, 6, 7, 8, 9, 11, and 12
Home wall with personal belongings	1
Low sill window	1
Sensors responding to movement of arms and legs for control	1, 6
Odour box	1, 7
Mobile furniture for relatives	1, 2, and 12
Workplace for relatives with ICT and Wi-Fi	1, 2
Moveable walls (privacy)	2
Flowers and plants	2, 3, and 5
Food and drinks services (for relatives)	2, 4, 5, 6, 8, 10, and 11
Devices and screens for online contacts (voice calls), chatting	2, 5, 6, 8, 9, 10, 11, and 12
Own choice for interior design	2
Wake-up call and good morning service	2, 4, 6
Atmosphere and homelikeness	2, 5, 7, 8, and 12
Moving experience ceiling	3
Lights, luminaires, sounds, and music	3, 4, 7, 8, 9, 11, and 12
Control buddy	3, 9
Mobile shower	3
Two-person bed	3, 5
Medical equipment unobtrusive	3
Robotics	4, 10, and 11
Smart window	4
Operable curtains	5, 6
Smart wardrobe	5
Doorbells, entrance control, and do-not-disturb button	5, 6, and 8
Mobile washbasin	5
Skylight	5
Mattress with temperature control/HVAC	5, 12
Bionic arms	6
Self-repetitive videos for restlessness	7
Wind machine	7
3D projector	7
Technology for sexual support	9
Planning assistant	10, 11
Control of technology based on eye movement	10
Need for face-to-face contact	11
Freedom to live where you want/mobile environment	12
Information glasses	12
Smart hat: control device for brain activity to steer locomotion	12

in order to think about improving products, environments, and services and, most of all, to involve nondesigning professionals in a design process. In this methodology, all participants have a role to play, whether it is a designer or engineer or a healthcare specialist. It is, therefore, a truly inclusive design process, but inclusive design in this sense does not pertain to inclusive design or design-for-all. In addition, the participants working in commerce can use the methodology to improve products being designed and produced within their own enterprises. The methodology can also be used for educational practices, for instance, in multi- or interdisciplinary classes [32, 33], for a large spectrum of design challenges, as is currently being done.

4.3. Reflection on the Methodology of the Study. In this study, older persons, nursing home residents, and actual bed-ridden persons were not included in the creative sessions. This means that any solution that comes to the fore does not necessarily reflect the actual needs of older, bed-ridden people. At the same time, the participating healthcare professionals could provide a foundation for the design solutions based on their practical knowledge. In future sessions, one could think of including informal or family carers or professional actors trained in playing nursing home residents, in order to obtain more accurate scenarios. The current cohort of participants, as was discussed in the methodology section, could have based their scenarios on stereotypes of bed-ridden residents or could have portrayed them as somewhat active and independently functioning older people, which does not match with the actual health status and abilities of bed-ridden nursing home residents. Moreover, the methodology chosen may lead to scenarios that are enacted in too playful a manner.

Another potential weakness of the study is that participants are not aware of all innovations in the field, of those that appear on the market or are being researched in research and development (R&D) facilities. This may give a skewed perspective on the scenarios, which are either too optimistic or somewhat out-of-date. In the current study, scenarios are enacted using simple, low fidelity prototypes. This also means that concepts are not being developed into real innovative products, which can, in turn, be tested in the nursing home. This means that no field-evidence is being gathered, although the scenarios themselves are based on practice-based evidence. The evidence-based and performance-based designs (van Hoof et al. [34]) are becoming important tools in optimizing the spatial layout and interior design of healthcare facilities. Marquardt and Motzek [35, page 116] stated that "*because architects and designers are often not trained in research methods, they may feel somewhat overwhelmed by the terms used in the description of the methodology of scientific papers. Therefore, when designing healthcare facilities, they may not feel confident discussing the evidence available from research studies with members of the medical professions, who often display a profound knowledge of research methods.*" When evidence of certain measures is absent, or when new innovations need to be designed, a qualitative approach based on performance ethnography and collaborative design may be a good step in exchanging ideas and come up with new innovative design solutions. The duration of an optimal session should be researched. In the current study, the 2–2.5-hour period was considered to be sufficient for writing the scenario, building the scene, and enacting the scenario.

4.4. Conclusive Remarks. In conclusion, the chosen methodology may help practitioners identify potential solutions that exist to support the challenges in nursing home care. Moreover, the results of this study can be used to adequately design the private rooms and bed environments of nursing home residents in accordance with personal preferences and needs and to stimulate innovations in product design which may become available on the marketplace in the future.

Appendix

Overview of Scenarios

Scenario 1 (3416). This room of the future revolves around the word "contact," as we think that residents of the future value being in touch with the world around them and that residents make choices on their own and have some degree of autonomy. The resident has a touch screen to control the room. As the resident will be in bed most of the times, this is an important feature of the room. The bed can be transformed into a chair. The bed is equipped with sensors to monitor the vital functions of the residents, such as heart rate, muscle tension, and blood pressure. The mattress can provide the resident with a massage. There are arm rests to the bed which are foldable and which allow the resident to sit down comfortably. The windows are positioned somewhat lower, so that people can look outside from the bed which is positioned next to the window. There is a seat next to the bed for relatives, so they can be close and make contact. In addition, there is a virtual wall on the opposite side of the bed, stretching across the wall from left to right, projecting images from the past, a holiday movie, or documentary about nature. This enables the resident to be in touch with things from the past as well as the present. In addition, the room is equipped with a virtual ceiling. As the resident is in such a position, lying on his back, looking towards the ceiling, there is actually something to experience on this ceiling. Moreover, there is an "odour box" installed, which emits scents from freshly baked bread, nature, and the sea. All senses should be stimulated, in order to get a complete experience of the world around the resident. In addition to the virtual wall and ceiling, there is the so-called "home wall." This wall offers space for personal belongings, ranging from books to a fish bowl, from picture frames to a plant or alarm clock. All furniture in the room is mobile and has been programmed in order to meet the needs of the visitors, of professionals, of the resident, as well as a day and night position. The resident has a freedom of choice if he wants to leave the room with his bed and drive towards the common living room. The furniture responds to software which can be operated through the touch screen from the bed and will move aside. There will be a family arrangement of the furniture or a work arrangement. It is also important to have a section in the room allocated to relatives, where they can sit down and work on their laptop as a flexible workplace. The one to one contact can sometimes be replaced by knowing that a relative is near, working in your room.

Scenario 2 (3417). Welcome to nursing home "All-I-Ever-Wanted." Mrs. Elisabeth Smith is 90 years old and has been living in the nursing home since a couple of months. She has dementia, morbid obesity (weighing 190 kg), diabetes, decubitus, and problems with her blood pressure. She has four children and 12 grandchildren, and five years ago she has lost her husband. They have moved abroad, but via a large screen in her room, she can keep track of their whereabouts and make digital contact with people far away. The room should create an atmosphere of safety and security, as well as homeliness, and with great lighting to create a healing environment. In the morning, the voice of her son living abroad wakes up Mrs. Smith. Whenever her children come to visit, they have to come from afar, and, therefore, a visit needs to be pleasant. Mrs. Smith values atmosphere and hospitality. Therefore, she has a small coffee corner in her room, which can be used by relatives. There are also small stools available next to the bed for children to sit on. Mrs. Smith can control and interact with movement program through moving her feet and hands and touch panels attached to her bed. This enables her to make use of the Internet, listen to the radio, and use the free Wi-Fi facilities in her room, together with a laptop for children. An LED panel behind her back provides feedback to her actions. Mrs. Smith can choose and select/program her own paintings of her liking. She is allowed to consult an interior architect in order to alter her room and change colours of the walls. The indoor climate can also be controlled according to personal preferences. The LED lighting and odours in the room can also be controlled from her bed. Mrs. Smith can alter the atmosphere of the room by changing the colours and shapes of the walls from her bed. A board placed below the bed monitors the vital functions of Mrs. Smith. As an additional feature, the bed has armrests. The bed itself is made of soft material and is positioned in an active posture: looking out over the entrance of the room. Mrs. Smith can turn the bed 360 degrees. This makes Mrs. Smith livelier and makes her more approachable to guests. Moreover, she herself can enjoy all features the room has to offer. She has a number of mobile panels in the room which can be lowered or raised in order to match privacy needs if other people are around. There are also flowers attached to the ceiling for Mrs. Smith to enjoy when she is lying on her bed. The digital era and independence are two key words of the concept.

Scenario 3 (3418). Welcome to Peter's "experience room." Peter is bed-ridden due to muscle problems. The most striking feature is the graciously moving ceiling. All around Peter, materials can change colour and shape. This ceiling can simulate various weather conditions through mild movement (for instance, through the wind), light, and sounds. Moreover, films can be played. Peter is confined to bed day-long, which always makes him be in the same environment. This concept, which can be operated through a Buddy, can give Peter the possibility to change his environment. The ceiling is connected to an interactive wall. This interactive wall has the same function as the ceiling. Through the interactive wall, Peter can make contact with his relatives and with Peter's personal Buddy. The Buddy reminds Peter of important personal things but can also provide counselling in the use of the system itself and other things. Peter's bed is equipped with numerous sensors for, among others, temperature, pressure, skin condition, movement, blood values, and sleep rhythm. Whenever there is something wrong, an alarm is sent to the tablet computer of the carer, who can then take action. There are plants near the bed. In the room, there is a mobile shower, which Peter can page whenever he wants to be showered. The shower turns the bed into a true Jacuzzi. This is enabled through a new innovative material the bed is made of, which can hold water, but which also drains the water with one push on the button. Thereafter, the bed can again be used as a bed. The bed also has various massage functions to alleviate Peter's physical pains. Whenever Peter's partner visits him, the bed can easily be extended into a two-person king-size bed. All medical devices are hidden away in the environment, in order for Peter not to be confronted with the fact he is residing in a nursing home all of the time.

Scenario 4 (3419). The resident lies in bed and slowly wakes up. An intelligent system called Service TV in the room recognizes and detects that the resident has woken up and adjusts to the room to the morning situation. The system can be used for communicating with care professionals and a virtual nursing aide. The system activates the sound of birds singing: this helps the resident to slowly wake up. Somewhat later, the system activates the Smart Window, a system which projects dynamic virtual images on an existing window, such as that of a forest with birds flying around and squirrels running from one tree to another. This could also be images from the former neighbourhood, which moves along with the direction of gazing by Mrs. Saunders. The intelligent system seeks contact with the resident when it detects more movement in the morning. "Good morning Mrs. Saunders," says the system, asking "Did you sleep well?" Mrs. Saunders talks to the smart system, which is a display at the end of the bed and asks the system to switch on the lights. The system asks if Mrs. Saunders wants to finish the movie she was watching the other night or to listen to some music. Mrs. Saunders opts for the music so she can wake up slowly. The system asks if Mrs. Saunders wants to have breakfast and tells, upon request, what is on today's menu. The screen displays the selection. Shortly after, breakfast is served. The bed is moving in an upright position so Mrs. Saunders is in a more convenient position to eat. James, the service robot, serves breakfast. This robot can also be used for transfers of the resident.

Scenario 5 (3406). Once upon a time, there was the nursing home of the future. Mr. Stevens is a resident of a somatic ward. One day, he wakes up and takes his touch screen device. His bed is moving into the upright position and Mr. Stevens opens the curtains. He sees the sunshine outside. The skylight above the bed can also be opened to let in a refreshing breeze. The touch screen can also be used to call a care professional, both by pushing a button or by speech. When the care professional stops by, she rings the doorbell and Mr. Stevens can open the door through his touch panel. He can see through the window who is in front of the door or through the camera of the touch screen. Mr. Stevens needs to get dressed, and his wardrobe is full of clothes. On the touch screen panel, he can browse through his outfits and let the care professional know what he would like to wear. Before getting dressed, Mr. Stevens need to be washed first. Because he is in a two-person king-sized bed, he can automatically move to the side with the help of a conveyor belt inside the bed. There, the care professional has better access to him. Mr. Stevens can also control a mobile wash basin next to his bed, which has sensors to dispense soap and make the water run. If Mr. Stevens prefers to be showered, the conveyor belt can move him to the other side of the mattress and place him onto a mobile shower seat. This seat can take him to the bathroom. Mr. Stevens is about to have visitors today, and their arrival is announced on the touch screen. Through the one-way-mirror-window, he sees a worker from the tax services standing in front. He leaves the door shut. His daughter, however, is most welcome. She brings flowers, which she puts in a vase next to a number of seats, put in place for visitors. Together, they go watch pictures, which his daughter has uploaded online, on a large screen hanging from the ceiling. The care professional joins in. Many functionalities are displayed on this screen, and together, Mr. Stevens and his daughter order a meal. The daughter wants to stay for the night, so the double bed comes in handy. The bed can be split into two separate beds. There are also movement sensors in the bed, also partly to prevent falls, so care professionals are alarmed and can have a look. The bed and mattress have temperature control. The bed frame itself is made of materials that give it a homelike appearance. Some of the technologies below the bed are covered with curtains and wood. The bed is preprogrammed in order to take on certain positions. The mattress itself makes movements to prevent decubitus. All measures contribute to the well-being of Mr. Stevens.

Scenario 6 (3406). "Let's have a look at what time it is. It's time to get up!" Mrs. Johnson is alarmed by her computer screen. She presses the do-not-disturb button. The bed moves into the upright position. With a swaying movement of her arms, Mrs. Johnson can open the curtains and let the sunshine in, as technology recognises the movement and turns it into action. "When I look outside, I have a beautiful view, and hopefully, good weather." Mrs. Johnson would like a cup of coffee, and a mobile drink machine/minibar pops up next to her bed. She orders breakfast via her tablet computer. On a large display hanging above her, Mrs. Johnson can see the views from the old pub she used to visit, the forest, the street in which the resident used to live, the home of friends, and even the evening news. This allows Mrs. Johnson to stay connected to the daily life of the old environment. In case the resident wants to lie down again, the screen can be raised once more so that it is visible from all corners. The screen itself can be controlled via a tablet computer which is at arm's length and has two sides, one side for functioning care and the other side for leisure and relaxation and leisure, including chatting. If Mrs. Johnson wants to go outside, the bed can be easily changed into a (wheel)chair. The middle piece of the bed can be disconnected, and the side frames remain standing. This allows Mrs. Johnson to ride outside independently. Taking a bath is difficult for Mrs. Johnson as he does not have sufficient strength in his arms. Therefore, bionic arms are put in place. These can be worn by Mrs. Johnson in order to be able to wash herself. In order to offer the best of the best to Mrs. Johnson there is a minibar and a combination oven next to the bed. Visitors can be catered with foods and drinks, which can be served by Mrs. Johnson herself.

Scenario 7 (3403). Anthony is a resident with late-stage dementia. He does not recognize himself and cannot express what he wants and needs. Anthony often gets restless and frightened. Therefore, a sensor has been placed onto the mattress, which registers the changes in behavioural patterns. The mattress is equipped with "pick sensors," which monitor hand picking movements being made onto the mattress. From analysis from Anthony's personal data, from a period before his late-stage dementia, we know what makes him more relaxed and at ease. One of these things are the personal videos about the family, which are displayed on a large screen, as well as Skype and music, in order to provide a sense of home. Next to the bed, there is a picture frame with digital pictures which shift from one picture to the other, whenever Anthony wants to see pictures of his wife and children. The music is tuned onto the mood of Anthony and the atmosphere. Because it is not desirable to call relatives ten times or more at night, because Anthony may be restless, there is a self-repetitive video image on display, which matches the needs of Anthony. In addition, there are numerous sensors in the mattress which measure vital functions, such as heart rate, blood pressure, muscle tension, respiration, and the amount of medication levels in one's blood. The sensors are self-learning. As you can see, Anthony is getting restless now, and that means his muscle tension is increasing, as well as his heart rate. We then know that he needs some medication to calm down. There are special luminaires mounted to the ceiling above Anthony, for projecting daylight, evening light, and so on. There is also a 3D projector, which has made images of Anthony's former home, living room, and bed room, which are projected onto the wall to make Anthony feel more at ease. There is also an odour dispenser, which emits the scent of Anthony's wife. Sounds of the sea, nature, and the city can be used to further make Anthony feel more at ease. There is also a wind machine to create a nice breeze. With this surround-system, the 3D projector becomes a 4D experience.

Scenario 8 (3403). Mary-Ann has chosen to wake up a little earlier because of television recordings. She put on her best dress, had her hair dressed, and put on her make-up. Of course, she needed help with this because she cannot do all this independently. To Mary-Ann, it is important to be the boss-in-her-own-bed. This means that through the use of a wide range of technological applications, she can control and decide about the things around her. For instance, via a control panel she can decide to open or shut curtains, watch television, and communicate with relatives or friends. Having a sense of autonomy is important to Mary-Ann. Mary-Ann also values the fact that her bed is in fact a "better-bed," a bed which can be transformed into a chair. "If anyone else can have a seat, why can't Mary-Ann?" This would call for additional adaptations, as Mary-Ann needs assistance with movement and the correction of her body. The new bed enables Mary-Ann to participate in daily activities in a sedentary way. Mary-Ann also cherishes things around her which contribute to the atmosphere, such as lighting, which can be either romantic, or functional for work processes, or suitable for the night so Mary-Ann can go sleep. She can control the lighting herself with the touch screen. In addition, when Mary-Ann is hungry, she wants a proper meal to be delivered. After ordering a meal via the screen, she is in touch with the catering service. When the meal is delivered, she asks the waiter to enter the room. Mary-Ann is also the boss-around-the-bed. Mary-Ann decided who she lets into her room. It is important to create a space in which Mary-Ann feels pleasant. Therefore, a virtual environment is created, in which Mary-Ann can call for functionalities which match her emotions. Although she now lives in a nursing home, she wants to be in touch with her former living room. With one push on a button, her former living room is projected around her, together with her own grandchildren. This makes her feel pleasant and comfortable. She can also bring the outdoor world indoors and see the outdoor weather displayed around her. Pictures, souvenirs, and hobbies can be displayed as well.

Scenario 9 (3403). The bed itself is made for persons with decubitus and is designed in such a way that it can be used to easily turn residents around in bed. This bed is full of sensors which can measure and detect body functions and health status and which should take actions to turn and move residents around the mattress. Moreover, the bed has a function that it can turn from a horizontal stretcher into an upright position, just like a wheelchair so people can easily get out of bed. The bed itself has wheels so it can be moved around. The bed can take action when it is needed for the health of the resident. Mr. Janssen is in this bed. He has a half-sided paralysis due to a stroke, and he has mild dementia. The first modification is related to odours: when these escape from the resident, or when others smell odours (urine, faeces, and wounds) on the corridor, this is considered to be unpleasant. An odour neutraliser should help stop the spread of unwanted odours. An "odour ring" can be placed near wounds to absorb the smell of wounds. There is an interactive ceiling, with projections of Dutch skies full of clouds, which has an effect on the circadian rhythm of the resident, with light being emitted that changes in intensity over the course of the day. Moreover, music and scents are being released by the ceiling. A suspended interactive multimedia screen (music, television, and chatting) is near the foot-end of the bed, which enables the resident to have contact with other rooms in which activities take place. This screen can be controlled via the "bunny toy." Residents can use this toy-like rabbit to steer the system via voice-control. The resident can thus give spoken commands. The bunny can be used for petting, it is easy to clean, and, in the future, it could be developed for sexual activities in combination with the screen.

Scenario 10 (3408). Mrs. Fontys has turned 50 years old and has been given a balloon flight for her birthday. This flight ended in a personal drama, in which Mrs. Fontys has got an injury high up in the spine. For two weeks, she has been in a rehabilitation ward of a nursing home, where staff is working hard on her recovery. Mrs. Fontys can still move her arms and head, but she no longer has any strength in her hands. The rehabilitation ward has been opened recently, and this offers a number of options. Today, Mrs. Fontys wakes up at 9 o'clock, and, fortunately, she has slept well last night. With the blink of her eyes she calls her Care4You: a large computerised screen. The options provided can be used throughout the day. First, Mrs. Fontys selects care services. On the online time line, she can select a number of times of day during which she receives help, for instance, when breakfast is served, when she is washed, and when she needs to go to the physiotherapist. She receives immediate feedback from the system when care professionals are available to stop by. Because it takes a while for breakfast to be served, Mrs. Fontys chooses on the care4You system to have a cup of coffee served. Bert, the catering robot, stops by and serves coffee via a straw. While enjoying her coffee, she wants to check how her daughter Karin is doing during her test week at school. Via the Care4You system, a connection with communication software is being made.

Scenario 11 (3408). Roderick wakes up and activates his tablet computer. Via a screen, which is projected on the wall, he can be woken up by his grandchild or a care professional. Via another functionality on his tablet, Roderick indicates he wants to go to the toilet. A robot comes to the rescue and is being used to help Roderick go to the toilet. The robot operates a hoist to lift Roderick out of bed and further guides him to the bathroom. The tablet computer can stay somewhere near the bed, as Roderick can control the robot via a Wi-Fi-operated voice control. When Roderick returns from his sanitary break, the robot helps him out of his bed. Roderick is now seated in a chair, ready for something to eat. Roderick takes the tablet computer again and activates a room service app and makes his selection for breakfast. Shortly after, breakfast is being served by a nursing aide. Apart from using technology, face-to-face contact with a care professional, who physically enters the room, remains very important. After his meal, Roderick seeks contact with the outside world. He makes online contact to his daughter's kitchen via the projection screen. This family is also finishing breakfast. Roderick and his family are exchanging the latest news. The projection screen also allows Roderick to seek contact with the common living area of the nursing home, where residents flock together, with whom he can exchange news. The projection screen also serves as a television to watch the news. These news items also serve as input for conversations. In the evening, Roderick is ready to go sleep. The robot is again activated, for instance, to go get a glass of water. Moreover, the robot can detect nocturnal restlessness or help Roderick go to the bathroom again. If Roderick has the strength to try walk around on his own, there is a night orientation light strip on the floor that helps guide him to the bathroom.

Scenario 12 (3408). Barbara cannot function without the help of her tablet computer. She has a critical character and wants to be in control and take care of her own business. Sometimes, she wants to watch television. When pressing her tablet computer, a television screen is lowered from the ceiling. At other times, she wants to go to the park or play cards. Barbara lives in iShell Park II, a cluster of three dwellings which are laid out in a circle, and which can be mutually exchanged for residence. Her personal iShell, a digitalised and mobile environment, is equipped with a large number of facilities: homeliness, a personalised ventilation and temperature control system, a comfortable chair for visitors, sound absorbing surroundings, and a music system, and she can steer around flexibly. These facilities can be controlled via the tablet computer. Her "information glasses" keep her up to date with the latest gossips. The multifunctional iWheel can take her "personal shell" out to the park. This is actually stimulated through the iShell meet and greet, so she can be in touch with others. Via the ShellBook app, Barbara stays in touch with her fellow residents through digital means. The iWheel is multifunctional and is, for instance, equipped with an agenda so she knows when her activities start. Barbara is wearing the so-called iShell cap, which monitors all of her movements and activity. In the future, it is expected that the iShell cap can take over her locomotion and motor skills.

Acknowledgments

All participants of the sessions are kindly thanked for their willingness to volunteer and share their views. Tom Raijmakers, Lotte Oude Weernink, Nakul Paricharak, Chris Hoedemakers, Josha Woudstra, Lisa van der Voort, Thomas van de Werff, and Bram van der Putten of the Department of Industrial Design of Eindhoven University of Technology are thanked for their support in the creative sessions. Mrs. Theresa Remmers-Kersten and Dr. Karen Cox of the Fontys School of People and Health Studies of Fontys University of Applied Sciences are thanked for hosting the sessions. The Municipality of Eindhoven (Gemeente Eindhoven) and Stichting Promotie Installatietechniek (PIT) are thanked for their financial support. The staff of Filmding B.V., Breda, Netherlands, are thanked for supporting the event by filming the scenarios.

References

[1] J. van Hoof, M. H. Wetzels, A. M. C. Dooremalen et al., "Technological and architectural solutions for Dutch nursing homes: results of a multidisciplinary mind mapping session with professional stakeholders," *Technology in Society*, vol. 36, no. 1, pp. 1–12, 2014.

[2] J. van Hoof and E. J. M. Wouters, *Het Verpleeghuis van de Toekomst is (een) Thuis*, Bohn Stafleu van Loghum, Houten, The Netherlands:, 2014.

[3] M. de Klerk, *Ouderen in instellingen. Landelijk overzicht van de leefsituatie van oudere tehuisbewoners*, Netherlands Institute for Social Research, The Hague, The Netherlands, 2005.

[4] M. Annemans, C. H. Van Audenhove, H. Vermolen, and A. Heylighen, "Being transported into the unknown: how patients experience the route to the operation room," in *Inclusive Designing: Joining Usability, Accessibility, and Inclusion*, P. M. Langdon, J. Lazar, A. Heylighen, and H. Dong, Eds., pp. 131–141, Springer, London, UK, 2014.

[5] S. van der Geest and G. Mommersteeg, "Beds and culture: introduction," *Medische Antropologie*, vol. 18, pp. 7–17, 2006.

[6] J. van Hoof, M. M. Verhagen, E. J. Wouters, H. R. Marston, M. D. Rijnaard, and B. M. Janssen, "Picture your nursing home: exploring the sense of home of older residents through photography," *Journal of Aging Research*, vol. 2015, Article ID 312931, 11 pages, 2015.

[7] N. Strating, R. van Herpen, and W. Zeiler, "Evacuatie van bedgebonden patiënten," *TVVL Magazine*, vol. 44, no. 2, pp. 46–48, 2015 (Dutch).

[8] J. van Hoof and M. J. Verkerk, "Developing an integrated design model incorporating technology philosophy for the design of healthcare environments: a case analysis of facilities for psychogeriatric and psychiatric care in The Netherlands," *Technology in Society*, vol. 35, no. 1, pp. 1–13, 2013.

[9] J. van Hoof, P. G. S. Rutten, C. Struck, E. R. C. M. Huisman, and H. S. M. Kort, "The integrated and evidence-based design of healthcare environments," *Architectural Engineering and Design Management*, vol. 11, pp. 243–263, 2015.

[10] C. Parker, S. Barnes, K. Mckee, K. Morgan, J. Torrington, and P. Tregenza, "Quality of life and building design in residential and nursing homes for older people," *Ageing and Society*, vol. 24, no. 6, pp. 941–962, 2004.

[11] D. Xu, R. L. Kane, and T. A. Shamliyan, "Effect of nursing home characteristics on residents' quality of life: a systematic review," *Archives of Gerontology and Geriatrics*, vol. 57, no. 2, pp. 127–142, 2013.

[12] P. Delhoofen, "Creativiteit en innovatie," in *Handboek Ontwerpen. Innovatie, Communicatie en Analyse bij het Ontwerpen van Producten*, chapter 11, Wolters-Noordhoff, Groningen, The Netherlands, 2nd edition, 2003.

[13] C. Argyris and D. A. Schön, "Participatory action research and action science compared: a commentary," *American Behavioral Scientist*, vol. 32, no. 5, pp. 612–623, 1989.

[14] M. Bilandzic and J. Venable, "Towards participatory action design research: adapting action research and design science research methods for urban informatics," *The Journal of Community Informatics*, vol. 7, no. 3, 2011.

[15] D. Madden, Y. Cadet-James, I. Atkinson, and F. Watkin Lui, "Probes and prototypes: a participatory action research approach to codesign," *CoDesign*, vol. 10, no. 1, pp. 31–45, 2014.

[16] M. Lahtinen, S. Nenonen, H. Rasila, J. Lehtelä, V. Ruohomäki, and K. Reijula, "Rehabilitation centers in change: participatory methods for managing redesign and renovation," *Health Environments Research & Design Journal*, vol. 7, no. 2, pp. 57–75, 2014.

[17] Z. Howard and M. M. Somerville, "A comparative study of two design charrettes: implications for codesign and participatory action research," *CoDesign*, vol. 10, no. 1, pp. 46–62, 2014.

[18] G. Malagon-Maldonado, "Qualitative research in health design," *Health Environments Research & Design Journal*, vol. 7, no. 4, pp. 120–134, 2014.

[19] E. B.-N. Sanders and P. J. Stappers, "Probes, toolkits and prototypes: three approaches to making in codesigning," *CoDesign*, vol. 10, no. 1, pp. 5–14, 2014.

[20] B. Laurel, "Design improvisation. Etnography meets theatre," in *Design Research: Methods and Perspectives*, B. Laurel, Ed., pp. 49–54, The MIT Press, Cambridge, Mass, USA, 2003.

[21] G. Triantafyllakos, G. Palaigeorgiou, and I. A. Tsoukalas, "Fictional characters in participatory design sessions: introducing the 'design alter egos' technique," *Interacting with Computers*, vol. 22, no. 3, pp. 165–175, 2010.

[22] P. Bate and G. Robert, *Bringing User Experience to Healthcare Improvement. The Concepts, Methods and Practices of Experience-Based Design*, Radcliffe Publishing, Oxford, UK, 2007.

[23] E. B.-N. Sanders and P. J. Stappers, "Co-creation and the new landscapes of design," *CoDesign*, vol. 4, no. 1, pp. 5–18, 2008.

[24] T. Miaskiewicz and K. A. Kozar, "Personas and user-centered design: how can personas benefit product design processes?" *Design Studies*, vol. 32, no. 5, pp. 417–430, 2011.

[25] F. Ferreira, N. Almeida, A. F. Rosa et al., "Elderly centered design for interaction—the case of the S4S medication assistant," *Procedia Computer Science*, vol. 27, pp. 398–408, 2014.

[26] P. Turner and S. Turner, "Is stereotyping inevitable when designing with personas?" *Design Studies*, vol. 32, no. 1, pp. 30–44, 2011.

[27] V. Braun and V. Clarke, "Using thematic analysis in psychology," *Qualitative Research in Psychology*, vol. 3, no. 2, pp. 77–101, 2006.

[28] K. Krippendorff, "Content analysis," in *International Encyclopedia of Communication*, E. Barnouw, G. Gerbner, W. Schramm, T. L. Worth, and L. Gross, Eds., vol. 1, pp. 403–407, Oxford University Press, New York, NY, USA, 1989.

[29] B. E. Carey-Smith, N. M. Evans, and R. D. Orpwood, "A user-centred design process to develop technology to improve sleep quality in residential care homes," *Technology and Disability*, vol. 25, no. 1, pp. 49–58, 2013.

[30] S. Martin, J. C. Augusto, P. McCullagh et al., "Participatory research to design a novel telehealth system to support the night-time needs of people with dementia: NOCTURNAL," *International Journal of Environmental Research and Public Health*, vol. 10, no. 12, pp. 6764–6782, 2013.

[31] S. Shortall, "Participatory action research," in *The A–Z of Social Research*, R. L. Miller and J. D. Brewer, Eds., pp. 225–227, Sage Publications, London, UK, 2003.

[32] J. van Hoof, R. A. Overdiep, C. M. M. Cox, M. L. L. Weymans, and L. J. Peeraer, "Health care and technology: a new approach to education and applied research," in *Everyday Technology for Independence and Care*, G. J. Gelderblom, M. Soede, L. Adriaens, and K. Miesenberger, Eds., pp. 222–224, IOS Press, Amsterdam, The Netherlands, 2011.

[33] J. van Hoof, E. L. M. Zwerts-Verhelst, M. E. Nieboer, and E. J. M. Wouters, "Innovations in multidisciplinary education in healthcare and technology," *Perspectives on Medical Education*, vol. 4, no. 3, pp. 146–148, 2015.

[34] J. van Hoof, P. G. S. Rutten, C. Struck, E. R. C. M. Huisman, and H. S. M. Kort, "The integrated and evidence-based design of healthcare environments," *Architectural Engineering and Design Management*, vol. 11, no. 4, pp. 243–263, 2015.

[35] G. Marquardt and T. Motzek, "How to rate the quality of a research paper: introducing a helpful algorithm for architects and designers," *Health Environments Research & Design Journal*, vol. 6, no. 2, pp. 119–127, 2013.

2

Clinical Correlates of Awareness for Balance, Function, and Memory: Evidence for the Modality Specificity of Awareness

Megan E. O'Connell,[1] Vanina Dal Bello-Haas,[2] Margaret Crossley,[1] and Debra Morgan[3]

[1] *Department of Psychology, Room 183 Arts Building, 9 Campus Drive, University of Saskatchewan, SK, Canada S7N 5A5*
[2] *School of Rehabilitation Science, McMaster University, Hamilton, ON, Canada L8S 1C7*
[3] *Canadian Centre for Health and Safety in Agriculture, University of Saskatchewan, SK, Canada S7N 5E5*

Correspondence should be addressed to Megan E. O'Connell; megan.oconnell@usask.ca

Academic Editor: F. Richard Ferraro

Awareness in dementia is increasingly recognized not only as multifactorial, but also as domain specific. We demonstrate differential clinical correlates for awareness of daily function, awareness of memory, and the novel exploration of awareness of balance. Awareness of function was higher for participants with mild cognitive impairment (aMCI and non-aMCI) than for those with dementia (due to Alzheimer disease; AD and non-AD), whereas awareness of memory was higher for both non-aMCI and non-AD dementia patients than for those with aMCI or AD. Balance awareness did not differ based on diagnostic subgroup. Awareness of function was associated with instrumental activities of daily living and caregiver burden. In contrast, awareness of balance was associated with fall history, balance confidence, and instrumental activities of daily living. Clinical correlates of awareness of memory depended on diagnostic group: associations held with neuropsychological variables for non-AD dementia, but for patients with AD dementia, depression and instrumental activities of daily living were clinical correlates of memory awareness. Together, these data provide support for the hypothesis that awareness and dementia are not unitary and are, instead, modality specific.

1. Introduction

Unawareness, lack of insight, or anosognosia refers to impaired awareness in persons with dementia [1–7]. Awareness is multifactorial and likely modular [4, 8–10], with each domain separable and potentially unique. Most of the literature on awareness in persons with dementia describes the clinical correlates of one awareness domain (reviews by [1, 4, 11]), but the few studies that have contrasted awareness for different domains have found differential patterns of clinical correlates [12–15]. This paper provides further support for the modality specific nature of awareness in dementia by contrasting the clinical correlates for awareness of balance in addition to more commonly measured awareness of day-to-day function and memory.

Awareness quantification remains elusive, and there is no consensus method for measuring awareness (e.g., [4, 9]). Awareness has been measured with clinician ratings [16, 17]; or based on discrepancy between self-report versus clinicians' impression [10] or versus informant report assessed with interview [10, 18] or questionnaires [7, 12, 14, 19–21]; or discrepancy between self-report and objective performance [21, 22], which, depending on the task, measures self-monitoring or metacognitive abilities [3]. Each assessment method has limitations: Clare et al. [21] detail difficulties with patient/informant discrepancies and the assumption that caregiver informants' or clinicians' reports are a better reflection of reality. Moreover, worry, anxiety, defensiveness, denial, or focus on "more important problems" can influence reflection for persons with dementia [9]. Caregivers' reports may be more highly correlated with objective measures of cognition than patient self-reports, suggesting there is value in using patient/informant discrepancies [7]. Nevertheless, caregiver/patient discrepancies may be a better measurement of patients' awareness of function, whereas clinician/patient discrepancies may be a better measure of patients' awareness of cognition [11].

Due, in part, to measurement challenges when assessing awareness, the literature on the clinical correlates of awareness in persons with dementia is contradictory [1]. Most, but not all, of the cumulative data suggest increasing dementia severity is associated with reduced awareness [1, 16, 18]. Others have found few group-based differences, but high individual variability in awareness declines when studied over one year [23], potentially because severity and awareness are mediated by cognitive reserve [24]. Other important clinical correlates of awareness include depression [18, 21, 22, 25], neuropsychiatric status [19–21, 26] caregiver burden [10, 11, 14, 26], activities of daily living [19], and neuropsychological status [12, 19, 20, 22, 27–29] which demonstrate variability in associations with awareness across domains and measurement methods [1].

Models of awareness suggest awareness is mediated by the frontal lobes [2, 3] or the right frontal lobe [30, 31], and lack of awareness is associated with other behavioural indicators of frontal dysfunction, such as increased apathy [32]. Localized imaging has implicated the orbitofrontal cortex [33], but most have implicated medial structures [34, 35], including the anterior [36] and posterior cingulate [35] in awareness. Despite converging evidence for prefrontal involvement in awareness, awareness may or may not be associated with tests of executive function (see review by [1]). Some studies demonstrate strong relationships between awareness and executive functioning [12, 19, 20, 27], with others reporting nonsignificant and trivial associations [19, 29]. Although clearly composite measures that rely on more basic cognitive functions, many summary scores from traditional tests of executive function are associated with the dorsolateral prefrontal circuit [37], and awareness has been associated with more midline [34–36] or orbitofrontal aspects of the prefrontal cortex [33].

Contradictory data on the clinical correlates of awareness is also due to the assumption that awareness is a unitary construct (see reviews by [4, 8]). Differential patterns of clinical correlates have been demonstrated for awareness of cognitive deficits versus awareness of behaviours [12–15], suggesting that awareness is modality specific.

The primary purpose of this paper is to describe the clinical correlates of awareness of balance in addition to the more commonly measured awareness of function in basic and instrumental activities of daily living (BADLs and IADLs, resp.) and awareness of memory. Awareness of balance is important in persons with dementia due to its relation with fall risk [38]. We hypothesize that awareness of balance will be associated with physical variables, such as gait, falls, and objectively measured balance. Based on the conceptualization of Markova and colleagues [39] and work suggesting differential clinical correlates for awareness of specific domains [13, 15], we hypothesize that awareness of functional abilities, memory, and balance will have differential patterns of clinical correlates.

A secondary purpose of this paper is to contrast awareness for balance, function, and memory for those diagnosed with mild cognitive impairment (MCI). Reduced awareness has been demonstrated for persons at high risk for dementia, and specifically for persons with amnestic MCI (aMCI) [40]. Moreover, since awareness appears to differ based on dementia subtype [28], awareness for balance, function, and memory could be differentially affected for participants diagnosed with dementia due to AD versus non-AD dementias. Therefore, the final comparison will explore awareness in groups of persons diagnosed with aMCI, non-amnestic MCI, AD, and non-AD dementias.

2. Method

2.1. Participants. Patients were from an interdisciplinary memory clinic established to provide early stage dementia differential diagnoses for rural persons [41]. For this IRB approved study, patients who were diagnosed with no cognitive impairment were excluded, and only patients who received a diagnosis of dementia or a variant of MCI were included. Diagnoses in this specialty clinic were consistent with the review of diagnostic guidelines provided by the Canadian Consensus on the Diagnosis and Treatment of Dementias [42] using recent comprehensive blood work, CT head scan, and interprofessional assessment data from neurology, neuropsychology, and physical therapy. The assessment procedures included standardized approaches (e.g., questionnaires, neuropsychological testing) and also family interviews for clinical history and interviews with the informal caregiver who accompanied patients to the clinic (families were strongly encouraged to attend the assessment and patients were asked to bring someone who knew them well. In the unusual circumstance when patients attended the clinic alone, telephone interviews were conducted with someone who knew them well, but questionnaire data were not collected). The sample consisted of 259 patients (in the clinic's 6th data release), and the vast majority (74%) reported their ancestry as European, 9% were First Nations or Metis, and 17% chose "other," rather than selecting one of the aforementioned categories, African or Asian ancestry. Table 1 includes descriptive information for the total clinical sample ($N = 259$ patients) and details the subgroups based on diagnosis. Patients with dementia due to AD was the most common diagnosis ($n = 113$), and another heterogeneous subgroup ($n = 100$) was created of patients with non-AD dementias (i.e., vascular dementias, mixed dementias, diffuse Lewy body disease, dementia due to Parkinsons' Disease, Huntington's dementia, variants of frontotemporal lobar degeneration, and dementias not otherwise specified). In addition, a third group included patients diagnosed with amnestic (single or multiple domain) mild cognitive impairment (aMCI; $n = 23$) and a fourth group included patients diagnosed with nonamnestic MCI (non-aMCI; $n = 23$; single or multiple domains, which included those with diagnoses of vascular cognitive impairment, no dementia [43]). Although most of the clinic data were focused on patients for diagnostic purposes, informal caregivers ($N = 244$) provided important collateral and personal information. Caregivers (M age = 61.40, SD = 14.63) were typically family members and most of many were females (64%): 33% were wives, 20% were husbands, 31% were daughters, 10% were

TABLE 1: Descriptive statistics for demographic, awareness, and clinical variables for each of the four diagnostic subgroups and for the overall sample.

	AD M (SD) *n*	Non-AD M (SD) *n*	aMCI M (SD) *n*	Non-aMCI M (SD) *n*	Overall M (SD) *n*
Age	75.81(7.51) 113	73.05 (10.15) 100	73.74 (8.87) 23	70.30 (11.06) 23	74.07 (9.18)[a] 259
Gender (% female)	67%	56%	70%	52%	62%
Education	10.16 (3.32) 108	10.57 (3.168) 87	11.13 (3.57) 23	11.05 (3.43) 23	10.48 (3.30) 240
Awareness of function	24.74 (3.53) 87	23.75 (3.91) 72	26.30 (3.06) 20	27.59 (3.02) 22	24.85 (3.76)[b] 201
Awareness of memory	2.13 (0.99) 88	2.69 (1.20) 61	2.55 (1.10) 22	3.10 (1.18) 21	2.46 (1.14)[c] 192
Awareness of balance	4.07 (0.99) 43	3.81 (0.92) 27	4.00 (0.91) 13	4.42 (0.79) 12	4.03 (0.94) 95
CDR-SOB	6.97 (3.45) 100	6.45 (3.58) 91	2.13 (1.310) 20	2.27 (1.22) 22	5.90 (3.66)[b] 233
IADL-patient	21.64 (5.05) 99	20.11 (5.47) 82	24.68 (2.71) 22	25.32 (2.73) 22	21.74 (5.14)[b] 225
FAQ-caregiver	15.52 (8.11) 109	15.36 (8.29) 94	7.82 (4.81) 22	6.65 (6.33) 23	13.96 (8.38)[b] 248
Bristol ADL-caregiver	8.90 (7.50) 102	10.97 (9.78) 89	2.96 (2.06) 23	4.04 (5.30) 23	8.63 (8.37)[b] 237
CESD overall	11.85 (9.46) 93	13.31 (9.10) 72	15.00 (8.54) 23	14.05 (7.86) 22	12.92 (9.08) 210
CESD depressed affect	2.91 (3.30) 93	2.89 (3.21) 72	3.70 (3.43) 23	2.68 (2.38) 22	2.97 (3.19) 210
CESD Lack of positive affect	2.75 (2.86) 93	3.35 (2.74) 72	4.00 (3.44) 23	3.41 (2.61) 22	3.16 (2.87) 210
CESD somatic/vegetative	5.08 (3.92) 93	5.96 (3.97) 72	5.96 (3.78) 23	6.73 (4.20) 22	5.65 (3.96) 210
CESD interpersonal	1.11 (1.77) 93	1.11 (1.44) 72	1.35 (1.90) 23	1.23 (1.66) 22	1.15 (1.65) 210
NPI-severity	8.70 (6.49) 103	9.24 (5.81) 84	15.50 (41.27)* 20	7.44 (8.03) 16	9.42 (13.64) 223
NPI-distress	10.08 (10.02) 103	10.57 (8.74) 82	14.45 (39.23)* 22	7.00 (11.96) 20	10.41 (15.18) 227
ZBI	13.76 (8.97) 107	14.25 (8.35) 89	11.73 (9.35) 22	10.35 (9.56) 23	13.43 (8.86) 241
BSI global severity	50.35 (10.05) 99	52.03 (9.30) 86	51.24 (10.51) 21	53.22 (11.34) 23	51.35 (9.93) 229
Fall history in past 6 months (no/yes)	65/25 90	45/36 81	12/8 20	10/12 22	132/81 213
Probability of falling (%)	38.00 (35.06) 76	56.02 (33.87) 63	32.84 (32.48) 17	39.45 (37.13) 14	44.28 (35.44) 170
ABC	80.95 (16.99) 44	74.40 (24.87) 29	86.15 (11.09) 13	72.92 (16.46) 12	78.72 (19.28) 98
BBS	46.44 (8.57) 77	41.97 (11.48) 64	49.53 (5.03) 17	49.14 (7.23) 14	45.30 (9.76)[d] 172
POMA	22.25 (4.85) 32	20.38 (5.54) 26	21.88 (4.70) 8	23.50 (4.09) 6	21.64 (5.05) 72
Stroop-interference	−0.90 (1.55) 79	−1.19 (1.64) 54	−0.43 (1.44) 21	0.21 (0.86) 18	−0.82 (1.55)[e] 172
TMT-B	−2.10 (1.26) 62	−2.32 (1.15) 48	−0.92 (1.00) 20	−1.68 (1.43) 17	−1.96 (1.29)[f] 147
Clock drawing	16.30 (4.28) 100	15.85 (4.79) 79	18.98 (1.86) 23	17.71 (4.43) 21	16.55 (4.39)[b] 223

Table 1: Continued.

	AD M (SD) n	Non-AD M (SD) n	aMCI M (SD) n	Non-aMCI M (SD) n	Overall M (SD) n
Phonemic fluency	−1.38 (1.00) 98	−1.93 (1.05) 75	−0.81 (1.05) 23	−1.52 (0.98) 22	−1.52 (1.07)[d] 218
Animal naming	−1.99 (0.78) 98	−2.01 (0.84) 77	−1.27 (1.02) 23	−1.26 (1.03) 22	−1.85 (0.90)[b] 220
DS-B	−1.04 (0.87) 98	−1.14 (0.82) 76	−0.31 (1.00) 23	−0.82 (0.81) 22	−0.98 (0.89)[b] 219
RBANS immed memory	57.47 (13.65) 98	65.59 (16.66) 73	75.48 (11.95) 23	82.95 (15.04) 22	64.73 (16.87)[g] 216
RBANS delayed memory	48.68 (9.35) 95	63.01 (19.13) 70	61.77 (16.89) 22	73.24 (22.74) 21	57.37 (17.71)[h] 208
RBANS language	78.00 (14.81) 98	78.96 (15.72) 74	94.30 (10.07) 23	94.29 (7.98) 21	81.65 (15.51)[b] 216
RBANS attention	74.98 (16.39) 91	70.20 (14.85) 64	86.68 (10.79) 22	77.15 (15.58) 20	74.95 (15.92)[i] 197
RBANS visuospatial/constructional	77.37 (17.60) 93	76.81 (15.83) 67	96.57 (14.83) 21	86.71 (12.79) 21	80.15 (17.38)[i] 202
RBANS total scale	61.16 (10.09) 83	66.03 (13.73) 59	77.41 (7.67) 22	78.79 (12.26) 19	66.51 (13.07)[b] 183

[a]AD group significantly older than non-aMCI group. [b]AD and non-AD dementia group similar, but significantly more impaired than the similar aMCI and non-MCI groups. [c]AD group similar to aMCI group, but more impaired than non-AD and non-aMCI groups. [d]Non-AD group more impaired than other groups. [e]non-aMCI group less impaired. [f]aMCI group less impaired. [g]AD group significantly more impaired than non-AD group and both more impaired than either MCI group. [h]AD group significantly more impaired than other groups. [i]AD group significantly lower than aMCI group. *outliers in these small samples.

sons of the patient, with a remaining 7% whose relationship status included grandchildren, nieces, nephews, or friends.

2.2. Measures

Clinical Correlates of Awareness Measures

(1) Assessment of Severity. The Clinical Dementia Rating (CDR) [44] is a standardized and psychometrically sound clinician-based rating scale (0 to 3; no impairment to severe impairment), but summing the box scores of the six rating areas of the CDR (CDR-SOB) provides a more detailed quantitative measure of global dementia severity and is more sensitive to detecting changes in dementia severity over time [45].

(2) Assessment of Activities of Daily Living. Patients rated their performance on the reliable and valid Lawton Instrumental Activities of Daily Living (IADL [46] higher scores indicating independent functioning). Patients' caregivers rated patients' performance of ADLs on two psychometrically strong scales: The Functional Assessment Questionnaire (FAQ) [47] and the Bristol ADL questionnaire [48] where higher scores indicate impaired performance.

(3) Assessment of Depression and Neuropsychiatric Symptoms. The Neuropsychiatric Inventory (NPI) is a well-researched and psychometrically strong caregiver rating of patients' behaviours and associated caregiver distress [49]. The Centre for Epidemiologic Studies of Depression (CESD), a reliable and valid screen of depression, was self-rated by patients [50], with four factors: (1) depressed affect (2) lack of positive affect (3) somatic/vegetative and (4) interpersonal measuring social disconnectedness.

(4) Assessment of Caregiver Psychological Distress and Burden. Self-report of caregiver burden was assessed with the short form of the Zarit Burden interview, which was shown to be psychometrically similar to the longer versions [51]. The Global Severity Index from the Brief Symptom Inventory (BSI) measured caregiver self-report of overall psychological distress [52].

(5) Assessment of Physical Variables. A comprehensivephysical therapy assessment included the psychometrically strong Berg Balance Scale (BBS) [53] and the Performance Oriented Mobility Assessment (POMA, which is a measure of gait and balance) [54]. Caregiver and patient reports of falls within the past 6 months were combined with BBS to estimate the probability of falling [55]. Patient self-report on the Activities-Specific Balance Confidence (ABC) scale [56] measured self-reported confidence in balance while doing a variety of day-to-day activities.

(6) Assessment of Neuropsychological Function. Each patient received a comprehensive neuropsychological assessment (see [57] for a review of the strong psychometric properties of these tests), and selected measures of executive function and working memory were analyzed. The ability to alternate attention was measured with the Trail Making Test Part B (TMT B) [58]. The ability to inhibit an automatic response was measured with the Stroop interference score [59].

Cognitive flexibility with speeded retrieval of language-based knowledge was measured using Animal Naming and phonemic fluency (Benton Oral Word Association Test [60]). The clock drawing test measured visual construction, abstraction, and inhibition [61]. Digit span backward subtest from the Wechsler Adult Intelligence Scale 3rd edition (WAIS-III) [62] measured working memory. Finally, the index scores from the Repeatable Battery for the Assessment of Neuropsychological Status (RBANS) [63] were analyzed.

(7) Awareness of Functional Deficits. Awareness of functional deficits (AF) was operationalized using patient/caregiver congruence on reports of the patient's ability to independently perform six IADLs: management of finances, use of telephone, use of transportation, shopping, meal preparation, and performance of housework (patient self-report version of the Lawton IADL Scale [46]; and caregiver report of patient's function from the Bristol ADL Scale [48]). For each IADL, congruence was ranked on a 5-point scale; the congruence ranking was summed across the six IADL items for a total of 30 possible points, with higher scores indicating greater awareness. Data were available for 201 participants, and as can be seen in Table 1, most patients had good awareness of their functional abilities. AF was significantly higher in the two MCI diagnostic groups when compared with the two groups with dementia diagnoses.

(8) Awareness of Memory. Awareness of memory (AM) was based on congruence between patient's self-reports of memory on a standardized scale (Self-Rating of Memory Scale) [64] and performance on a neuropsychological test of new learning (Repeatable Battery for Assessment of Neuropsychological Status; RBANS delayed memory index score [63]). The delayed memory measure was chosen since it best captured consolidation difficulties asked about in the Self-Rating of Memory Scale. Both the self rating of memory standardized scores and the RBANS index scores were transformed into a linear ranked scale from 1 to 5, with 1 indicating the lowest self-rating of memory and the lowest memory performance. The AM score was created based on the congruence in ranking between self-reported and objectively measured memory, with 5 indicating perfect congruence. Complete data were available for 192 participants. As can be seen in Table 1, most participants' AM was at the mid-point of the scale, but the AD and the aMCI subgroups reported significantly lower AM than the non-AD dementia and non-aMCI groups.

(9) Awareness of Balance. Awareness of balance (AB) was based on congruence between patients' ratings of balance confidence on the ABC scale [56] and the probability of falling [55]. The ABC and probability of falling were each transformed into ranked scores with 1 indicating low confidence or high probability of falling and 4 representing high confidence or low probability of falling. The AB score was created based on the congruence in ranking between self-reported balance confidence and objectively measured probability of falling, with 1 indicating low congruence and 4 indicating perfect congruence. Perfect congruence between balance confidence and objective measurement may not be sufficient for stability; rather underestimation of balance (i.e., less confidence than objective measurement would support) has been shown to be associated with greater stability (e.g., [38, 65]). Consistent with this premise, AB ranking of 5 represented an underestimation of balance confidence relative to objectively measured balance. Complete data were available to create AB for 95 participants. Approximately one third of the sample (36%) reported equivalent balance confidence to measured stability, 27% reported greater balance confidence than would be supported by objective measurement (i.e., reduced awareness), and 37% reported an underestimation of balance, which may be appropriate awareness for maximal stability (e.g., [38, 65]). Although the sample size was relatively small, AB was high for all groups and did not differ significantly for patients with diagnoses of aMCI, non-aMCI, AD, or non-AD dementias (see Table 1).

2.3. Statistical Procedure. Zero-order correlations were completed separately for AF (Table 2), AM (Table 3), and AB (Table 4). Only variables with significant correlations were used to minimize specification errors (potential over- or undercorrection) as predictors in simultaneous multiple regression equations. Variables with variance inflation factors over 5.0 were excluded due to concerns about multicollinearity. For each measure of awareness, analyses were conducted for the overall sample, but also for each of the four diagnostic groups. Descriptors of magnitude of association were consistent with guidelines for small, medium, and large effect sizes provided by Cohen [66].

3. Results

3.1. Evidence for Validity of Awareness Measures. As can be seen in Table 2, AF was highly correlated with caregiver report of ADLs (FAQ and Bristol ADL each large magnitude associations). The correlation with patient report of IADL was a moderate magnitude. Together these data suggest AF was highly associated, but not redundant, with more comprehensive measures of day-to-day function.

Similarly, AM was highly associated, but not redundant with the measures used to create it. As can be seen in Table 3, these associations were strong for the non-AD dementia and two MCI groups but trivial for the AD group.

Finally, AB also demonstrated moderate, but nonredundant, associations with the variables used to create it. As can be seen in Table 4, the association with the ABC scale was a moderate magnitude overall and for all diagnostic groups except the non-aMCI group. Also seen in Table 4, AB was associated with both fall history in the past 6 months for the larger samples and overall. AB was associated with probability of falling only for specific diagnostic groups and the overall sample. The cell sizes for the POMA were below 10 for the MCI groups, but the small association was significant for the overall sample.

Overall, the correlations provide evidence for the convergent validity for each of the derived awareness measures.

TABLE 2: Clinical correlates of awareness of function (AF) for each diagnostic group.

	AD r_s, n	Non-AD r_s, n	aMCI r_s, n	Non-aMCI r_s, n	Overall r_s, n
CDR-SOB	−0.443, 78**	−0.292, 69*	−0.177, 17	−0.121, 21	−0.435, 185**
IADL-patient	0.274, 87*	0.276, 72*	0.688, 20**	0.575, 22**	0.406, 201**
FAQ-caregiver	−0.543, 87**	−0.454, 72**	−0.517, 20*	−0.624, 22**	−0.583, 201**
Bristol ADL-caregiver	−0.651, 87**	−0.513, 72**	−0.651, 20**	−0.632, 22**	−0.655, 201**
CESD overall	−0.005, 79	0.012, 62	0.218, 20	0.338, 21	0.076, 182
CESD depressed affect	−0.023, 79	−0.081, 62	0.303, 20	−0.032, 21	0.007, 182
CESD lack pos affect	−0.071, 79	0.191, 62	0.120, 20	0.496, 21*	0.092, 182
CESD somatic/vegetative	0.064, 79	−0.109, 62	0.335, 20	0.231, 21	0.043, 182
CESD interpersonal	0.070, 79	0.113, 62	0.104, 20	0.127, 21	0.088, 182
NPI-severity	−0.202, 83	−0.073, 64	−0.210, 17	−0.511, 15	−0.236, 179**
NPI-distress	−0.276, 83*	0.020, 61	−0.106, 19	−0.436, 19	−0.270, 182**
ZBI	−0.321, 86**	−0.055, 70	−0.437, 20	−0.453, 22*	−0.305, 198**
BSI global severity	−0.037, 78	0.022, 69	−0.087, 19	−0.003, 22	−0.003, 188
Fall history in past 6 months	−0.011, 73	−0.146, 62	0.144, 18	−0.668, 21**	−0.078, 174
Probability of falling (%)	−0.012, 62	−0.160, 48	0.036, 15	−0.815, 14**	−0.188, 139*
ABC	−0.046, 37	−0.127, 24	0.232, 12	0.538, 12	−0.025, 85
BBS	0.028, 63	0.136, 49	0.263, 15	0.640, 14*	0.213, 141*
POMA	0.277, 25	0.177, 22	—	—	0.253, 59
Stroop-interference	−0.006, 65	−0.060, 45	−0.164, 18	0.257, 17	0.147, 145
TMT-B	0.086, 51	−0.020, 43	−0.074, 17	0.015, 16	0.135, 127
Clock drawing	0.188, 81	0.172, 63	0.166, 20	0.350, 20	0.304, 184**
Phonemic fluency	0.099, 79	0.080, 61	−0.102, 20	0.075, 21	0.128, 181
Animal naming	0.022, 79	0.017, 63	−0.114, 20	0.205, 21	0.128, 183
DS-B	0.092, 81	0.037, 62	0.043, 20	−0.357, 21	0.071, 184
RBANS immed memory	0.063, 80	0.091, 60	0.130, 20	−0.096, 21	0.164, 181*
RBANS delayed memory	0.182, 77	0.065, 57	−0.360, 19	0.147, 20	0.125, 173
RBANS language	0.244, 80*	0.106, 60	−0.047, 20	0.365, 20	0.287, 180**
RBANS attention	0.006, 74	0.196, 51	−0.012, 19	0.020, 19	0.104, 163
RBANS visuospatial/constructional	0.110, 75	0.166, 53	0.328, 19	−0.184, 20	0.205, 167**
RBANS total scale	0.137, 66	0.202, 48	0.023, 19	0.039, 18	0.246, 151**

*$P < 0.05$ but > 0.01. **$P < 0.01$.

Of interest, each measure of awareness appeared orthogonal: awareness of function was not associated with either awareness of memory ($r_s = 0.026$, $P > 0.05$, trivial magnitude) or balance ($r_s = 0.207$, $P > 0.05$, small magnitude), and the latter two measures of awareness are similarly not well associated ($r_s = 0.153$, $P > 0.05$, small magnitude).

3.2. Clinical Correlates for Awareness Measures

3.2.1. Awareness of Function. Zero-order correlations for AF are provided in Table 2. For the overall sample, regression diagnostics suggested the Bristol ADL-caregiver, NPI-Distress, and RBANS immediate and total scale indices were multicollinear, so these variables were excluded from the regression equation. The remaining predictors of CDR-SOB, IADL-Patient, FAQ-caregiver, NPI-severity, ZBI, probability of Falling, BBS, clock drawing, RBANS language, and visuospatial/constructional Indices accounted for a large proportion of AF variance ($R = 0.688$, $P < 0.001$). Not all predictors were equally predictive, however, and only the FAQ-caregiver ($t = -4.64$, $P < 0.001$) and ZBI ($t = -3.06$, $P = 0.003$) were significant predictors of AF. Equivalent regression procedures were conducted separately for the four diagnostic subgroups, and across these analyses only measures of function were significant predictors of AF (AD group FAQ-caregiver $t = -3.29$, $P = 0.002$; non-AD group FAQ-caregiver $t = -3.03$, $P = 0.004$; aMCI group IADL-patient $t = 2.30$, $P = 0.035$; and non-aMCI group BADL-caregiver $t = -2.37$, $P = 0.029$).

3.2.2. Awareness of Memory. Awareness of memory demonstrated a different pattern of zero-order correlations (see Table 3), and the results of the regression analyses also suggested that the clinical correlates of AM clearly

Table 3: Clinical correlates of awareness of memory (AM) for each diagnostic group.

	AD r_s, n	Non-AD r_s, n	aMCI r_s, n	Non-aMCI r_s, n	Overall r_s, n
CDR-SOB	0.034, 83	0.067, 59	0.208, 19	−0.218, 20	−0.058, 181
IADL-patient	−0.293, 85**	−0.062, 60	−0.221, 22	−0.253, 20	−0.163, 187*
FAQ-caregiver	0.185, 88	−0.053, 61	0.011, 21	0.264, 21	0.009, 191
Bristol ADL-caregiver	0.079, 82	0.087, 57	0.022, 22	0.120, 21	0.032, 182
CESD overall	0.537, 83**	0.226, 58	−0.023, 22	0.071, 20	0.333, 183**
CESD depressed affect	0.326, 83**	0.021, 58	−0.085, 22	0.188, 20	0.172, 183*
CESD lack of positive affect	0.522, 83**	0.179, 58	−0.054, 22	−0.061, 20	0.276, 183**
CESD somatic/vegetative	0.450, 83**	0.265, 58*	−0.094, 22	0.191, 20	0.330, 183**
CESD interpersonal	0.343, 83**	0.218, 58	0.249, 22	0.120, 20	0.272, 183**
NPI-severity	0.163, 84	0.108, 55	0.457, 19*	0.460, 15	0.211, 173**
NPI-distress	0.201, 88	0.123, 59	0.443, 21*	0.018, 21	0.171, 189*
ZBI	−0.002, 88	0.242, 59	0.149, 21	0.147, 21	0.092, 189
BSI global severity	0.278, 81*	0.517, 58**	−0.135, 20	0.042, 21	0.303, 180**
Fall history in past 6 months	0.059, 68	0.039, 46	−0.114, 19	−0.173, 20	0.080, 153
Probability of falling (%)	0.020, 58	−0.154, 36	−0.045, 16	−0.568, 12	−0.010, 122
ABC	−0.112, 34	0.134, 21	−0.555, 13*	0.182, 11	−0.097, 79
BBS	−0.010, 58	0.213, 37	0.001, 16	0.723, 12**	0.090, 123
POMA	0.064, 22	0.309, 16	—	—	0.229, 51
Stroop-interference	−0.081, 71	0.175, 44	0.298, 20	−0.177, 17	0.112, 152
TMT-B	−0.129, 55	0.428, 43**	−0.040, 19	−0.087, 16	0.111, 133
Clock drawing	−0.123, 86	0.202, 58	0.118, 22	0.270, 20	0.078, 186
Phonemic fluency	−0.065, 84	0.153, 59	0.159, 22	0.135, 21	0.010, 186
Animal naming	0.025, 83	0.306, 60*	0.182, 22	0.523, 21*	0.209, 186**
DS-B	−0.133, 87	0.023, 60	0.239, 22	0.087, 21	0.009, 190
RBANS immed memory	−0.089, 88	0.294, 61*	0.273, 22	0.737, 21**	0.232, 192**
RBANS delayed memory	0.005, 85	0.547, 58**	0.450, 21*	0.710, 20**	0.381, 184**
RBANS language	−0.102, 87	0.192, 60	0.065, 22	0.248, 20	0.107, 189
RBANS attention	−0.182, 79	0.347, 52*	0.038, 21	0.217, 19	0.053, 171
RBANS visuospatial/constructional	0.130, 81	0.397, 54**	0.023, 20	0.328, 20	0.252, 175**
RBANS total scale	−0.079, 74	0.527, 49**	0.359, 21	0.768, 18**	0.334, 162**

*$P < 0.05$ but > 0.01. **$P < 0.01$.

differed from those of AF. For the overall sample, the initial regression diagnostics resulted in removal of NPI-severity and distress in addition to the RBANS total scale index score due to multicollinearity. The overall model accounted for a large proportion of variance in AM ($R = 0.736$, $P < 0.001$), but of the predictors (IADL-Patient, CESD overall, CESD depressed affect, CESD somatic/vegetative, CESD interpersonal, BSI global severity, animal naming, and RBANS immediate memory were excluded) only the CESD-Lack of positive affect ($t = 3.19$, $P = 0.002$), the RBANS visuospatial/constructional index ($t = 2.63$, $P = 0.01$), and the RBANS delayed memory index ($t = 8.65$, $P < 0.001$) remained significant. The regression equations for the diagnostic groups differed from the predictors for the overall group. For the non-aMCI group the overall model was nonsignificant (likely due to only 9 participants having all variables complete). For the non-AD dementia group the RBANS delayed memory index was the only significant predictor of AM ($t = 2.32$, $P = 0.028$), but for the few aMCI patients with all predictors complete the delayed memory was not significant ($t = 2.22$, $p = 0.053$). Perhaps most salient was the radically different associations between AM and the clinical correlates for the AD group. Here, only the IADL-Patient ($t = -2.15$, $P = 0.035$) and CESD lack of positive affect ($t = 2.32$, $P = 0.024$) predicted AM.

3.2.3. *Awareness of Balance.* The zero-order correlations that drove the regression equations for AB are shown in Table 4. The regression equations for the overall sample were less plagued by small sample size problems than the two MCI groups. The clinical correlates of probability of falling, POMA, and the BBS were excluded, however, due to multicollinearity. The remaining predictors were all significant: FAQ-caregiver ($t = -4.77$, $P < 0.001$), the ABC scale

TABLE 4: Clinical correlates of awareness of balance (AB) for each diagnostic group.

	AD	Non-AD	aMCI	Non-aMCI	Overall
	r_s, n	r_s, n	r_s, n	r_s, n	r_s, n
CDR-SOB	−0.001, 37	−0.024, 24	−0.606, 10	−0.543, 11	−0.176, 82
IADL-patient	0.268, 39	−0.222, 24	−0.464, 13	0.063, 12	0.013, 88
FAQ-caregiver	−0.261, 41	−0.142, 26	−0.027, 13	−0.614, 12*	−0.253, 92*
Bristol aDL-caregiver	0.003, 41	−0.036, 26	−0.064, 13	−0.440, 12	−0.138, 92
CESD overall	−0.021, 38	0.345, 22	0.268, 13	−0.099, 12	0.109, 85
CESD depressed affect	−0.022, 38	0.063, 22	0.403, 13	−0.182, 12	0.070, 85
CESD lack of positive affect	0.006, 38	0.339, 22	−0.295, 13	0.090, 12	0.069, 85
CESD somatic/vegetative	0.051, 38	0.316, 22	0.182, 13	0.159, 12	0.139, 85
CESD interpersonal	−0.079, 38	0.296, 22	0.061, 13	−0.064, 12	0.028, 85
NPI-severity	−0.114, 39	−0.083, 26	0.149, 12	—	−0.064, 86
NPI-distress	−0.061, 38	−0.017, 25	0.244, 12	−0.400, 10	−0.073, 85
ZBI	−0.238, 41	0.171, 25	0.074, 13	−0.416, 12	−0.196, 91
BSI global severity	−0.033, 37	0.271, 23	−0.292, 12	−0.168, 12	−0.002, 84
Fall history in past 6 months	−0.570, 43**	−0.569, 27**	−0.331, 13	−0.544, 12	−0.512, 95**
Probability of falling (%)	−0.549, 43**	−0.372, 27	−0.428, 13	−0.612, 12*	−0.501, 95**
ABC	−0.368, 43*	−0.480, 27*	−0.554, 13*	−0.109, 12	−0.392, 95**
BBS	0.310, 43*	0.049, 27	0.326, 13	0.593, 12*	0.289, 95**
POMA	0.324, 24	0.101, 17	—	—	0.316, 54*
Stroop-interference	−0.201, 35	0.203, 22	0.164, 12	−0.152, 12	0.076, 81
TMT-B	0.118, 19	0.051, 11	0.294, 10	−0.116, 10	0.063, 50
Clock drawing	−0.129, 39	0.077, 25	0.029, 13	0.144, 12	0.006, 89
Phonemic fluency	−0.126, 38	−0.033, 25	0.247, 13	0.257, 12	0.009, 88
Animal naming	−0.157, 39	0.133, 25	−0.035, 13	0.680, 12*	0.020, 89
DS-B	0.073, 37	−0.077, 24	0.077, 13	−0.030, 12	0.044, 86
RBANS immed memory	−0.109, 37	−0.091, 24	−0.027, 13	0.271, 12	0.016, 86
RBANS delayed memory	−0.130, 36	−0.056, 21	0.077, 12	0.723, 12**	−0.001, 81
RBANS language	−0.277, 37	0.113, 23	0.362, 13	0.129, 12	0.035, 85
RBANS attention	0.133, 37	0.125, 20	−0.342, 12	0.228, 12	0.072, 81
RBANS visuospatial/constructional	0.047, 37	−0.366, 20	−0.101, 11	0.050, 12	0.012, 80
RBANS Total Scale	−0.022, 34	0.052, 20	0.067, 12	0.583, 11	0.114, 77

*$P < 0.05$ but > 0.01. **$P < 0.01$.

($t = 6.61$, $P < 0.01$), and fall history in Last 6 Months (coded yes/no, $t = -8.01$, $P < 0.001$) and together accounted for a large proportion of variance in AB ($R = 0.757$, $P < 0.001$). When compared across the diagnostic groups, the two regression equations for the MCI groups were not statistically significant, likely due to small sample sizes. For both dementia groups the ABC scale was a significant predictor of AB (AD group $t = 4.61$, $P = 0.038$, non-AD $t = -2.34$, $P = 0.014$) but, in addition, for the non-AD group the fall history in Last 6 Months was significant ($t = -3.81$, $P = 0.001$).

4. Discussion

These data support the hypothesis that awareness for different domains, specifically awareness of function, memory, and balance, would differentially relate to clinical correlates. This is in keeping with early work on awareness demonstrating differential clinical correlates for specific awareness domains [12–15] and provides support for the assertion by Markova and colleagues [39] that awareness must be conceptualized as specific to the domain being measured, and that research on one domain cannot be generalized to another domain. In addition to finding differential patterns of clinical correlates across domains of awareness, these data suggest that diagnostic group is also an important consideration in the clinical correlates of awareness. This was most evident in the clinical correlates for the AD group versus the non-AD and aMCI groups for awareness of memory. Here, the relationship between specific symptoms of depression and awareness of memory was only evident for the AD group. In contrast, the clinical correlates for the other groups remain restricted to measures of memory. These data suggest the assertion by Markova et al. [39] regarding caution in cross-domain generalization is not sufficient, and diagnostic grouping is another important consideration, at least for some domains of awareness.

Moreover, awareness for specific domains was shown to vary across the diagnostic groups. Awareness of function was lower for the groups diagnosed with dementia than those with MCI whereas awareness of memory was lower for the group with AD dementia and the group with aMCI, often considered a precursor to AD [67], than for the non-AD dementia or non-aMCI groups. Awareness of balance did not appear to differ across the diagnostic subgroups.

Our data suggest that awareness of specific domains was orthogonal: awareness of function was not associated with awareness of memory or awareness of balance. This was in contrast to the findings by Ott and colleagues [12] who found moderate correlations between awareness of memory and awareness of function. Our method for measuring awareness of function was similar to that used by Ott and colleagues (namely, patient/caregiver discrepancy), but we used a discrepancy between performance and self-report to assess memory and balance awareness, which may account for these inconsistent findings.

Evidence for the modality specific nature of awareness is provided by the differential patterns of clinical correlates depending on domain measured. We found that the relation between caregiver burden and distress depended on the modality of awareness measured: reduced awareness of function was associated with increased caregiver reports of burden, which is consistent with findings from previous research [10, 11, 14]. Balance awareness was the only awareness measure associated with physical variables such as past history of falls and self-reported balance confidence. The relation between balance awareness and falls is consistent with previous research demonstrating a strong relationship between proprioception and balance [65] or falls [38]. Differential patterns of awareness were also shown for relations with neuropsychological variables. Balance awareness was not related to any measure of neuropsychological functioning, despite previously reported relationships between risk of falls and measures of executive function [68]. Similarly, awareness of function was not associated with neuropsychological variables. Although none of the domains of awareness were associated with measures of executive function, awareness of memory was associated with neuropsychological variables of the delayed memory index and the visuospatial/constructional indices from the RBANS. The associations with neuropsychological variables differed, however, when the diagnostic groups were considered separately. Interestingly, awareness of memory was not associated with the delayed memory scores for the AD group. A floor effect in the delayed memory score appears to have created problems with heteroscedasticity in the bivariate memory awareness relationship, which may have attenuated any associations. The possible floor effect in memory measures did not, however, impact the association between depressive symptoms and awareness of memory, only for the AD group.

The findings of differential clinical correlates for awareness of memory based on diagnostic group may speak to some of the most contradictory findings regarding correlates of awareness. Neuropsychological function is inconsistently related to awareness [1, 12, 19, 20, 27, 29], and the relationship between awareness in dementia and depression is complicated, with clinical lore and empirical data supporting the notion that increased awareness is associated with more symptoms of depressed mood [18, 25], but increased awareness and depression may only be related to subclinical (or dysthymia) rather than major depression [1]. Our data suggest that in addition to modality of awareness being considered when measuring associations of neuropsychological and depressive symptoms with awareness, diagnostic group is an additional important consideration. Patients with dementia due to AD appear to have differential clinical correlates for awareness of memory versus patients with non-AD dementia, for example.

Although the prediction of differential clinical correlates for the different domains of awareness was supported, some of our predictions regarding these clinical correlates were contrary to previous research. In zero-order associations, severity was associated with awareness of function, but with no other domain of awareness. Moreover, severity did not account for sufficient unique variance in awareness of function and was, therefore, not a significant predictor. This finding is in contrast to the cumulative cross-sectional data demonstrating an association between severity of cognitive impairment and awareness (see [1] for a thorough review) and is contrary to the more compelling longitudinal data demonstrating decreasing awareness with increasing cognitive impairment [16, 18]. These contrasting findings likely speak to the orthogonal and domain-specific nature of the construct of awareness. Aalten and colleagues' [18] and McDaniel and colleagues' [16] prospective studies measured awareness by clinician ratings based on an interview with patient and caregiver regarding the patient's history of cognitive deficits and their impact on function.

Finally, all measures of awareness were associated with some measure of independence in daily function, particularly instrumental activities of daily living which is evidence against modality specificity. Assessment of functional abilities as a clinical correlate for measures of awareness is not often reported in the literature, but the few studies that do exist suggest that decreased awareness is associated with increased functional limitations [19], which is consistent with our data.

Despite adding to the converging research on the modality-specific nature of awareness [4, 8–10], these data are limited by the inconsistency in the measurement methods used for each modality of awareness. Measurement of awareness of function was based on caregiver/patient discrepancy, whereas awareness of memory and of balance was based on discrepancy between self-report and objective measures of performance. If awareness is a true construct, it should not be highly dependent on how it is measured. If, for example, awareness of function differs greatly when measured with caregiver/patient discrepancy versus patient/observation discrepancy, then this would not be a construct at all and would be considered an artifact of measurement [69]. If awareness is an artifact of measurement, future research measuring awareness of different modalities of awareness with different methods for measuring awareness will find markedly different clinical correlates than those presented here.

Another more problematic limitation of these data is the fact that this sample is derived from a specialty clinic. Specialty clinic patients have been postulated to have higher awareness than the general dementia population due to the referral process for specialty clinics [70]. It is unclear how having higher awareness may have impacted the differential patterns of clinical correlates for these multiple domains of awareness.

Although replication is required, these data demonstrate differential patterns of clinical correlates for awareness of function and memory. In addition, this study provides a novel contribution by describing the clinical correlates for awareness of balance. These data provide evidence for modality specific relations between awareness and clinical correlates in a database with a wide range of standardized measures of clinical correlates including severity, function, neuropsychiatric symptoms, depression, caregiver burden and distress, and a comprehensive assessment of neuropsychological status. Differing patterns of clinical correlates for awareness of function, awareness of memory, and awareness of balance provide support for the modality specific uniqueness of awareness measures for each of these domains. Data demonstrating different patterns of awareness based on diagnostic group (namely, aMCI, non-aMCI, AD, and non-AD dementia diagnoses) provides further evidence for the modality specific nature of awareness. Modality specificity, if replicated in different populations, for example, stroke patients, could have implications for rehabilitation. These data would suggest that rehabilitation needs to be targeted to a domain of awareness since awareness is not a unitary construct. Future research is needed on the clinical course and implications for day-to-day care associated with impairments in specific modalities of awareness for persons with dementia.

Conflict of Interests

The authors declare that there is no conflict of interests regarding the publication of this paper.

Acknowledgments

There is no conflicts of interests for any of the authors that would impact this paper. The Rural and Remote Memory Clinic was funded by a New Emerging Team Grant from the Canadian Institutes for Health Research (CIHR) Institute of Aging, CIHR Institute of Health Services and Policy Research, CIHR Rural and Northern Health Initiative, Saskatchewan Health Research Foundation, University of Saskatchewan, Alzheimer Society of Saskatchewan, and Telehealth Saskatchewan (in part).

References

[1] P. Aalten, E. van Valen, L. Clare, G. Kenny, and F. Verhey, "Awareness in dementia: a review of clinical correlates," *Aging and Mental Health*, vol. 9, no. 5, pp. 414–422, 2005.

[2] E. Ecklund-Johnson and I. Torres, "Unawareness of deficits in Alzheimer's disease and other dementias: operational definitions and empirical findings," *Neuropsychology Review*, vol. 15, no. 3, pp. 147–166, 2005.

[3] S. Cosentiono and Y. Stern, "Metacognitive theory and assessment in dementia: do we recognize our areas of weakness?" *Journal of the International Neuropsychological Society*, vol. 11, no. 7, pp. 910–919, 2005.

[4] I. S. Marková and G. E. Berrios, "Insight in clinical psychiatry. A new model," *The Journal of nervous and mental disease*, vol. 183, no. 12, pp. 743–751, 1995.

[5] D. C. Mograbi, R. G. Brown, and R. G. Morris, "Anosognosia in Alzheimer's disease—the petrified self," *Consciousness and Cognition*, vol. 18, no. 4, pp. 989–1003, 2009.

[6] K. P. Rankin, E. Baldwin, C. Pace-Savitsky, J. H. Kramer, and B. L. Miller, "Self awareness and personality change in dementia," *Journal of Neurology, Neurosurgery and Psychiatry*, vol. 76, no. 5, pp. 632–639, 2005.

[7] S. E. Starkstein, R. Jorge, R. Mizrahi, and R. G. Robinson, "A diagnostic formulation for anosognosia in Alzheimer's disease," *Journal of Neurology, Neurosurgery and Psychiatry*, vol. 77, no. 6, pp. 719–725, 2006.

[8] L. Clare, I. Marková, F. Verhey, and G. Kenny, "Awareness in dementia: a review of assessment methods and measures," *Aging and Mental Health*, vol. 9, no. 5, pp. 394–413, 2005.

[9] P. Howorth and J. Saper, "The dimensions of insight in people with dementia," *Aging and Mental Health*, vol. 7, no. 2, pp. 113–122, 2003.

[10] A. L. Snow, M. P. Norris, R. Doody, V. A. Molinari, C. A. Orengo, and M. E. Kunik, "Dementia deficits scale: rating self-awareness of deficits," *Alzheimer Disease and Associated Disorders*, vol. 18, no. 1, pp. 22–31, 2004.

[11] A. L. Snow, D. P. Graham, V. A. Molinari et al., "Factors affecting deficit awareness in persons with dementia," *Dementia and Geriatric Cognitive Disorders*, vol. 20, no. 2-3, pp. 133–139, 2005.

[12] B. R. Ott, G. Lafleche, W. M. Whelihan, G. W. Buongiorno, M. S. Albert, and B. S. Fogel, "Impaired awareness of deficits in Alzheimer disease," *Alzheimer Disease and Associated Disorders*, vol. 10, no. 2, pp. 68–76, 1996.

[13] R. Migliorelli, A. Teson, L. Sabe et al., "Anosognosia in Alzheimer's disease: a study of associated factors," *Journal of Neuropsychiatry and Clinical Neurosciences*, vol. 7, no. 3, pp. 338–344, 1995.

[14] B. Seltzer, J. J. Vasterling, J. Yoder, and K. A. Thompson, "Awareness of deficit in Alzheimer's disease: relation to caregiver burden," *Gerontologist*, vol. 37, no. 1, pp. 20–24, 1997.

[15] S. E. Starkstein, L. Sabe, E. Chemerinski, L. Jason, and R. Leiguarda, "Two domains of anosognosia in Alzheimer's disease," *Journal of Neurology Neurosurgery and Psychiatry*, vol. 61, no. 5, pp. 485–490, 1996.

[16] K. D. McDaniel, S. D. Edland, A. Heyman et al., "Relationship between level of insight and severity of dementia in Alzheimer disease," *Alzheimer Disease and Associated Disorders*, vol. 9, no. 2, pp. 101–104, 1995.

[17] B. R. Ott and B. S. Fogel, "Measurement of depression in dementia: self vs clinician rating," *International Journal of Geriatric Psychiatry*, vol. 7, no. 12, pp. 899–904, 1992.

[18] P. Aalten, E. van Valen, M. E. de Vugt, R. Lousberg, J. Jolles, and F. R. J. Verhey, "Awareness and behavioral problems in dementia patients: a prospective study," *International Psychogeriatrics*, vol. 18, no. 1, pp. 3–17, 2006.

[19] Y. Kashiwa, Y. Kitabayashi, J. Narumoto, K. Nakamura, H. Ueda, and K. Fukui, "Anosognosia in Alzheimer's disease: association with patient characteristics, psychiatric symptoms and cognitive deficits," *Psychiatry and Clinical Neurosciences*, vol. 59, no. 6, pp. 697–704, 2005.

[20] C. A. Mangone, D. B. Hier, P. B. Gorelick et al., "Impaired insight in Alzheimer's disease," *Journal of Geriatric Psychiatry and Neurology*, vol. 4, no. 4, pp. 189–193, 1991.

[21] L. Clare, B. A. Wilson, G. Carter, I. Roth, and J. R. Hodges, "Assessing awareness in early-stage Alzheimer's disease: development and piloting of the memory awareness rating scale," *Neuropsychological Rehabilitation*, vol. 12, no. 4, pp. 341–362, 2002.

[22] C. H. Y. Wong, L. C. W. Lam, V. W. C. Lui, H. F. K. Chiu, S. S. M. Chan, and C. W. C. Tam, "Subjective complaints and self-evaluation of memory test performancen in questionable dementia," *International Journal of Geriatric Psychiatry*, vol. 21, no. 10, pp. 937–944, 2006.

[23] L. Clare and B. A. Wilson, "Longitudinal assessment of awareness in early-stage Alzheimer's disease using comparable questionnaire-based and performance-based measures: a prospective one-year follow-up study," *Aging and Mental Health*, vol. 10, no. 2, pp. 156–165, 2006.

[24] M. B. Spitznagel, G. Tremont, L. B. Brown, and J. Gunstad, "Cognitive reserve and the relationship between depressive symptoms and awareness of deficits in dementia," *Journal of Neuropsychiatry and Clinical Neurosciences*, vol. 18, no. 2, pp. 186–190, 2006.

[25] D. G. Harwood, D. L. Sultzer, and M. V. Wheatley, "Impaired insight in Alzheimer disease: association with cognitive deficits, psychiatric symptoms, and behavioral disturbances," *Neuropsychiatry, Neuropsychology and Behavioral Neurology*, vol. 13, no. 2, pp. 83–88, 2000.

[26] A. Vogel, F. B. Waldorff, and G. Waldemar, "Impaired awareness of deficits and neuropsychiatric symptoms in early Alzheimer's disease: the Danish Alzheimer Intervention Study (DAISY)," *Journal of Neuropsychiatry and Clinical Neurosciences*, vol. 22, no. 1, pp. 93–99, 2010.

[27] A. Michon, B. Deweer, B. Pillon, Y. Agid, and B. Dubois, "Relation of anosognosia to frontal lobe dysfunction in Alzheimer's disease," *Journal of Neurology Neurosurgery and Psychiatry*, vol. 57, no. 7, pp. 805–809, 1994.

[28] E. Salmon, D. Perani, F. Collette et al., "A comparison of unawareness in frontotemporal dementia and Alzheimer's disease," *Journal of Neurology, Neurosurgery and Psychiatry*, vol. 79, no. 2, pp. 176–179, 2008.

[29] A. Vogel, S. G. Hasselbalch, A. Gade, M. Ziebell, and G. Waldemar, "Cognitive and functional neuroimaging correlates for anosognosia in mild cognitive impairment and Alzheimer's disease," *International Journal of Geriatric Psychiatry*, vol. 20, no. 3, pp. 238–246, 2005.

[30] D. G. Harwood, D. L. Sultzer, D. Feil, L. Monserratt, E. Freedman, and M. A. Mandelkern, "Frontal lobe hypometabolism and impaired insight in Alzheimer disease," *American Journal of Geriatric Psychiatry*, vol. 13, no. 11, pp. 934–941, 2005.

[31] M. F. Mendez and J. S. Shapira, "Loss of insight and functional neuroimaging in frontotemporal dementia," *Journal of Neuropsychiatry and Clinical Neurosciences*, vol. 17, no. 3, pp. 413–416, 2005.

[32] S. E. Starkstein, S. Brockman, D. Bruce, and G. Petracca, "Anosognosia is a significant predictor of apathy in Alzheimer's disease," *Journal of Neuropsychiatry and Clinical Neurosciences*, vol. 22, no. 4, pp. 378–383, 2010.

[33] K. Shibata, J. Narumoto, Y. Kitabayashi, Y. Ushijima, and K. Fukui, "Correlation between anosognosia and regional cerebral blood flow in Alzheimer's disease," *Neuroscience Letters*, vol. 435, no. 1, pp. 7–10, 2008.

[34] M. Mimura, "Memory impairment and awareness of memory deficits in early-stage Alzheimer's disease," *Tohoku Journal of Experimental Medicine*, vol. 215, no. 2, pp. 133–140, 2008.

[35] M. L. Ries, B. M. Jabbar, T. W. Schmitz et al., "Anosognosia in mild cognitive impairment: relationship to activation of cortical midline structures involved in self-appraisal," *Journal of the International Neuropsychological Society*, vol. 13, no. 3, pp. 450–461, 2007.

[36] H. Hanyu, T. Sato, T. Akai et al., "Neuroanatomical correlates of unawareness of memory deficits in early Alzheimer's disease," *Dementia and Geriatric Cognitive Disorders*, vol. 25, no. 4, pp. 347–353, 2008.

[37] D. T. Stuss and B. Levine, "Adult clinical neuropsychology: lessons from studies of the frontal lobes," *Annual Review of Psychology*, vol. 53, pp. 401–433, 2002.

[38] N. Kamata, Y. Matsuo, T. Yoneda, H. Shinohara, S. Inoue, and K. Abe, "Overestimation of stability limits leads to a high frequency of falls in patients with Parkinson's disease," *Clinical Rehabilitation*, vol. 21, no. 4, pp. 357–361, 2007.

[39] I. S. Markova, L. Clare, M. Wang, B. Romero, and G. Kenny, "Awareness in dementia: conceptual issues," *Aging and Mental Health*, vol. 9, no. 5, pp. 386–393, 2005.

[40] A. Vogel, J. Stokholm, A. Gade, B. B. Andersen, A.-M. Hejl, and G. Waldemar, "Awareness of deficits in mild cognitive impairment and Alzheimer's disease: do MCI patients have impaired insight?" *Dementia and Geriatric Cognitive Disorders*, vol. 17, no. 3, pp. 181–187, 2004.

[41] D. G. Morgan, M. Crossley, A. Kirk et al., "Improving access to dementia care: development and evaluation of a rural and remote memory clinic," *Aging and Mental Health*, vol. 13, no. 1, pp. 17–30, 2009.

[42] A. Robillard, "Clinical diagnosis of dementia," *Alzheimer's and Dementia*, vol. 3, no. 4, pp. 292–298, 2007.

[43] K. Rockwood, "Vascular cognitive impairment and vascular dementia," *Journal of the Neurological Sciences*, vol. 203-204, pp. 23–27, 2002.

[44] J. C. Morris, "The clinical dementia rating (CDR): current version and scoring rules," *Neurology*, vol. 43, no. 11, pp. 2412–2414, 1993.

[45] S. E. O'Bryant, S. C. Waring, C. M. Cullum et al., "Staging dementia using clinical dementia rating scale sum of boxes scores: a Texas Alzheimer's Research Consortium Study," *Archives of Neurology*, vol. 65, no. 8, pp. 1091–1095, 2008.

[46] M. P. Lawton, M. Moss, M. Fulcomer, and M. H. Kleban, "A research and service oriented multilevel assessment instrument," *Journals of Gerontology*, vol. 37, no. 1, pp. 91–99, 1982.

[47] R. I. Pfeffer, T. T. Kurosaki, C. H. Harrah, J. Chance, and S. Filos, "Measurement of functional activities in older adults in the community," *Journals of Gerontology*, vol. 37, no. 3, pp. 323–329, 1982.

[48] R. S. Bucks, D. L. Ashworth, G. K. Wilcock, and K. Siegfried, "Assessment of activities of daily living in dementia: development of the Bristol activities of Daily Living Scale," *Age and Ageing*, vol. 25, no. 2, pp. 113–120, 1996.

[49] J. L. Cummings, M. Mega, K. Gray, S. Rosenberg-Thompson, D. A. Carusi, and J. Gornbein, "The neuropsychiatric inventory: comprehensive assessment of psychopathology in dementia," *Neurology*, vol. 44, no. 12, pp. 2308–2314, 1994.

[50] P. M. Lewinsohn, J. R. Seeley, R. E. Roberts, and N. B. Allen, "Center for epidemiologic studies depression scale (CES-D) as a screening instrument for depression among community-residing older adults," *Psychology and Aging*, vol. 12, no. 2, pp. 277–287, 1997.

[51] N. O'Rourke and H. A. Tuokko, "Psychometric properties of an abridged version of the Zarit Burden Interview within a representative Canadian caregiver sample," *Gerontologist*, vol. 43, no. 1, pp. 121–127, 2003.

[52] L. Derogatis, *Brief Symptom Inventory*, Clinical Psychometric Research, Baltimore, Md, USA, 1975.

[53] K. Berg, S. Wood-Dauphinee, J. I. Williams, and D. Gayton, "Measuring balance in the elderly: preliminary development of an instrument," *Physiotherapy Canada*, vol. 41, no. 6, pp. 304–311, 1989.

[54] M. E. Tinetti, "Performance-orientated assessment of mobility problems in elderly patients," *Journal of the American Geriatrics Society*, vol. 34, no. 2, pp. 119–126, 1986.

[55] A. Shumway-Cook, M. Baldwin, N. L. Polissar, and W. Gruber, "Predicting the probability for falls in community-dwelling older adults," *Physical Therapy*, vol. 77, no. 8, pp. 812–819, 1997.

[56] L. E. Powell and A. M. Myers, "The Activities-specific Balance Confidence (ABC) Scale," *Journals of Gerontology A*, vol. 50, no. 1, pp. M28–M34, 1995.

[57] E. Strauss, E. M. S. Sherman, and O. Spreen, *A Compendium of Neuropsychological Tests: Administration, Norms, and Commentary*, Oxford University Press, New York, NY, USA.

[58] R. M. Reitan and D. Wolfson, *The Halstead-Reitan Neuropsycholgical Test Battery: Therapy and Clinical Interpretation*, Neuropsychological Press, Tucson, AZriz, USA, 1985.

[59] M. R. Trennery, B. Crosson, J. DeBoe, and W. R. Leber, *Stroop Neuropsychological Screening Test*, Psychological Assessment Resources, Fla, USA, 1989.

[60] H. Goodglass and E. Kaplan, *The Assessment of Aphasia and Related Disorders*, Lea & Febiger, Philadelphia, PA, 2nd edition, 1983.

[61] H. Tuokko and M. E. O'Connell, "A review of quantified approaches to the qualitative assessment of clock drawing," in *The Quantified Process Approach to Neuropsychological Assessment*, A. M. Poreh, Ed., pp. 173–206, Taylor & Francis, New York, NY, USA, 2006.

[62] D. Wechsler, *Wechsler Adult Intelligence Scale*, Psychological Corporation, San Antonio, Tex, USA, 3rd edition, 1997.

[63] C. Randolph, *Repeatable Battery for the Assessment of Neuropsychological Status Manual*, Psychological Corporation, San Antonio, Tex, USA, 1998.

[64] L. R. Squire and J. A. Zouzounis, "Self-ratings of memory dysfunction: different findings in depression and amnesia," *Journal of Clinical and Experimental Neuropsychology*, vol. 10, no. 6, pp. 727–738, 1988.

[65] S. N. Robinovitch and T. Cronin, "Perception of postural limits in elderly nursing home and day care participants," *Journals of Gerontology A*, vol. 54, no. 3, pp. B124–B131, 1999.

[66] J. Cohen, *Statistical Power Analysis for the Behavioral Sciences*, Lawrence Erlbaum Associates, Mahwah, NJ, USA, 2nd edition, 1988.

[67] M. S. Albert, S. T. DeKosky, D. Dickson et al., "The diagnosis of mild cognitive impairment due to Alzheimer's disease: recommendations from the National Institute on Aging and Alzheimer's Association workgroup," *Alzheimer's and Dementia*, 2011.

[68] T. Herman, A. Mirelman, N. Giladi, A. Schweiger, and J. M. Hausdorff, "Executive control deficits as a prodrome to falls in healthy older adults: a prospective study linking thinking, walking, and falling," *Journals of Gerontology A*, vol. 65, no. 10, pp. 1086–1092, 2010.

[69] J. Michell, "Quantitative science and the defination of measurement in psychology," *British Journal of Psychology*, vol. 88, no. 3, pp. 355–383, 1997.

[70] C. Helmer, K. Pérès, A. Pariente et al., "Primary and secondary care consultations in elderly demented individuals in France: results from the three-city study," *Dementia and Geriatric Cognitive Disorders*, vol. 26, no. 5, pp. 407–415, 2008.

3

Learning from "Knocks in Life": Food Insecurity among Low-Income Lone Senior Women

Rebecca J. Green-LaPierre,[1] Patricia L. Williams,[1,2] N. Theresa Glanville,[1] Deborah Norris,[3] Heather C. Hunter,[4] and Cynthia G. Watt[4]

[1] *Department of Applied Human Nutrition, Mount Saint Vincent University, Halifax, NS, Canada B3M 2J6*
[2] *Atlantic Health Promotion Research Centre, Dalhousie University, Halifax, NS, Canada B3H 3J5*
[3] *Department of Family Studies and Gerontology, Mount Saint Vincent University, Halifax, NS, Canada B3M 2J6*
[4] *Participatory Food Costing Project, Mount Saint Vincent University, Halifax, NS, Canada B3M 2J6*

Correspondence should be addressed to Patricia L. Williams, patty.williams@msvu.ca

Academic Editor: Joseph R. Sharkey

Building on earlier quantitative work where we showed that lone senior households reliant on public pensions in Nova Scotia (NS), Canada lacked the necessary funds for a basic nutritious diet, here we present findings from a qualitative study involving in-depth interviews with eight low-income lone senior women living in an urban area of NS. Using a phenomenological inquiry approach, in-depth interviews were used to explore lone senior women's experiences accessing food with limited financial resources. Drawing upon Bronfenbrenner's Ecological Systems Theory, we explored their perceived ability to access a nutritionally adequate and personally acceptable diet, and the barriers and enablers to do so; as well in light of our previous quantitative research, we explored their perceptions related to adequacy of income, essential expenses, and their strategies to manage personal finances. Seven key themes emerged: world view, income adequacy, transportation, health/health problems, community program use, availability of family and friends, and personal food management strategies. World view exerted the largest influence on seniors' personal perception of food security status. The implications of the findings and policy recommendations to reduce the nutritional health inequities among this vulnerable subset of the senior population are considered.

1. Introduction

In 2008, we published unique work addressing the question of whether Canada's public pensions, Old Age Security[1] and the Canada Pension Plan[2], provide adequate income for four hypothetical senior households living in Nova Scotia (NS) to afford a basic nutritious diet [1]. This was the first published study using food costing[3] data to investigate the sufficiency of public financial programs targeted at seniors. Results showed that single-member households in NS in 2008 lacked the necessary funds, with monthly deficits estimated to be as high as $224.18 if they were to purchase a basic nutritious diet.

The province of NS is home to the oldest population in Canada, with 16.5% of its residents over the age of 65 years; the majority of which are women [2]. As elsewhere [3], senior women in NS are disproportionally impacted by poverty. In 2006, almost one-third of lone senior women lived below the before-tax low-income Cutoff (LICO)[4] Canada's unofficial poverty line, compared to one in five men who lived alone [4]. In NS, 74% of seniors living below the LICO are women [4].

2. Purpose

The purpose of this paper is to explore the phenomenon of food insecurity for low-income lone senior women living in NS. This study used in-depth interviews to explore lone senior women's experiences accessing food with limited financial resources. We explored their perceived ability to access a nutritionally adequate and personally acceptable diet, and the barriers and enablers to do so; as well in light of our previous quantitative research [1], we explored their perceptions related to adequacy of income, essential expenses, and their strategies to manage personal finances.

3. Background

The United Nations' Food and Agricultural Organization states that "food security exists when all people, at all times, have physical and economical access to sufficient, safe, and nutritious food that meets their dietary needs and food preferences for an active and healthy life" [6, page 1560]. An assured ability to acquire acceptable foods in socially acceptable ways is also considered a key component of being food secure [7]. The easiest way to understand food insecurity is lack of financial resources to purchase food needed and wanted; however, in some of the pioneering research, which came out of Cornell University, on hunger and food insecurity, Radimer and colleagues [8] found that two dimensions of food insecurity existed: an individual dimension and a household dimension with each dimension containing four components: quantitative, qualitative, psychological, and social.

The quantitative and qualitative components of food insecurity are the most easily measured: experiencing hunger, going without food, or having to eat less food than usual, and consumption of nutritionally inadequate meals. Individuals reporting food insecurity are significantly more likely to consume less energy and other key nutrients than those self-reporting as having sufficient food [9, 10]. The psychological component to food insecurity is exemplified by an individual's anxiety over their food situation, such as wondering where their next meal will come, while the social component is manifested by socially or culturally less normative patterns of eating (e.g., skipping meals), and acquiring food in socially unacceptable ways (e.g., using a food bank) [8]. While these characteristics have been documented among senior populations in the US by Wolfe et al. [5], they also found that having the right foods for health and anxiety over not having these specific health-related foods are phenomena within the qualitative and psychological components of food insecurity that are unique to seniors.

Other food security research focusing on seniors has also found that finances are not the only limiting factor for seniors to access acceptable and adequate food. Upon analyzing in-depth interviews with 145 adults, age 70 years and older, living in rural North Carolina, Quandt and Rao [11] revealed that barriers to food security in rural American seniors were associated with material (e.g., low-income), social (e.g., limited family network), and health (e.g., presence of disease or disability) related factors. Dean et al. [12] report that among older and senior adults in a largely rural area of central Texas, food insecurity is associated with diminished social capital (limited access to community and familial resources) and perceptions of personal disparity in comparison with others. Single, widowed, or divorced persons also reported higher levels of food insecurity, related in part to limited familial social capital [12]. Reliance on others for help with food-related activities such as grocery shopping and meal preparation can influence food intake and can be considered part of the concept of food insecurity among older adults [13].

There is also the "generational lens" through which seniors view the world. Other work completed by Quandt and colleagues [14] suggests that pride, self-sufficiency, and "you cannot always get what you want" attitude are aspects of the generational lens that colour the nature of food security for seniors. These "senior-relevant" factors highlighted by researchers in the US suggest that what food security means to seniors, and therefore how they manage their ability to access food is different than younger populations' views of food security. However, Canadian research in this area is lacking. Given the different history and health and social systems in the US, it is not clear whether pride and a self-sufficient attitude would play the same role in a Canadian senior's meaning of food security.

These newer "senior-relevant" factors also suggest the possibility that Canada's current food security measurement tools, which focus on low-income as the most significant determinant of food insecurity [15], may not accurately capture the other major enablers and barriers seniors face in accessing sufficient, quality foods in socially acceptable ways. It is possible we are not understanding and therefore not capturing the full picture of food insecurity among seniors.

The negative relationship between food insecurity and one's ability to access a nutritious diet and mitigate risk for chronic disease is well understood. Chronic diseases commonly impacting seniors such as cardiovascular disease and cancer are used to exemplify the relationship between insufficient access to nutritious food and the resulting poor health outcomes [16–18]. Therefore, understanding how a particular group of seniors—lower income senior women living alone in Nova Scotia—attempt to maintain food security, can provide insights to the necessary policies and programs needed to reduce the nutritional health inequities among this vulnerable subset of the senior population.

4. Theoretical Framework

An ecological model was used to frame the participants' perceived realities regarding their ability to access a nutritionally adequate and personally acceptable diet, the barriers and enablers to do so; as well their perceptions related to adequacy of income, essential expenses, and their strategies to manage personal finances, guiding our approach to addressing our research purpose. Ecological models reveal that individual behaviours such as food procurement patterns are influenced by biological, demographic, psychological, social/cultural, environmental, and policy variables. Bronfenbrenner's Ecological Systems Theory [19, 20] was used as a framework to examine the many different areas in the seniors' environment where these variables exert their influence.

Three key themes characterize ecological systems theory. First, individuals are characterized as embodied within a system comprising a nested arrangement of structures.

The first of these structures, the microsystem refers to the face-to-face interactions within immediate settings such as home, neighbourhood, and informal social networks. The mesosystem comprises the relationships between and among the immediate settings, for example, family, seniors' centres, and community facilities. The exosystem consists of the social structures, both formal and informal, removed from the individual but yet functioning at the local level to regulate and control their everyday lives within the *microsystem*. These structures include the major institutions within society rendered visible through the implementation of policies and practices at the local level. Examples include mass media, government agencies, and social networks. *Macrosystems* may be defined as the overarching meaning systems, conveyed symbolically through culture. Macrosystems such as religious, political, legal, economic, health, and social systems are understood in ecological theory not just as reified structures but also as carriers of ideology that construct a "world view" that, both implicitly and explicitly, shapes experience at all other levels of the environment [21, 22].

Second, the conceptualization of the levels of the environment as a *nested* arrangement of structures implies that they are not mutually exclusive. Rather, it is assumed that a system cannot be understood when broken into its component parts or when separated from its context. Transactions flow bidirectionally from the outer level (*macrosystem*) inward, and conversely, from the inner level (*microsystem*) outward. These reciprocal exchanges are vital to maintaining the equilibrium of individuals, a proposition that has significance for this research.

Third, ecological theory brings into view the *interdependencies* that exist between immediate environments and broader systems. Change in one part of the system will stimulate changes in other parts. An ecological approach facilitates and emphasizes consideration of the impact of multiple and overlapping influences in addressing food security issues.

5. Methods

5.1. Data Collection and Sampling. Eligible participants were women 65 years of age or older, who lived by themselves in a noninstitutionalized setting (i.e., independent) in urban NS, and who were in receipt of the Guaranteed Income Supplement (GIS)[5]. Women living by themselves who had a spouse in a nursing home, hospital, or other type of institution were ineligible to participate. Interviews took place over the course of four months between June and September 2007. Lone senior women were the focus of this research as national statistics show this subgroup of the senior population at greatest risk for poverty and the most likely to not access all the financial benefits available [4, 23], and our previous research suggest seniors living alone are more likely to be unable to afford a nutritious diet than those living with a partner [1]. Sampling was done using purposive and snowball methods, using site-based recruitment through health care agencies and seniors' centres. Data collection and analysis continued concurrently until theoretical saturation was reached at eight participants.

Women participated in semistructured face-to-face interviews. The interview guide used to facilitate the interview was formulated using Radimer's conceptualization of food insecurity and hunger with its individual and household dimensions and four components: quantitative, qualitative, psychological, and social [8]. The intent was to use this framework to draw out health and world view as distinguishing features of food security in the elderly. The interview guide also contained questions developed by the Institute for Research on Poverty [24] dealing with how study participants procured and prepared food, their typical daily food routine, and asked questions about a time (if relevant) when they had difficulty getting enough food. Lastly, the interview guide asked participants to review hypothetical affordability scenarios comparing monthly income to expenses constructed in our earlier work [1] to gain their perspective on adequacy of Canadian public pensions to afford the food they needed and wanted, as well as other essential expenses. Broad, open-ended, semi-structured questions with probes were used.

Interviews took place in participants' homes or a location of the participant's choosing. Interviews were conducted in English, lasted between 60 and 120 minutes, were digitally recorded and transcribed verbatim. Journal and field notes were also recorded directly following the interviews. All participants were offered the opportunity to review their transcript. Study procedures were approved by Mount Saint Vincent University's Ethics Review Board.

5.2. Data Analysis. During the analysis, a phenomenological approach [25], in combination with a conceptual framework based on Bronfenbrenner's ecological model [20], was used to explore senior women's perceptions of their lived realities. Phenomenology is used to uncover the meaning behind a phenomenon, it goes beyond simply describing an experience, seeking to arrive at a structural description of the experience and expose the underlying and precipitating factors that account for what is being experienced [26].

Transcribed interviews, journal and field notes were imported into NVivo 7.0, a qualitative data analysis software program (QSR International, 2007). One of the authors (RGL) analyzed transcripts by systematically coding text, informed by the interview guide topics and themes that emerged from the data corresponding to environmental levels in Brofenbrenner's Ecological Systems Theory (microsystem, mesosystem, exosystem, and macrosystem) [19, 20]. Later, findings and links to the conceptual framework were strengthened through investigator triangulation.

6. Results

6.1. The Participants. Of the eight women who participated, four were 65–74 years of age and four were 75 years or older. All women rented their dwelling: one lived in a duplex, one in a townhouse complex, one in an apartment building, and five lived in senior-geared apartments. Seven of the eight women lived in subsidized housing, meaning their rent was based on a percentage of their income, while the eighth participant paid market rent for her duplex. One woman was never married while the other participants lived alone because they were either widowed or divorced. All women received the basic OAS pension and GIS. Four women received a Canada Pension, the result of their contribution to the Pension Plan when they were previously employed. Two women received survivor's benefit through the CPP. Only one woman reported receiving a private pension, although it only amounted to $73/month after working almost 25 years. None of the women owned a car; health reasons and finances were the main impetuses for "giving up" their vehicle.

As the women talked about their experiences managing finances, accessing the food they needed and wanted, and how they viewed their situation, seven main themes emerged depicting their perception of their food security status. These themes can be placed within the four interconnected layers of the seniors' environment as defined by Bronfenbrenner: (1) at the macrosystem level, *world view,* (2) within the exosystem, *income adequacy*, (3) at both the exo- and mesosystems levels, *transportation related factors,* (4) at both the exo- and microsystem levels, *health/health problems,* (5) within the mesosystem, *community program use*, (6) at the meso- and microsystems, *availability of family and friends,* and (7) within the microsystem, *personal food management strategies.* Figure 1 provides a visual map of the meaning of food security to these women, organized according to Bronfenbrenner's Ecological Framework.

6.2. World View (Macrosystem Factor). All of the women in this study met the criteria (according to its definition) to be classified as food insecure. They all used various coping skills to bring food into the house, such as accessing food banks, stretching meals, relying on credit; however, interestingly, none of them perceived themselves to be food insecure. At one or more points in the interview, participants were asked if they could recall a time in their life since they were a senior and living on their own when they had difficulty getting the food they needed and wanted. Some shared stories of going hungry in the past, such as when they were caring for their children or when they were first on their own without their spouse, but none considered their current situation as food insecure. A world view, or generational lens, develops as a result of past life experiences, cultural and religious beliefs and personal belief systems, and contribute, to the women's self-perceived food security status.

These women had a general contentedness about their diet, their life, and general circumstances. As stated by one participant: "*No, because as I say I've been doing good the way I've been doing now for many years and I've got no complaints with any of it. I've got a roof over my head and I've got food to put in my stomach and my doctors tell me I'm doing good so there's nothing else I could want. I mean there's a lot of people that can't say that.*" Although this woman was content with her life, she accessed a nearby food bank frequently, sometimes weekly. Despite needing to access food in a socially unacceptable way on a regular basis she perceived nothing problematic with her situation—due to her resourcefulness she did not lack food. A sense of resilient self-sufficiency was detected in the women interviewed, as most spoke about needing to be vigilant about their spending to assure that bills could be paid and assuring they had enough for the expenses they needed versus what they wanted. It was evident in talking with them that they had been through a lot and could manage most things that might come their way. "*I had a hard time bringing up my children, and you learn from your knocks in life eh? Don't want to go through those again, I got to look after me, and I am, I'm looking after me.*"

The lives all of these women were impacted in some way by the Depression and World War II so they understood the need to be resourceful and not wasteful. Some were lone parents, as were these two participants: "*No I've never ever went hungry, the only time I've ever went hungry when I was with my children*". "*Because I went for quite a few years where I didn't get enough to eat because I had to make sure my children were eating.*" Experiencing hunger earlier in life shaped how they saw their current situations; by definition, the participants experienced food insecurity within the quantitative component.

All eight women acknowledged factors hindering their access to food; however, they perceived the strategies they took to overcome the obstacles as either acceptable or just a fact of life; just something you do if you're old, poor, and so forth. None of the participants identified themselves as living in poverty or being in great need, or even want. The generational lens through which they viewed their situation allowed them to compare their current situation to situations in the past where they faced extreme financial difficulties; relative to more difficult times, they perceived their current income to be adequate, in other words, their perspectives were colored by their prior experiences and resultant world view.

6.3. Adequacy of Income (Exosystem Factor). As the women reviewed the affordability scenarios created in our previous work that compared monthly income to monthly basic expenses for two hypothetical lone senior households [1], the women were very candid in disclosing how much income they received each month and what bills their income went towards. The biggest lesson from their stories was the role of GIS and income-geared housing in protecting the funds remaining for food, and the importance of a "med-alert" type device and cable TV, two expenses which the participants deemed to be essential.

In general, the women were appreciative of the pensions they received, they were thankful to have a reliable monthly income; however, there were notions that they could use a bit more. "*Old Age Pensions and that? Well I tell ya, they could be more. They could be more. Of course, now this is a God send, what I get now compared to what I got then...when I was on mothers' allowance.*" Another participant shared: "*Oh, I'm always just about at the end of it at the end of the month... nobody's gonna get rich when I go, there'll be no fighting over my money!*" Public Pensions programs exist at the exosystem level, they are formal programs removed from the individual, but yet functioning at the local level to regulate and control their everyday lives and ability to access food.

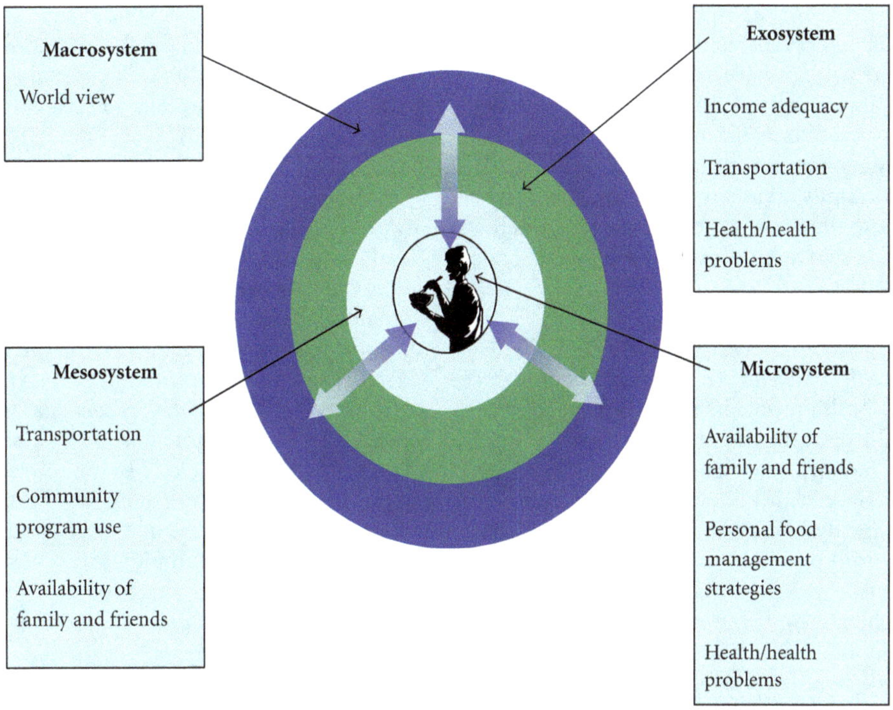

Figure 1: How low-income lone senior women living in NS experience food security, organized according to Bronfenbrenner's Ecological Framework.

Another significant example of a social structure directly impacting seven of the eight interviewed women's lives was the provincial senior social housing program. Two of the participants explain: "*Every year you have to call Ottawa and get them to send you a letter saying exactly what you're getting then you give that to Housing and they figure out 30% of it, they take. And the rest you've got for your TV and your phone and your groceries and to live on. It doesn't leave you a lot... Before you get your Old Age pension you only pay 25% of what you're getting, but once you hit 65 you pay 30% ...*"

"*[Housing] always take a third because that's their share of the rent. Every time rent comes up they take a third of that, whatever you get, so they can't put any more on for rent, because it's subsidized housing.*" This controlled rent expense meant despite the adequacy or inadequacy of their overall income, seven of the eight women never had to pay a disproportionate amount on shelter; thus their funds could be better distributed to other necessary expenses.

While none of the women conveyed that their food intake suffered because of inadequate income, due to their various coping strategies, what did seem to suffer was their social life. For example, participants commented, "*Like I never go to movies, the last time I went to a movie I took my children by their hands to see Herbie The Love Bug. They're now 46 and 43. Because I can't afford to go to movies.*" or "*No I can't afford to go out [to dinner], unless one of my children, my daughter she generally takes me out on Mother's Day and on Christmas I generally go down to her place... but no I eat by myself.*"

Although admittedly it wasn't a necessity, cable TV was viewed as an important component of their daily routine and helped to address the isolation these women experienced. Many watched television while eating their meals alone, and many would watch their favourite shows to help pass the time. "*If you don't have cable you can't watch TV ... like I've got digital cable because I can't go out. I mean the girls will come in to play cards and sometimes we'll go to Bingo every once and a while but that [cable] is the only enjoyment I have, know what I mean?*" Within the context of these low-income lone seniors' lives, cable was essential to help them cope with their situation, to help improve their quality of life.

6.4. Transportation (Exo- and Mesosystem Factor). The cost and feasibility of transportation was a major reoccurring theme during all interviews. None of the women owned cars, many had mobility issues, and all depended on family, friends, or neighbours to access grocery stores, medical appointments, or church.

Even the municipal accessible bus service did not meet the needs of some of the participants to access the foods they needed and wanted. Changes in the bus routes and a policy stating the accessible bus would only venture a certain number of meters off the urban transit (nonaccessible) route meant one participant could no longer rely on this service. Another participant noted how far in advance she would have to schedule the bus. "*You have to give exactly two weeks notice and then they'll work you in. So therefore you have to make your appointments [well in advance] ... And you [referring to interviewer] can get up in the morning and say I think I'll go get groceries today... we can't do that.*"

Within the mesosystem layer of the women's environment, family and friends provided the transportation to enable access to food for six of the eight women. The senior woman is involved in her mesosystem environment albeit not as intensely, as she will not have as much control at this level because it will always involve influence from another party (e.g., the family member or friend). While family and friends were the primary source of transportation for six of the women, for others family members were dispersed across the country, or of those that lived nearby some were unable or unwilling to provide this service for the participants on a consistent, reliable basis.

6.5. Health and Health Problems (Exo- and Microsystem Factor). A myriad of health problems affected this group of women: five suffered from arthritis or joint pain, four had Type 2 diabetes, four had hypertension, three had some type of digestive disorder, three had full or partial dentures, two were on medication for dyslipidemia, and two were cancer survivors. Stroke, thyroid problems, cardiovascular disease, and severe food allergies were reported once each. Overall, the main health problems contributing to food insecurity were physical and mobility limitations. The participants' multiple health issues required various medications, thus resulting in these women being regulated by drug plan policies. For six of the women enrolled in the provincial seniors' Pharmacare[6] program, they greatly benefited from the policy that exempted all seniors in receipt of the GIS from paying the annual premium associated with Pharmacare. The copayment policy also protected them from paying extreme costs at the pharmacy—the plan is structured so seniors pay a certain percentage of the total prescription cost at the pharmacy up to a maximum amount of (at the time of study) $30 for each prescription, with an annual maximum of $382. One participant explains: "*We gotta pay 30% ... it doesn't matter how much my medication comes to, you still only pay $30. Now this here [referring to a prescription], it's $96.95 but you still only pay $30. And same with my cholesterol pills, you still only pay $30. Those cholesterol pills are $133.82. But I still only pay $30. It doesn't matter if they were $500, you'd still only pay $30.*"

Saving money on medications and health benefits was important so that money could be better distributed to other parts of the budget, despite loss of services. One of the participants, formerly with her deceased husband's employer's insurance company, shared that once she turned 65 years of age and was eligible for Pharmacare she took advantage of the cheaper drug insurance plan, despite losing some health services. "*Yeah, I dropped Blue Cross; the thing was costing me a lot of money. But I used to be able to get some therapy for my arthritis, they'd pay for that but Pharmacare don't pay for that.*"

Throughout the interviews, as the women reviewed the affordability scenarios created in our previous work [1], an emergency response-type service was often mentioned as an essential expense, where the client wears a button, as a pendant or bracelet, which activates a speakerphone putting them in touch with the operator who in turn phones a first responder. A couple of the participants shared stories of how this service has alleviated the fear of having a fall when living alone. "*I call it my panic button. Oh I've used it a lot.*" One woman was adamant that it should be built into the Pharmacare program. "*I think not enough have it. I think that should be a basic thing that you should have to have. Some before they turn 65 if they have any type of medical problem and it should be required when you turn 65.*"

Grocery stores were another social structure which the women had minimal control over as store location and layout greatly impacted their food access. While grocery shopping had previously been viewed as a social outing for some of the women, mobility limitations turned it into a chore. "*Oh it's too much walking around. The stores are too big and my foot's too sore, I could never get around it. You know, just like going to the mall, you know, the mall is so awful, you know about that, the mall, it's so big by the time you get around and get home it's just like, ahhhh. You feel like you're dead. And grocery stores are just the same, they're too big and I don't want to get in no wheelchair, where am I gonna put the groceries at?*"

Health and health problems were also a direct part of the women's microsystem, a part of their everyday experiences interacting with their diet. For example, needing to avoid food because of allergies, sensitivities or because it was contraindicated with a medication was an issue for some of the women. One participant had nine different ingredients listed on her allergy information card, meaning sometimes she was left with little choice for meal options available through the congregate dining program at her seniors' manor. "*Your only choice is take it or leave it. A lot of foods I'm allergic to and they used to substitute but now the new the director's decided no no, no more substitution.... I'm allergic to many, many foods. I'm allergic to hamburg, which (participants of the congregate dining program) eat a lot. And things like peas, and carrots and bananas, and all kinds of nuts...*" The reality for this particular woman was that her health issues dictated whether she could participate in a meal or not, thus comprising her nutritional intake, her social interactions from being part of a congregate dining program, and her finances as she lived at a manor where she opted for her monthly rent to include the dining program.

6.6. Community Program Use (Mesosystem Factor). All eight women described how they regularly accessed community-based food resources, including food banks, congregate seniors' dining programs, and meal delivery programs. While home-delivered meal programs have potential to make a significant contribution to the nutrient intake of seniors, it was common for the women in this study to stretch one meal to make it into two, as this participant shared: "*Well at first when I first was getting [a home meal delivery service] they were wonderful. And I always had the soup for my lunch and I could make the dinner do two dinners.*"

Three of our participants regularly accessed a food bank, these women talked casually about their use of food banks with no sense of shame detected, perhaps attributable to life experiences and "world view." They spoke accolades about the staff and volunteers at the food banks they attended and were so appreciative of the food they received. Not only could they receive food when in need, their food banks also delivered to them, which was considered a "God-send" for one participant who had difficulty walking. "*Well sometimes like if I need, say if I need onions or anything like that, I'll phone up and see if they've got any and if they have well [volunteer] will bring it down*". They were careful to point out that they only received food when it really needed it and took strides to make their food last as long as possible. "*I just get the food once a month, they give me quite a bit, it lasts, I'm not that big of an eater... they give me stuff that I make on my own, and I make enough that it lasts me for almost the week...*" Throughout the interviews it was clear these women used community food resources when needed and were thankful for the increased access to food they provided.

6.7. Availability of Family and Friends (Meso- and Microsystem Factor). All participants were asked what the biggest factor in their lives was influencing their ability to access food; four of the women immediately responded with "family". The role that family members played varied amongst the participants, but critical roles were seen in providing transportation to shopping and medical appointments, housework, caring for them if they were sick, tending to legal matters, paying certain bills if necessary, and offering love and company.

One of the women when asked what was the biggest factor influencing her ability to access food she quickly responded "neighbours with cars," she explains: "*Well actually I'm in a very lucky situation, because a downstairs neighbour takes another neighbour for groceries every month and she said to me one day I might as well get your groceries while I'm walking around with her. And I just give her my debit card and my list and she does my shopping... And she not only goes and gets my groceries, but she brings them back and she puts them away for me.*" It was unclear if this strong trust between these two individuals existed prior to the woman being unable to shop for her own groceries, or if the trusting relationship was created out of necessity so the participant could bring food into her house.

Three of the women had no family close by. One brought up the point several times throughout the interview that when you have no family, no one to fall back on, you have to be financially prepared for the unexpected. "*It's good to have a little bit of money, it doesn't matter how young you are [and] it don't matter how old you are, you don't know what's going to come up that you're not counting on, and then when you've got nobody to come back on. [I've made wise choices] with the money, it's because I've got nobody to come back on. You've got to have some money or somebody to help you out you know.*"

Social capital, the number of people who can be expected to provide support and the resources those people have at their disposal [27], seemed essential for all women to help them complete various activities of daily living. As age brought about increases in health and mobility issues, reliance on others also increased.

6.8. Personal Food Management/Coping Strategies (Microsystem Factor). Additional to using organized community-based programs, the women in this study employed other food management strategies at the individual level to buffer food insecurity. Strategies included tight budgeting, "stretching" food, stock-piling nonperishables, eating poor quality (old) produce, purchasing food or medications on credit, and using various resources available at grocery stores. A unique shopping practice carried out by one of the women included asking produce department staff to chop or peel vegetables, particularly hard root vegetables like squash and turnip. She would also request staff to cut whole vegetables in half. For example, she knew she couldn't eat a whole bunch of celery and didn't want to pay for something that was going to rot in her fridge. "*I'll say (to produce department staff) I really don't want to buy that great big bunch of celery, because it'll rot on me. And he'll say, So? And I'll say, cut it in half! And if I buy a squash I'll say will you cut my squash, and he'll say how do you want it? And I'll say in quarters. And they'll cut it for me. And if I buy a turnip because my hands can't do it anymore and I'll say will you cut that? How do you want it? Cut it in chunks so I can just peel it and that's what I do... I thought, what's the sense of me buying it if I can't cut it?... Yeah, when you're a senior and you're living alone you got to, economically you got to do it. I got sick of throwing vegetables out. Well I'm not doing it anymore, because I don't have the money.*" The women interviewed were all very resourceful, and perhaps due to their past experiences, current financial restraints and "world view", they have developed unique strategies to cope with hunger.

7. Discussion

The purpose of this work was to explore the phenomenon of food insecurity for low-income lone senior women living in NS. To help us examine the meanings behind these women's experiences of accessing food, Bronfenbrenner's Ecological Systems Theory provided a model to observe the women in their immediate environments and then examine their situations more broadly so as to determine how their everyday actions (e.g., food acquisition and consumption) are mediated by more distal aspects of their physical and social milieus.

Of particular interest was the generational lens that was cast over all the participants' perceptions of their food security status. Despite participants clearly meeting criteria for food insecurity, for example, some reported having difficulty accessing food because they are in too much pain to shop, needing to use food banks or other charitable food models, or having difficulty accessing food that meets special dietary requirements. They also reported needing to make sacrifices such as switching insurance plans or sacrificing social outings so that they can maintain enough self-sufficiency to consider themselves food secure. Yet overwhelmingly, the participants did not self-identify as having any real problem accessing food. This finding may be a product of their world view, a macrosystem factor, which reflects their experiences of living through more difficult, or food insecure periods of life.

In contrast to findings by Hamelin et al. [28] and our previous work with low-income lone mothers [29–31], the shame often associated with food insecurity and accessing food banks does not seem to be part of the experience for these senior women. American researchers have suggested that experiences are colored by the world view or generational lens which enables seniors to endure hardships, this may be due to the impact of remembering the Great Depression or the World Wars [32, 33]. Similar to findings among seniors in the US, our research suggests that while food insecurity among lone senior women in Canada does exist, senior women's self-perceptions of food insecurity are influenced by a macrosystem cultural lens from an older generation, which may be at odds with current cultural understandings of food insecurity. The finding that senior women in this study have skills and perceptions that enable them to cope with food insecurity raises questions about how future generations will experience food insecurity and how this will impact their health and well-being if they do not share a similar world view or generational lens then that of their parents or grandparents. While an argument can be made that senior women of the future will not be as vulnerable to food insecurity because many more will have worked (may have greater access to CPP or personal savings) and can drive (may not be as isolated), there is a risk that food insecurity among seniors will become a more prominent social issue if we do not have the proper mechanisms in place to support seniors' ability to access a nutritious diet.

At the exosystem level, the participants identified several policies and programs such as OAS, CPP, and Pharmacare that influenced access to food. Consistent with findings of our previous research [1], participants described the protective effect of the GIS, the OAS program for low-income seniors. If a low-income senior has no other source of income besides the OAS basic pension (i.e., did not pay into CPP or have a private pension plan), they can receive up to an additional $738.96 (effective July 2012) in monthly income on top of the basic OAS pension [34], this additional GIS benefit is nontaxable income. As of July 2012, the average monthly GIS benefit received by a single senior is $492.23 [35]. Canada's universal health care has a protective effect on the food security status of seniors. In NS, no senior need absorb the full cost of their medications because of the compulsory drug insurance plan, Pharmacare. Recipients of the GIS also do not have to pay the annual premium associated with the insurance plan. Although Pharmacare is an exosystem factor its existence speaks to Canadians' values and beliefs at the macrosystem level that healthcare should be accessible to every citizen [36].

Unfortunately, a recent evaluation of the GIS shows that many seniors who are eligible to receive GIS are not doing so; it is speculated that a large proportion of eligible nonrecipients consists of seniors in vulnerable communities, such as aboriginal people, homeless or near homeless, and immigrants [23]. While increasing the accessibility of GIS would help to address food insecurity among vulnerable seniors, the findings from our provincial food costing research consistently show that even with the GIS, not a great deal of money is left at the end of the month, which can leave lone seniors vulnerable to food insecurity if emergency or unforeseen expenses arise [1, 37, 38].

Also at the exosystem level, is the protective role subsidized housing plays on freeing up money to be made available for food. Seven of the eight participants lived in subsidized housing; affordable and accessible housing is necessary to help low-income persons, including seniors, achieve food security [39]. Our findings suggest that housing costs absorb the "lion's share" of seniors' monthly pensions; this has been shown in other research in NS [1, 37] and elsewhere [38]. Finding and maintaining housing on limited income can be a major challenge for seniors, as heard in two of the stories from the women interviewed who spoke of excessively long wait lists to get an apartment in a seniors' manor in urban NS. In 2006, 4% of seniors in NS were able to access the provincial government's Seniors Rental Housing program [4]; many more seniors would benefit from the income-protection subsidized housing offers but there are not enough spaces allocated for the 11% of seniors (13,715), living below the low-income cutoff [4]. It could be speculated that the voices of seniors paying market rent would reflect more food insecure experiences than the women interviewed here.

At a more local level, social supports for seniors may be dwindling. Our qualitative results suggest that reliable and accessible transportation is an issue for senior women in urban NS. Statistics Canada shows that relatively few seniors use public transit [40], and our participants clearly shared their challenges with transit systems. Most seniors in NS live in areas without public transit [4] meaning volunteer drivers, private transportation services, and reliance of family and friends become more and more important to help gain access to groceries. Unfortunately, the trend in NS is migratory as youth and adults leave the province in search of employment [41] and as the volunteer sector dwindles [42]. It is quite plausible the NS senior's microsystem is shrinking as the structures with which the senior has direct contact become fewer and fewer [43]. This is of concern in light of the "world view," we notice today's seniors working within; will seniors in need reach out to community resources if they've been raised to weather hard times? Who, if not a family member, will notice a lone senior women stretching or skipping meals, or eating nutritionally inadequately?

The finding that seniors may be experiencing food insecurity, relying heavily on social networks and personal coping strategies suggests existing data of food insecurity in seniors may not be comprehensive; current indicators and measures do not capture the whole experience of how seniors experience food insecurity. In addition, with their generational lens and experience of previous hardships such as the Great Depression and World Wars, food insecurity amongst seniors is not viewed as a serious problem by seniors themselves. This may help to explain why rates of food insecurity among seniors in Canada are reported to be low (3.2%) [44], while poverty rates as determined by the LICO are much higher (11.8%) [45]. It is unclear whether food insecurity among seniors is truly being captured by current means of data collection. If the results from this study are any indication,there may be a great many seniors with similar generational views who are silently "coping", effectively rendering the issue of food insecurity among seniors invisible.

The results from this study are timely, as in Canada, policies in place to protect vulnerable populations such as seniors may be at risk. During the announcement of Canada's Economic Action Plan 2012 (the Federal Budget), significant changes to the OAS program were proposed: starting in 2023, the age of entitlement for all OAS benefits would gradually increase by two years from 65 to 67, with full implementation by 2029. This proposed policy change may mean more seniors will be relying on provincial social assistance and disability programs longer, especially given that statistics are showing that the Canadian population is aging, with population projections suggesting that by 2051 seniors will form 24.7% of the Canadian population compared to 14.4% in 2011, and 9.6% in 1981 [46]. In light of this, our findings raise concerns that the risk of poverty and food insecurity among lone senior women may be significant into the future.

These findings and our earlier work [1] suggest that OAS and GIS benefits are essential to ensuring food security for seniors. However, even with these public pensions, seniors incorporate a variety of strategies to ensure access to food, as observed by the eight women interviewed. Given the anticipated increase in the aging population in Canada, as well as the changing *world view* of the next generation, the coping strategies employed by these women may be lost and thus, food insecurity rates in future generations will likely increase. This demonstrates the importance of ensuring that progressive and sustainable social policies are implemented at multiple levels.

We close with the following recommendations to better monitor and address food insecurity in the Canadian senior population; however, lessons learned can be extended beyond our political borders.

(i) Currently, tools used to capture the prevalence of food insecurity, for example, the Food Security Survey Module used as part of the Canadian Community Health Survey since 2004 only use *income* security as an indicator for *food* security. Other indicators such as health status, social inclusion, availability of affordable and accessible housing and transportation are important influencers on seniors' ability to achieve food security and therefore measurement tools which incorporate consideration of these factors should be developed and validated.

(ii) Adequate funding should be allocated to community programs that provide nutritious food to seniors (e.g., meals on wheels, etc.) to better protect those seniors from malnutrition who are unable to cook or travel due to health/mobility limitations and those with unavailable personal social supports.

(iii) Accessible and affordable housing (e.g., subsidized housing) must be available and reflective of the level of need among community dwelling seniors.

(iv) Accessible municipal transportation, with adequate scheduling and routes, should be available in urban centres, with various methods of community input available to ensure the system is meeting the needs of its users/community residents.

(v) In terms of further reaching policy implications, federal and provincial governments in Canada should develop and implement a poverty reduction strategy that aims to lift people out of poverty. In relation to seniors, this would include continuing to review and implement changes to public pension systems to ensure income adequacy among Canadian seniors and increasing access and awareness of programs, services, and support, such as Guaranteed Income Supplement for low-income seniors.

Endnotes

1. The Old Age Security (OAS) program is the cornerstone of Canada's retirement income system. At age 65, it provides seniors with a modest pension (average of $510.17/month in July 2012) [35] if they have lived in Canada for at least 10 years [47].
2. Nearly all Canadians between the ages of 18–70 years who are employed (including self-employed individuals) earning more than $3500 a year contribute to the CPP and are entitled to a retirement pension once they turn 60 years of age [48]. The age at which a senior decides to start collecting his/her pension affects the amount payable to the contributor.
3. Food costing, conducted in towns and cities across Canada, involves using the National Nutritious Food Basket to monitor the cost and affordability of a basic nutritious diet [49].
4. The LICO is an income threshold below which a family will devote 20% more of its income on the necessities of food, shelter, and clothing than the average Canadian family living in a similar-sized community [50].
5. The Guaranteed Income Supplement (GIS) is a part of the Old Age Security (OAS) benefits for lower-income seniors. To be eligible, seniors must be receiving an OAS basic pension and meet other certain income requirements. The monthly amount available depends on the applicant's marital status and income. Seniors must apply for their GIS, generally through the income tax system, and this benefit is not taxable [51].
6. The Nova Scotia Seniors Pharmacare Program is a provincial drug insurance program that helps seniors with the cost of their prescription drugs. GIS recipients are not required to pay the annual premium [52].

References

[1] R. J. Green, P. L. Williams, C. S. Johnson, and I. Blum, "Can Canadian seniors on public pensions afford a nutritious diet?" *Canadian Journal on Aging*, vol. 27, no. 1, pp. 69–79, 2008.

[2] "Population by sex and age group, by province and territory," CANSIM table 051-0001, 2011, http://www.statcan.gc.ca/tables-tableaux/sum-som/l01/cst01/demo31f-eng.htm.

[3] "Persons in low income before tax. [in percent, 2006 to 2010]," CANSIM table 202-0802 and catalogue no. 75-202-X, Government of Canada, Ottawa, Canada, 2012, http://www.statcan.gc.ca/tables-tableaux/sum-som/l01/cst01/famil41a-eng.htm?sdi=low%20income.

[4] Nova Scotia Department of Seniors, "Seniors statistical profile 2009," Communications Nova Scotia, 2009.

[5] W. S. Wolfe, E. A. Frongillo, and P. Valois, "Understanding the experience of food insecurity by elders suggests ways to improve its measurement," *Journal of Nutrition*, vol. 133, no. 9, pp. 2762–2769, 2003.

[6] Food and Agriculture Organization, "Rome declaration on world food security and world food summit plan of action," Tech. Rep. W3613/E, Rome, Italy, 1996.

[7] American Dietetic Association, "Position of the American dietetic association: food insecurity and hunger in the United States," *Journal of the American Dietetic Association*, vol. 106, pp. 446–458, 2006.

[8] K. L. Radimer, C. M. Olson, and C. C. Campbell, "Development of indicators to assess hunger," *Journal of Nutrition*, vol. 120, no. 11, pp. 1544–1548, 1990.

[9] E. A. Frongillo, B. S. Rauschenbach, C. M. Olson, A. Kendall, and A. G. Colmenares, "Questionnaire-based measures are valid for the identification of rural households with hunger and food insecurity," *Journal of Nutrition*, vol. 127, no. 5, pp. 699–705, 1997.

[10] D. Rose and V. Oliveira, "Nutrient intakes of individuals from food-insufficient households in the United States," *American Journal of Public Health*, vol. 87, no. 12, pp. 1956–1961, 1997.

[11] S. A. Quandt and P. Rao, "Hunger and food security among older adults in a rural community," *Human Organization*, vol. 58, no. 1, pp. 28–35, 1999.

[12] W. R. Dean, J. R. Sharkey, and C. M. Johnson, "Food insecurity is associated with social capital, perceived personal disparity, and partnership status among older and senior adults in a largely rural area of central Texas," *Journal of Nutrition in Gerontology and Geriatrics*, vol. 30, no. 2, pp. 169–186, 2011.

[13] H. H. Keller, "Reliance on others for food-related activities of daily living," *Journal of Nutrition for the Elderly*, vol. 25, no. 1, pp. 43–59, 2006.

[14] S. A. Quandt, T. A. Arcury, J. McDonald, R. A. Bell, and M. Z. Vitolins, "Meaning and management of food security among rural elders," *Journal of Applied Gerontology*, vol. 20, no. 3, pp. 356–376, 2001.

[15] "Household food insecurity in Canada in 2007-2008: key statistics and graphics," Government of Canada, 2011, http://www.hc-sc.gc.ca/fn-an/surveill/nutrition/commun/insecurit/key-stats-cles-2007-2008-eng.php#d.

[16] N. T. Vozoris and V. S. Tarasuk, "Household food insufficiency is associated with poorer health," *Journal of Nutrition*, vol. 133, no. 1, pp. 120–126, 2003.

[17] R. Iqbal, S. Anand, S. Ounpuu et al., "Dietary patterns and the risk of acute myocardial infarction in 52 countries: Results of the INTERHEART study," *Circulation*, vol. 118, no. 19, pp. 1929–1937, 2008.

[18] Health Canada, *Eating Well with Canada's Food Guide: A Resource for Educators and Communities*, Government of Canada, Ottawa, Canada, 2011.

[19] U. Bronfenbrenner, "Ecology of the family as a context for human development: research perspectives," *Developmental Psychology*, vol. 22, no. 6, pp. 723–742, 1986.

[20] U. Bronfenbrenner, *The Ecology of Human Development. Experiments by Nature and Design*, Harvard University Press, Cambridge, Mass, USA, 1979.

[21] U. Bronfenbrenner, "Toward an experimental ecology of human development," *American Psychologist*, vol. 32, no. 7, pp. 513–531, 1977.

[22] K. R. McLeroy, D. Bibeau, A. Steckler, and K. Glanz, "An ecological perspective on health promotion programs," *Health Education Quarterly*, vol. 15, no. 4, pp. 351–377, 1988.

[23] Human Resources and Skills Development Canada, "Evaluation of the guaranteed income supplement take-up measures and outreach-February 2010," Government of Canada, Ottawa, Canada, 2010.

[24] C. M. Olson, A. Kendall, W. S. Wolfe, and E. A. Frongillo Jr., "Understanding the measurement of hunger and food insecurity in the elderly," Tech. Rep. 1088-96, Institute for Research on Poverty, Madison, Wis, USA, 1996.

[25] M. Q. Patton, *Qualitative Evaluation and Research Methods*, Sage, Newbury Park, Calif, USA, 2nd edition, 1990.

[26] C. Moustakas, *Phenomenology Science and Psychotherapy*, University College of Cape Breton, Cape Breton, Canada, 1988.

[27] E. A. W. Boxman, P. M. De Graaf, and H. D. Flap, "The impact of social and human capital on the income attainment of Dutch managers," *Social Networks*, vol. 13, no. 1, pp. 51–73, 1991.

[28] A. M. Hamelin, M. Beaudry, and J. P. Habicht, "Characterization of household food insecurity in Québec: food and feelings," *Social Science and Medicine*, vol. 54, no. 1, pp. 119–132, 2002.

[29] P. L. Williams, L. McIntyre, and N. T. Glanville, "Milk insecurity: accounts of a food insecurity phenomenon in Canada and its relation to public policy," *Journal of Hunger and Environmental Nutrition*, vol. 5, no. 2, pp. 142–157, 2010.

[30] L. McIntyre, P. Williams, and N. T. Glanville, "Milk as metaphor: low-income lone mothers' characterization of their challenges acquiring milk for their families," *Ecology of Food and Nutrition*, vol. 46, no. 3-4, pp. 263–279, 2007.

[31] P. L. Williams, R. MacAulay, B. Anderson, K. Barro, D. E. Gillis, C. Johnson et al., "'I would have never thought that I would be in such a predicament': voices from women experiencing food insecurity in Nova Scotia, Canada," *Journal of Hunger and Environmental Nutrition*, vol. 7, no. 2-3, pp. 253–270, 2012.

[32] M. Nord, "Measuring the food security of elderly persons," *Family Economics and Nutrition Review*, vol. 15, no. 1, pp. 33–46, 2003.

[33] L. I. Vailas, S. A. Nitzke, M. Becker, and J. Gast, "Risk indicators for malnutrition are associated inversely with quality of life for participants in meal programs for older adults," *Journal of the American Dietetic Association*, vol. 98, no. 5, pp. 548–553, 1998.

[34] Service Canada, "Table of benefit amounts by marital status and income level: old age security pension, guaranteed income supplement [GIS] allowance, allowance for the survivor," Goverment of Canada, Ottawa, Canada, 2012.

[35] "Old age security payment amounts: July–September 2012," Government of Canada, Ottawa, Canada, 2012, http://www.servicecanada.gc.ca/eng/isp/oas/oasrates.shtml.

[36] L. I. Reutter, G. Veenstra, M. J. Stewart et al., "Public attributions for poverty in Canada," *Canadian Review of Sociology and Anthropology*, vol. 43, no. 1, pp. 1–22, 2006.

[37] Mount Saint Vincent University and Nova Scotia Food Security Network, "Can Nova Scotians afford to eat healthy?" Report of 2010 Food Costing, Halifax, Canada, 2011.

[38] National Advisory Council on Aging, *Seniors on the Margins: Aging in Poverty in Canada*, Minister of Public Works and Government Services Canada, Ottawa, Canada, 2005.

[39] S. I. Kirkpatrick and V. Tarasuk, "Housing circumstances are associated with household food access among low-income

urban families," *Journal of Urban Health*, vol. 88, no. 2, pp. 284–296, 2011.

[40] M. Turcotte, "Profile of seniors' transportation habits," Statistics Canada Catalogue 11-008-X, Statistics Canada, Ottawa, Canada, 2012.

[41] "Canada-Nova Scotia labour market agreement. 2009-2010," Annual Report, Govermment of Canada, 2011.

[42] Nova Scotia Department of Health Promotion and Protection, "Talking with volunteers. . .Recommendations for government action," Nova Scotia—Canada Volunteerism Initiative Report, Government of Nova Scotia, Halifax, Canada, 2008.

[43] D. Cloutier-Fisher, K. Kobayashi, and A. Smith, "The subjective dimension of social isolation: a qualitative investigation of older adults' experiences in small social support networks," *Journal of Aging Studies*, vol. 25, no. 4, pp. 407–414, 2011.

[44] "Household food insecurity, by age group and sex, Canada, provinces, territories, health regions [2007 boundaries] and peer groups," CANSIM table 105-0547, 2010, http://www5.statcan.gc.ca/cansim/a05?lang=eng&id=1050547.

[45] "Persons in low income before tax [in percent, 2005 to 2009]," CANSIM table 202-0802, 2011, http://www.statcan.gc.ca/tables-tableaux/sum-som/l01/cst01/famil41a-eng.htm.

[46] "Canadians in context—aging population," Government of Canada, 2012, http://www4.hrsdc.gc.ca/.3ndic.1t.4r@-eng.jsp?iid=33.

[47] "Old Age Security [OAS] program," Government of Canada, 2012, http://www.servicecanada.gc.ca/eng/isp/oas/oastoc.shtml.

[48] "General information about the Canada pension plan," Government of Canada, 2011, http://www.servicecanada.gc.ca/eng/isp/oas/oastoc.shtml.

[49] "National nutritious food basket," Health Canada, 2009, http://www.hc-sc.gc.ca/fn-an/surveill/basket-panier/index-eng.php.

[50] "Low income cut-offs," Government of Canada, 2009, http://www.statcan.gc.ca/pub/75f0002m/2009002/s2-eng.htm.

[51] "Guaranteed income supplement," Government of Canada, Ottawa, Canada, 2012, http://www.servicecanada.gc.ca/eng/sc/oas/gis/guaranteeddincomesupplement.shtml.

[52] Nova Scotia Pharmacare Programs, *Senior's Pharmacare Information Booklet*, Government of Nova Scotia, 2010.

4

Factors Affecting Mortality in Elderly Patients Hospitalized for Nonmalignant Reasons

Teslime Ayaz,[1] Serap Baydur Sahin,[2] Osman Zikrullah Sahin,[3] Ozlem Bilir,[4] and Halil RakJcJ[5]

[1] *Department of Internal Medicine, Faculty of Medicine, Recep Tayyip Erdogan University, Rize 53100, Turkey*
[2] *Department of Endocrinology, Faculty of Medicine, Recep Tayyip Erdogan University, Rize 53100, Turkey*
[3] *Department of Nephrology, Faculty of Medicine, Recep Tayyip Erdogan University, Rize 53100, Turkey*
[4] *Department of Emergency, Faculty of Medicine, Recep Tayyip Erdogan University, Rize 53100, Turkey*
[5] *Department of Gastroenterology, Faculty of Medicine, Recep Tayyip Erdogan University, Rize 53100, Turkey*

Correspondence should be addressed to Teslime Ayaz; drthess@hotmail.com

Academic Editor: Johannes Grillari

Elderly population is hospitalized more frequently than young people, and they suffer from more severe diseases that are difficult to diagnose and treat. The present study aimed to investigate the factors affecting mortality in elderly patients hospitalized for nonmalignant reasons. Demographic data, reason for hospitalization, comorbidities, duration of hospital stay, and results of routine blood testing at the time of first hospitalization were obtained from the hospital records of the patients, who were over 65 years of age and hospitalized primarily for nonmalignant reasons. The mean age of 1012 patients included in the study was 77.8 ± 7.6. The most common reason for hospitalization was diabetes mellitus (18.3%). Of the patients, 90.3% had at least a single comorbidity. Whilst 927 (91.6%) of the hospitalized patients were discharged, 85 (8.4%) died. Comparison of the characteristics of the discharged and dead groups revealed that the dead group was older and had higher rates of poor general status and comorbidity. Differences were observed between the discharged and dead groups in most of the laboratory parameters. Hypoalbuminemia, hypertriglyceridemia, hypopotassemia, hypernatremia, hyperuricemia, and high TSH level were the predictors of mortality. In order to meet the health necessities of the elderly population, it is necessary to well define the patient profiles and to identify the risk factors.

1. Introduction

Life expectancy increases each year due to the improvements in living conditions and advances in medicine resulting in an incremental increase in elderly population [1, 2]. Physiological, psychological, and social problems of the elderly require different approaches and this necessitates the physicians being ready for the increasing population of the elderly. Many factors including aging-associated diseases, chronic diseases and comorbidities, multiple drug use, functional disability, and feeding problems make health care difficult in the elderly. In addition, symptoms and signs vary in the elderly and are usually atypical [2]. It is known that physiological processes show variations in the elderly as compared to young individuals; many biomarkers alter with age, and within this context, laboratory reference range values also differ in elderly population [3, 4].

Elderly population is hospitalized more frequently and for a longer period of time as compared to young population and they suffer from more severe diseases that are difficult to diagnose and treat [5]. Patients aged 65 years or over have been reported to be hospitalized approximately 3 times more frequently than young individuals [6]. Additionally, it has been reported that one-third of them are discharged with lower functional capacity than they admitted with and that approximately 5% die during hospital stay, whereas 20%–30% die within one year following hospital discharge [6]. It has been reported that some known traditional risk factors causing poor prognosis may vary in the elderly and even some may act opposite to the expected effect. In a study conducted in a very elderly population, low body mass index (BMI), low diastolic blood pressure, and low cholesterol levels (which indicate reverse metabolic syndrome) were found to be significant predictors of mortality [7]. In the light of this information, comprehensive studies are needed to better understand the factors that influence mortality in elderly population.

The present study aimed to investigate the factors affecting mortality in elderly patients hospitalized for nonmalignant reasons and to determine the relation between laboratory parameters measured routinely in clinical practice and in-hospital mortality, as well as to determine the predictors of mortality.

2. Methods

This is a retrospective cohort study of hospitalized patients followed during hospitalization.

Records of the patients hospitalized in the Internal Medicine Clinic of our hospital between September 2010 and September 2012 were retrospectively reviewed. Patients over the age of 65 years and hospitalized primarily for nonmalignant reasons were included in the study. Surgery or trauma patients were excluded. Study participants comprised also the patients who had comorbid malignant diseases, as well as the patients treated for malignancy who were cured or in remission. Demographic data, reasons for hospitalization, comorbidities, duration of hospital stay, and results of the routine blood tests at the time of first hospitalization were obtained from the hospital records. The study was conducted in accordance with the ethical rules for human experimentation that are stated in the Declaration of Helsinki. These inpatients' privacy and confidentiality are guaranteed.

TABLE 1: General characteristics of the patients.

Characteristics	
Age, years	77.8 ± 7.6
Gender	
Female	592 (58.5)
Male	420 (41.5)
Reason for hospitalization	
Poor general status	169 (16.7)
Diabetes mellitus	185 (18.3)
Cardiovascular diseases	67 (6.6)
Pulmonary diseases	96 (9.5)
Gastrointestinal diseases	95 (9.4)
Renal diseases	157 (15.5)
Infection	77 (7.6)
Anemia	124 (12.3)
Rheumatologic diseases	9 (0.9)
Electrolyte imbalance	25 (2.5)
Other	8 (0.8)
Presence of at least one comorbidity	914 (90.3)
Comorbidity	
Cardiovascular disease	412 (40.7)
Hypertension	610 (60.3)
Diabetes mellitus	389 (38.4)
Chronic renal failure	65 (6.4)
Malignant diseases	91 (9.0)
Cirrhosis	23 (2.3)
Other	200 (19.8)
Duration of hospital stay, days	7.7 ± 5.9

Values are presented as mean ± standard deviation or number (%), where appropriate.

2.1. Statistical Analysis. Data were analyzed using the Statistical Package for the Social Sciences (SPSS, Inc., Chicago, IL, USA) version 15.0 for Windows program. Descriptive statistics were expressed as cross-tables for categorical variables and as mean ± standard deviation for numerical variables. Independent categorical variables were compared using chi-square test. In the event that chi-square assumption was not met, Fisher's exact test was used for paired group comparison. Paired group comparisons were performed using independent samples t-test for normally distributed numerical variables or using Mann-Whitney U test for nonnormally distributed numerical variables. Risk factors were identified by backward method and logistic regression analysis. A P value of <0.05 was considered statistically significant.

3. Results

The present study included 1012 patients, of whom 592 were female with a mean age of 78.4 ± 7.8 years and 420 were male with a mean age of 77.0 ± 7.1 years. The most common reason for hospitalization was diabetes mellitus (DM), followed by poor general status and kidney diseases. Of the patients, 90.3% had at least a single comorbidity. The most frequently observed comorbidities were hypertension and cardiovascular diseases. Demographic characteristics of the patients and information about hospitalization are summarized in Table 1.

Whilst 927 (91.6%) of the hospitalized patients were discharged from the hospital (discharged group), 85 (8.4%) died (dead group).

Evaluation of the general characteristics of the discharged and dead groups revealed that the dead group was older and that poor general status at the time of hospitalization, comorbidities of DM, malignant disease and cirrhosis, and presence of at least a single comorbidity were significantly more prevalent in this group (Table 2).

Comparison of the discharged and dead groups in terms of laboratory results revealed that the mean values of platelets, iron, total iron-binding capacity (TIBC), albumin, calcium, total cholesterol, low-density lipoprotein (LDL) cholesterol, and high-density lipoprotein (HDL) cholesterol were significantly lower in the dead group. The mean values of mean platelet volume (MPV), erythrocyte sedimentation rate (ESR), urea, uric acid, creatinine, alanine aminotransferase (ALT), aspartate aminotransferase (AST), sodium, triglyceride, and C-reactive protein (CRP) were significantly higher in the dead group (Table 3).

TABLE 2: General characteristics of the discharged and dead groups.

Characteristics	Discharged group (n = 927)	Dead group (n = 85)	P
Age, years	77.6 ± 7.5	80.7 ± 7.7	**<0.001**
Gender			
Female	540 (58.3)	52 (61.2)	0.601
Male	387 (41.7)	33 (38.8)	
Reason for hospitalization			
Poor general status	114 (12.3)	55 (64.7)	**<0.001**
Diabetes mellitus	182 (19.6)	3 (3.5)	—
Cardiovascular diseases	64 (6.9)	3 (3.5)	—
Pulmonary diseases	93 (10.0)	3 (3.5)	—
Gastrointestinal diseases	90 (9.7)	5 (5.9)	—
Renal diseases	147 (15.9)	10 (11.8)	0.318
Infection	75 (8.1)	2 (2.4)	—
Anemia	121 (13.1)	3 (3.5)	—
Rheumatologic diseases	9 (1.0)	0 (0.0)	—
Electrolyte imbalance	24 (2.6)	1 (1.2)	—
Other	8 (0.9)	0 (0.0)	—
Presence of at least one comorbidity	831 (89.6)	83 (97.6)	**0.017**
Comorbidity			
Cardiovascular disease	371 (40.0)	41 (48.2)	0.140
Hypertension	555 (59.9)	55 (64.7)	0.383
Diabetes mellitus	346 (37.3)	43 (50.6)	**0.016**
Chronic renal failure	62 (6.7)	3 (3.5)	0.256
Malignant diseases	68 (7.3)	23 (27.1)	**<0.001**
Cirrhosis	18 (1.9)	5 (5.9)	**0.037**
Other	188 (20.3)	12 (14.1)	0.172
Duration of hospital stay, days	7.7 ± 5.8	8.0 ± 6.7	0.449

In the discharged and dead groups, the rates of patients with normal laboratory values were compared with those of patients with values lower or higher than the normal laboratory values. The rates of patients with a low hemoglobin level, thrombocytopenia, a high ESR, a low TIBC, uremia, hyperuricemia, hypercreatininemia, hypoalbuminemia, a high AST level, a high ALT level, hypernatremia, hypopotassemia, hyperpotassemia, hypocalcemia, hypertriglyceridemia, a low HDL level, a low thyroid stimulating hormone (TSH) level, a high CRP level, and a positive HBsAg were significantly higher in the dead group. The rate of patients with hypercholesterolemia and the rate of those with a high LDL were significantly lower in the dead group (Table 4).

In order to identify the risk factors for mortality, analysis was performed in a model including the following variables: gender, age, poor general status, renal disease diabetes mellitus, cardiovascular disease, pulmonary disease, gastrointestinal disease, infections, anemia, rheumatologic disease and electrolyte imbalance as the reason for hospitalization, presence of DM, hypertension, cardiovascular disease, malignancy, chronic renal failure and cirrhosis as comorbidities, duration of hospital stay, CRP, HBsAg, anti-HCV antibody, anti-HIV antibody, hemoglobin, platelet, MPV, ESR, iron, TIBC, MCV, glucose, urea, uric acid, creatinine, albumin, ALT, AST, sodium, potassium, calcium, cholesterol, triglyceride, HDL cholesterol, LDL cholesterol, and TSH. Poor general status as the reason for hospitalization, presence of malignancy or cirrhosis as comorbidity, hypoalbuminemia, hypertriglyceridemia, hypopotassemia, hypernatremia, hyperuricemia, and high TSH were found to be the significant risk factors for mortality (Table 5).

4. Discussion

In the present study, the rate of in-hospital mortality was found to be 8.4% in the hospitalized patients over 65 years of age. To the best of our knowledge, there are very few studies performed on this subject in elderly patients. In addition, different patient populations having different reasons for hospitalization, differences in the lower age limit of the participants, and differences in duration of hospital stay require attention when comparing the results. The rate of in-hospital mortality among elderly patients has been reported to be 12% [8], 14.9% [9], and 16.4% [10] in various studies.

In addition to common parameters, different risk factors have also been reported in the limited number of studies

TABLE 3: Laboratory values of the discharged and dead groups at the time of hospitalization.

Characteristics	Discharged group (n = 927)	Dead group (n = 85)	P
Hemoglobin (g/dL)	11.3 ± 2.2	10.9 ± 1.9	0.069
MCV (fL)	85.0 ± 8.0	84.9 ± 7.3	0.964
PLT (K/μL)	267.9 ± 123.4	239.9 ± 144.1	**0.002**
MPV (fL)	8.5 ± 1.7	9.1 ± 2.2	**0.009**
ESR (mm/h)	48.1 ± 34.2	61.0 ± 37.5	**0.001**
Iron (μg/dL)	46.3 ± 42.1	35.9 ± 31.7	**0.003**
TIBC (μg/dL)	197.8 ± 93.7	152.3 ± 89.3	**<0.001**
Glucose (mg/dL)	159.7 ± 103.5	167.6 ± 135.4	0.905
Urea (mg/dL)	84.1 ± 57.8	127.7 ± 75.5	**<0.001**
Uric acid (mg/dL)	6.6 ± 2.7	9.1 ± 3.9	**<0.001**
Creatinine (mg/dL)	2.0 ± 1.9	2.4 ± 1.8	**0.010**
Albumin (g/dL)	3.4 ± 0.6	2.7 ± 0.6	**<0.001**
ALT (U/L)	27.0 ± 66.8	43.8 ± 107.3	**0.027**
AST (U/L)	30.1 ± 53.7	66.7 ± 130.4	**0.001**
Sodium (mmol/L)	137.9 ± 6.4	140.4 ± 9.6	**0.022**
Potassium (mmol/L)	4.5 ± 0.8	4.5 ± 1.1	0.313
Calcium (mg/dL)	8.8 ± 0.9	8.3 ± 1.0	**<0.001**
Triglyceride (mg/dL)	134.1 ± 73.1	155.0 ± 89.8	**0.045**
Total cholesterol (mg/dL)	170.9 ± 49.5	147.5 ± 62.5	**<0.001**
LDL cholesterol (mg/dL)	105.7 ± 38.7	91.0 ± 53.4	**<0.001**
HDL cholesterol (mg/dL)	36.0 ± 13.8	25.2 ± 16.1	**<0.001**
TSH (μIU/mL)	1.5 ± 3.2	2.1 ± 5.0	0.196
CRP (mg/dL)	6.1 ± 8.2	10.6 ± 10.9	**<0.001**

MCV: mean corpuscular volume; PLT: platelet; MPV: mean platelet volume; ESR: erythrocyte sedimentation rate; TIBC: total iron-binding capacity; ALT: alanine aminotransferase; AST: aspartate aminotransferase; LDL: low-density lipoprotein; HDL: high-density lipoprotein; TSH: thyroid stimulating hormone; CRP: C-reactive protein.

investigating general risk factors for mortality in the hospitalized elderly. Ponzetto et al. [9] investigated the risk factors affecting mortality in 987 hospitalized patients aged ≥70 years and determined functional impairment, medical condition-related disability, cerebrovascular disease, cancer, an albumin level of 3–3.4 g/dL, a creatinine level of 1.5–3 mg/dL, a creatinine level of >3 mg/dL, and a fibrinogen level of ≥452 mg/dL as the independent risk factors for in-hospital mortality. Sousa et al. [8] evaluated 158 hospitalized patients aged >70 years and found a subjective medical evaluation at the beginning of the hospital admission, a low Barthel score, a low serum albumin, and a high white blood cell (WBC) count to be correlated with high mortality. Silva et al. [10] evaluated 856 patients aged between 60 and 104 years and determined that delirium, cancer, immobility, low albumin levels, elevated creatinine levels, history of heart failure, and advanced age were associated with increased mortality. In a study conducted to investigate known cardiovascular risk factors that influence mortality in elderly population, Zhang et al. [11] found that left ventricular ejection fraction (LVEF), LDL and HDL cholesterol levels, albumin level, and creatinine clearance rate (CCR) were significantly lower and the incidence of atrial fibrillation was higher in the patients with all-cause mortality than in the survived patients. Moreover, they reported LVEF, atrial fibrillation, LDL cholesterol, albumin, and CCR to be significant and independent predictors for mortality in multivariate Cox regression model. Buurman et al. [12] evaluated 639 hospitalized patients aged ≥65 years in terms of risks for functional decline; of the patients, 27% were at low risk, 33% were at intermediate risk, and 40% were at high risk for developing new disability. High risk patients were also reported to be at high risk for mortality. Fontana et al. [13] assessed the relation between 17 biomarkers and mortality in 594 hospitalized elderly patients. They reported blood levels of insulin-like growth factor (IGF-1), triiodothyronine (T3), CRP, ESR, WBC and lymphocyte counts, iron, albumin, total cholesterol, and LDL cholesterol to be associated with mortality. They also determined in multivariate Cox proportional hazard model that IGF-1, CRP, hemoglobin, and glucose were the biomarkers that most strongly predicted the mortality. Moreover, studies have reported malnutrition [14], red blood cell distribution width (RDW) [15], advanced age (≥85 years) [16], medical adverse events [17], high serum vitamin B12 level [18], and arrhythmia [19] among the parameters associated with mortality in hospitalized elderly patients.

In the present study, comparison of the characteristics of the discharged and dead groups demonstrated that general condition was poor and comorbidity was higher in the dead group, and laboratory parameters varied between the two patient groups. In the risk factor analysis, poor general status as the reason for hospitalization, presence of malignancy or cirrhosis as comorbidity, hypoalbuminemia, hypertriglyceridemia, hypopotassemia, hypernatremia, and a high TSH level were determined to be the predictors of mortality.

Among the risk factors affecting mortality, the presence of comorbidity was 89.6% in the discharged group, whereas it was significantly higher in the dead group with a rate of 97.6%. The most common comorbidities were cardiovascular diseases, DM, and hypertension. Ahluwalia et al. [20] determined the prevalence of comorbidity to be higher in the hospitalized patients than in the nonhospitalized patients in a population aged over 65 years and having heart failure (n = 201130) and found that comorbidity was associated with an increased risk for mortality in the whole population. They reported myocardial infarction, DM, chronic kidney disease, chronic obstructive pulmonary disease, dementia, depression, hip fracture, stroke, colorectal cancer, and lung cancer to be significantly associated with the risk for mortality in hospitalized patients. In the present study, malignancy (OR = 4.381) and cirrhosis (OR = 9.628) were the comorbidities determined as risk factors for mortality.

Hypoglycemia can occur during hospital stay regardless of the presence of DM. Kagansky et al. [21] reported that

TABLE 4: Abnormal laboratory results at the time of hospitalization in the discharged and dead groups.

Problem	Definition	Discharged group (n = 927)	Dead group (n = 85)	P
Low hemoglobin	Hb < 12.2 g/dL	593 (64.0)	65 (76.5)	**0.021**
Thrombocytopenia	PLT < 142 K/μL	90 (10.7)	18 (22.5)	**0.002**
High ESR	ESR E: > 20 K: > 30 mm/h	614 (66.3)	69 (81.2)	**0.005**
Low TIBC	<120 μg/dL	182 (19.8)	31 (36.5)	**<0.001**
Uremia	Urea > 43 mg/dL	687 (74.4)	79 (92.9)	**<0.001**
Hyperuricemia	Uric acid > 6 mg/dL	490 (54.4)	65 (78.3)	**<0.001**
Hypercreatininemia	Creatinine > 1.1 mg/dL	506 (56.3)	59 (72.0)	**0.006**
Hypoalbuminemia	Albumin < 3.5 mg/dL	466 (50.4)	76 (89.4)	**<0.001**
High ALT	ALT > 55 U/L	56 (6.0)	13 (15.3)	**0.001**
High AST	AST > 34 U/L	180 (19.4)	29 (34.5)	**0.001**
Hypernatremia	Sodium > 145 mmol/L	41 (6.1)	21 (33.3)	**<0.001**
Hypopotassemia	Potassium < 3.5 mmol/L	73 (9.7)	15 (24.2)	**<0.001**
Hyperpotassemia	Potassium > 5.1 mmol/L	174 (20.4)	23 (32.9)	**0.014**
Hypocalcemia	Calcium < 8.4 mg/dL	269 (29.9)	41 (49.4)	**<0.001**
Hypertriglyceridemia	Triglyceride > 149 mg/dL	292 (31.5)	41 (48.2)	**0.002**
Hypercholesterolemia	Total cholesterol > 199 mg/dL	228 (24.6)	12 (14.1)	**0.030**
High LDL cholesterol	LDL > 100 mg/dL	492 (53.1)	31 (36.5)	**0.003**
Low HDL cholesterol	HDL < 35 mg/dL	424 (46.4)	64 (76.2)	**<0.001**
Low TSH	TSH < 0.35 μIU/mL	169 (18.9)	31 (39.2)	**<0.001**
High TSH	TSH > 4.94 μIU/mL	31 (4.1)	6 (11.1)	**0.030**
High CRP	CRP > 0.8 mg/dL	639 (68.9)	70 (82.4)	**0.010**
HBsAg positivity		11 (1.2)	4 (4.7)	**0.031**

Hb: hemoglobin; PLT: platelet; ESR: erythrocyte sedimentation rate; TIBC: total iron-binding capacity; ALT: alanine aminotransferase; AST: aspartate aminotransferase; LDL: low-density lipoprotein; HDL: high-density lipoprotein; TSH: thyroid stimulating hormone; CRP: C-reactive protein.

hypoglycemia was determined at a rate of 5.2% in the hospitalized patients over the age of 70 years and that mortality was two times higher in the hypoglycemic patients than in the nonhypoglycemic patients. Nevertheless, in the same study, sepsis, a low albumin level, and malignancy, but not hypoglycemia, were found to be independent predictors of mortality by multivariate analysis. In the present study, hyperglycemia and hypoglycemia were determined in about 60% and 10% of the patients, respectively; there was no difference between the discharged and dead groups in this respect.

A low albumin level has been associated with mortality in the hospitalized elderly patients [8, 10, 11, 18, 21]. In the present study, hypoalbuminemia was more frequent in the dead group (89.4 versus 50.4), and it was also found to be a significant risk factor (OR = 3.818).

Electrolyte imbalance, mainly due to DM and diuretics, is a common problem in elderly population. The frequency of mild electrolyte disorder has been reported to be 15% in the general population aged over 55 years [22]. Electrolyte imbalance is one of the conditions necessary to be monitored closely because of its life-threatening character [22]. Hyponatremia and hypernatremia are among the most frequently encountered electrolyte disorders in hospitalized patients and are associated with increased mortality [23]. In a study in which sodium concentration was measured in 3182 patients (mean age, 53 ± 21 years) admitted to the emergency room, hyponatremia and hypernatremia were determined at the rates of 4% and 13%, respectively, and the patients with hyponatremia were reported to be older [24]. In another study, hyponatremia was determined in 14.5% of 98411 adult hospitalized patients, hyponatremic patients were reported to be older and to have more comorbidity, and hyponatremia was found to be associated with increased in-hospital mortality [25]. In the present study, we also found the frequency of hypernatremia to be significantly higher in the dead group than in the discharged group (33.3% versus 6.1%). Although the frequency of hyponatremia was higher in the dead group, the difference was not statistically significant as compared to the discharged group (34.4% versus 28.4%). In the present study, hypernatremia was found effective on mortality in the risk factor analysis (OR = 3.5).

Severe hyperkalemia (hyperpotassemia) is known to be a life-threatening electrolyte imbalance. Hyperkalemia in hospitalized patients is encountered at a rate between 1% and 10% [26]. In a study conducted in 923 adult patients with severe hyperkalemia, the rate of in-hospital mortality was found to be 30.7% despite appropriate and aggressive treatment. In addition to the contribution of comorbidities to the increased mortality, hyperkalemia itself has been reported to have a role [27]. In the present study, the rates of hyperpotassemia (32.9% versus 20.4%) and hypopotassemia (24.2% versus 9.7%) were significantly higher in the dead

TABLE 5: Risk factor analysis for mortality.

	P	OR	95.0% CI	
			Lower bound	Upper bound
Poor general status as the reason for hospitalization	**<0.001***	7.964	4.435	14.299
Presence of malignancy as comorbidity	**<0.001***	4.381	2.179	8.810
Presence of cirrhosis as comorbidity	**0.001***	9.628	2.653	34.938
Low hemoglobin	0.078	1.825	0.934	3.564
Uremia	0.060	2.658	0.959	7.366
Hypoalbuminemia	**0.001***	3.818	1.699	8.583
High ALT	0.066	2.128	0.952	4.756
Sodium (normal)	0.001	1		
Hyponatremia	0.235	0.677	0.355	1.290
Hypernatremia	**0.002***	3.500	1.596	7.675
Potassium (normal)	0.038	1		
Hypopotassemia	**0.018***	2.582	1.178	5.658
Hyperpotassemia	0.144	1.631	0.846	3.146
Uric acid (normal)	0.040	1		
Hypouricemia	0.421	1.988	0.374	10.573
Hyperuricemia	**0.011***	2.366	1.216	4.605
Hypertriglyceridemia	**0.020***	1.935	1.108	3.381
TSH (normal)	0.005	1		
Low TSH	0.485	1.249	0.670	2.328
High TSH	**0.001***	6.166	2.048	18.568

OR: odds ratio; CI: confidence interval; ALT: alanine aminotransferase; TSH: thyroid stimulating hormone.
*$P < 0.05$ is statistically significant.

group as compared to the discharged group. Nevertheless, in the risk factor analysis, only hypopotassemia was found to be a significant risk factor (OR = 2.582).

Studies have demonstrated an association between thyroid hormones and mortality in elderly population [28, 29]. De Alfieri et al. [30] investigated thyroid hormone as a predictor of mortality in the hospitalized very old patients (mean age, 84 years). They emphasized that low T3 syndrome contributed to in-hospital mortality; however, hormone levels were influenced by comorbidities, drug interactions, and nutritional status; therefore, the results should be cautiously interpreted. Iglesias et al. [31] investigated the relation between in-hospital mortality and thyroid functions in 447 patients aged >60 years and reported alterations in thyroid function tests in 74.3% of the patients as well as a positive association between the presence of these alterations and the age of the patients and in-hospital mortality. They also reported the decrease in free-T3 value to be a powerful predictor of in-hospital mortality in elderly patients. In the present study, the rates of both low TSH (39.2% versus 18.9%) and high TSH levels (11.1% versus 4.1%) were higher in the dead group as compared to the discharged group. The risk factor analysis revealed that high TSH significantly influenced the mortality (OR = 6.166).

In conclusion, in order to meet the health necessities of the elderly population, which is gradually increasing worldwide, it is necessary to well define the patient profiles and to identify the risk factors, and further studies are required to collect more data on this subject.

Conflict of Interests

The authors declare that there is no conflict of interests regarding the publication of this paper.

References

[1] E. E. Tung, C. Y. Y. Chen, and P. Y. Takahashi, "Common curbsides and conundrums in geriatric medicine," *Mayo Clinic Proceedings*, vol. 88, no. 6, pp. 630–635, 2013.

[2] H. Arai, Y. Ouchi, M. Yokode et al., "Toward the realization of a better aged society: messages from gerontology and geriatrics," *Geriatrics and Gerontology International*, vol. 12, no. 1, pp. 16–22, 2012.

[3] L. Carlsson, L. Lind, and A. Larsson, "Reference values for 27 clinical chemistry tests in 70-year-old males and females," *Gerontology*, vol. 56, no. 3, pp. 259–265, 2010.

[4] I. Ryden, L. Lind, and A. Larsson, "Reference values of thirty-one frequently used laboratory markers for 75-year-old males and females," *Upsala Journal of Medical Sciences*, vol. 117, no. 3, pp. 264–272, 2012.

[5] R. M. Palmer, "Acute hospital care of the elderly: making a difference," in *Caring for the Hospitalized Elderly: Current Best Practice and New Horizons*, pp. 4–7, Society of Hospital Medicine, 2004.

[6] C. S. Landefeld, "Improving health care for older persons," *Annals of Internal Medicine*, vol. 139, no. 5, pp. 421–424, 2003.

[7] U. M. Vischer, M. E. Safar, H. Safar et al., "Cardiometabolic determinants of mortality in a geriatric population: is there a

"reverse metabolic syndrome"?" *Diabetes and Metabolism*, vol. 35, no. 2, pp. 108–114, 2009.

[8] S. Sousa, M. F. Moraes, V. Beato et al., "Predictive in-hospital and 6-month morbidity and mortality factors in elderly hospitalized patients," *Acta Medica Portuguesa*, vol. 15, no. 3, pp. 177–184, 2002.

[9] M. Ponzetto, B. Maero, P. Maina et al., "Risk factors for early and late mortality in hospitalized older patients: the continuing importance of functional status," *Journals of Gerontology A: Biological Sciences and Medical Sciences*, vol. 58, no. 11, pp. 1049–1054, 2003.

[10] T. J. A. Silva, C. S. Jerussalmy, J. M. Farfel, J. A. E. Curiati, and W. Jacob-Filho, "Predictors of in-hospital mortality among older patients," *Clinics*, vol. 64, no. 7, pp. 613–618, 2009.

[11] Y. Zhang, A. D. Protogerou, P. Iaria, M. E. Safar, Y. Xu, and J. Blacher, "Prognosis in the hospitalized very elderly: the PROTEGER study," *International Journal of Cardiology*, vol. 168, no. 3, pp. 2714–2719, 2013.

[12] B. M. Buurman, J. G. Hoogerduijn, E. A. van Gemert, R. J. de Haan, M. J. Schuurmans, and S. E. de Rooij, "Clinical characteristics and outcomes of hospitalized older patients with distinct risk profiles for functional decline: a prospective cohort study," *PLoS ONE*, vol. 7, no. 1, Article ID e29621, 2012.

[13] L. Fontana, F. Addante, M. Copetti et al., "Identification of a metabolic signature for multidimensional impairment and mortality risk in hospitalized older patients," *Aging Cell*, vol. 12, no. 3, pp. 459–466, 2013.

[14] S. Rasheed and R. T. Woods, "Malnutrition and associated clinical outcomes in hospitalized patients aged 60 and older: an observational study in rural Wales," *Journal of Nutrition in Gerontology and Geriatrics*, vol. 32, no. 1, pp. 71–80, 2013.

[15] N. Martínez-Velilla, B. Ibáñez, K. Cambra, and J. Alonso-Renedo, "Red blood cell distribution width, multimorbidity, and the risk of death in hospitalized older patients," *Age*, vol. 34, no. 3, pp. 717–723, 2012.

[16] J. S. Saczynski, C. E. Darling, F. A. Spencer, D. Lessard, J. M. Gore, and R. J. Goldberg, "Clinical features, treatment practices, and hospital and long-term outcomes of older patients hospitalized with decompensated heart failure: The Worcester heart failure study," *Journal of the American Geriatrics Society*, vol. 57, no. 9, pp. 1587–1594, 2009.

[17] C. Szlejf, J. M. Farfel, J. A. Curiati, E. D. B. Couto Juniorde, W. Jacob-Filho, and R. S. Azevedo, "Medical adverse events in elderly hospitalized patients: a prospective study," *Clinics*, vol. 67, no. 11, pp. 1247–1252, 2012.

[18] S. Tal, V. Guller, Y. Shavit, F. Stern, and S. Malnick, "Mortality predictors in hospitalized elderly patients," *QJM*, vol. 104, no. 11, pp. 933–938, 2011.

[19] C. Vesin, A. D. Protogerou, A. Lieber et al., "Predictive factors for all-cause mortality in the hospitalized elderly subject: the importance of arrhythmia," *Atherosclerosis*, vol. 207, no. 2, pp. 507–513, 2009.

[20] S. C. Ahluwalia, C. P. Gross, S. I. Chaudhry et al., "Impact of comorbidity on mortality among older persons with advanced heart failure," *Journal of General Internal Medicine*, vol. 27, no. 5, pp. 513–519, 2012.

[21] N. Kagansky, S. Levy, E. Rimon et al., "Hypoglycemia as a predictor of mortality in hospitalized elderly patients," *Archives of Internal Medicine*, vol. 163, no. 15, pp. 1825–1829, 2003.

[22] G. Liamis, E. M. Rodenburg, A. Hofman, R. Zietse, B. H. Stricker, and E. J. Hoorn, "Electrolyte disorders in community subjects: prevalence and risk factors," *The American Journal of Medicine*, vol. 126, no. 3, pp. 256–263, 2013.

[23] G.-C. Funk, G. Lindner, W. Druml et al., "Incidence and prognosis of dysnatremias present on ICU admission," *Intensive Care Medicine*, vol. 36, no. 2, pp. 304–311, 2010.

[24] S. Arampatzis, A. Exadaktylos, D. Buhl, H. Zimmermann, and G. Lindner, "Dysnatraemias in the emergency room: undetected, untreated, unknown?" *Wiener Klinische Wochenschrift*, vol. 124, no. 5-6, pp. 181–183, 2012.

[25] S. S. Waikar, D. B. Mount, and G. C. Curhan, " Mortality after hospitalization with mild, moderate, and severe hyponatremia," *The American Journal of Medicine*, vol. 122, no. 9, pp. 857–865, 2009.

[26] B. A. Mahoney, W. A. Smith, D. S. Lo, K. Tsoi, M. Tonelli, and C. M. Clase, "Emergency interventions for hyperkalaemia," *Cochrane Database of Systematic Reviews*, no. 2, Article ID CD003235, 2005.

[27] J. N. An, J. P. Lee, H. J. Jeon et al., "Severe hyperkalemia requiring hospitalization: predictors of mortality," *Critical Care*, vol. 16, no. 6, article R225, 2012.

[28] A. W. Van Den Beld, T. J. Visser, R. A. Feelders, D. E. Grobbee, and S. W. J. Lamberts, "Thyroid hormone concentrations, disease, physical function, and mortality in elderly men," *Journal of Clinical Endocrinology and Metabolism*, vol. 90, no. 12, pp. 6403–6409, 2005.

[29] A. C. van de Ven, R. T. Netea-Maier, M. Medici et al., "Underestimation of effect of thyroid function parameters on morbidity and mortality due to intra-individual variation," *The Journal of Clinical Endocrinology and Metabolism*, vol. 96, no. 12, pp. E2014–E2017, 2011.

[30] W. De Alfieri, F. Nisticò, T. Borgogni et al., "Thyroid hormones as predictors of short- and long-term mortality in very old hospitalized patients," *The Journals of Gerontology. Series A, Biological Sciences and Medical Sciences*, vol. 68, pp. 1122–1128, 2013.

[31] P. Iglesias, A. Muñoz, F. Prado et al., "Alterations in thyroid function tests in aged hospitalized patients: prevalence, aetiology and clinical outcome," *Clinical Endocrinology*, vol. 70, no. 6, pp. 961–967, 2009.

5

Differential Item Functioning Related to Age in the Reading Subtest of the Test of Functional Health Literacy in Adults

Raymond L. Ownby[1] and Drenna Waldrop-Valverde[2]

[1] *Department of Psychiatry and Behavioral Medicine, Nova Southeastern University, Fort Lauderdale, FL 33318, USA*
[2] *Emory University, Atlanta, GA 30322, USA*

Correspondence should be addressed to Raymond L. Ownby; ro71@nova.edu

Academic Editor: F. Richard Ferraro

Differential item functioning (DIF) occurs when items in a measure perform in ways that are different for members of a target group when the different performance is not related to the individual's overall ability to be assessed. DIF may arise for a number of reasons but is often evaluated in order to ensure that tests and measures are fair evaluations of a group's abilities. Based on observations when administering the test, we developed the hypothesis that some items on the reading comprehension subtest of the Test of Functional Health Literacy (TOFHLA) might be differentially more difficult for older adults and the elderly due to its use of the cloze response format, in which the participant is required to determine what word, when placed in a blank space in a sentence, will ensure that the sentence is intelligible. Others have suggested that the cloze response format may make demands on verbal fluency, an ability that is reduced with the increasing age. Our analyses show that age-related DIF may present in a nearly one-half of reading comprehension items of the TOFHLA. Results of this measure in older persons should be interpreted cautiously.

1. Introduction

Health literacy has assumed increasing importance over the past decade as research has continued to accumulate showing that patients' levels of it have important relations to their health, use of health services, and health outcomes [1, 2]. Health literacy is defined as "... *the degree to which individuals have the capacity to obtain, process, and understand basic health information and services needed to make appropriate health decisions* [3]." It has been related to a number of variables reflecting patients' ability to obtain and use information to reach their desired state of health, including use of preventive health services, indices of disease control such as glycosylated hemoglobin in diabetes, risk for hospitalization, and even increased likelihood for death [1, 4].

One especially important finding in health literacy research has been the fact that racial and ethnic minorities and the elderly perform at lower levels on several measures of health literacy compared to the general population [5, 6]. One widely cited study, for example, was the National Assessment of Adult Literacy (NAAL) which included a health literacy scale [5]. The study, based on a nationally representative sample, showed that blacks, Hispanics, and the elderly had lower levels of health literacy on the NAAL health literacy scale. Studies with other measures, including the widely used Test of Functional Health Literacy in Adults (TOFHLA) [7], have also found similar differences. Given the link between health literacy and health status and the common finding of disparities in health among racial and ethnic minorities, several authors have suggested that differences in health literacy may be a factor in health disparities [6].

Although studies have often treated health literacy as a unitary characteristic of the persons assessed, studies have used a number of different measures to assess it [4]. It is not clear, however, whether various measures of health literacy assess the same abilities and skills. The TOFHLA, for example, includes two subtests that assess reading comprehension and numeracy skills. An issue that may limit the usefulness of the TOFHLA is the response format in the reading comprehension subtest. The TOFHLA uses the cloze procedure [8] to assess reading comprehension. In this approach, comprehension is tested by asking the person evaluated to demonstrate their understanding by supplying a word missing in a sentence (e.g., "The sky is —"). This strategy may create items that are differentially more difficult for older persons as it taps abilities known to decline with increasing age [8, 9].

Another widely used measure, the Rapid Estimate of Adult Literacy in Medicine, or REALM [10], assesses health literacy only regarding the person's ability to read a list of health-related words aloud. Other measures of health literacy may evaluate still other abilities using other response formats. The Rapid Estimate of Adult Literacy in Medicine, or REALM [10], only assesses health literacy regarding patients' ability to correctly pronounce a series of health-related words (e.g., anatomical terms and the names of diseases and condition) and thus does not directly assess their ability to understand what they read. The REALM does not assess numeracy skills, consistently shown to be an important aspect of health literacy [11]. The Newest Vital Sign [12] only assesses patients' comprehension of a single food label, and thus it only taps a very narrow range of skills. Further, the psychometric characteristics of most measures are not well known, as noted by Jordan et al. [13]. One important task for health literacy researchers is to better understand the currently available measures of health literacy and to address concerns about scale characteristics in developing new measures [14].

In a previous study, we used the TOFHLA with elderly patients who were being treated with medications for memory problems [15, 16]. In pilot testing of the study assessment battery, it became apparent that many elderly patients had difficulty with the cloze format of the TOFHLA reading comprehension, appearing to not understand the task even after multiple explanations and finding it difficult to produce responses even when able to choose from multiple available choices. By contrast, younger persons commonly have little or no difficulty with the response format. These observations led us to evaluate the possibility that the TOFHLA response format might be differentially more difficult for older compared to younger individuals.

Other authors have suggested that the cloze format may be difficult for older adults due to its demands on cognitive abilities known to decline with increasing age, including verbal fluency working memory and psychomotor speed [17]. Further, Ackerman et al. showed that cloze performance modified the relation between age and general cognitive ability [8]. If cloze items are in fact differentially more difficult for older adults due to changes in their basic cognitive abilities, then a health literacy measure that uses this response format might produce results suggesting that elders' health literacy skills are lower than they actually are. One strategy to evaluate this possibility is to assess whether the items are associated with *differential item functioning* (DIF) [18]. DIF is said to exist for a particular item in a measure when its difficulty is not the same for individuals of equal ability. In the case of health literacy measures like the TOFHLA that use the cloze procedure [8], the result would be that some items would be more difficult for older individuals than for younger individuals with same overall health literacy ability, not because of actual differences in health literacy but because the item requires a cognitive ability (e.g., verbal fluency) that is lower in the older individuals. The item would thus tap two abilities (health literacy and verbal fluency) while ostensibly assessing only one (health literacy). Since the second ability differs between the two groups, the item will appear to be more difficult for older individuals, but not because they actually have lower health literacy. The purpose of this paper was thus to evaluate whether the cloze items on the TOFHLA presented evidence of age-related DIF. We hypothesized that the response format of the measure would result in evidence of age-related DIF.

2. Method

2.1. Participants. Data for this study were drawn from a study of cognition and medication adherence in persons treated for HIV [19]. Participants were recruited from several local clinics in South Florida, USA, and were referred by healthcare providers or as a result of their having seen flyers that publicized the study. All were 18 years of age or older and were judged as requiring treatment for HIV infection. Participants were screened for serious neurological or psychiatric impairment and indicated that they had not used illicit drugs during the past 12 months. The full testing procedure required no more than 2 hours for completion, and subjects were paid $50 for their participation.

2.2. Measures. As part of a battery of measures, the reading comprehension portion of the TOFHLA was administered. This measure comprises three health-related paragraphs of increasing reading difficulty, beginning with instructions on how to prepare for a radiographic study and concluding with an informed consent for a surgical procedure. Words are removed from sentences with a blank substituted, and possible correct options are listed below each blank. The total number of responses for the all paragraphs is 50. Participants were tested according to the standard directions for the measure [7] and were given 20 minutes to complete the questions. Their responses were categorized as right or wrong according to the test's administration instructions [7].

2.3. Procedures. Sample sizes required for stable estimates via parametric item response theory (IRT) are large. Most experts suggest that sample size should be in the range of 1,000 [18]. Because of our small sample size, data analyses were completed using a nonparametric item response theory (IRT) strategy using the TestGraf software (http://www.psych.mcgill.ca/misc/fda/downloads/testgraf/), a package that is freely available for download [20]. In addition to providing nonparametric IRT plots of the relation of participants' overall ability to their probability of obtaining a correct answer, this software package calculates a measure of overall DIF, *beta*, for each item. Based on extensive simulation modeling, Zumbo and Witarsa [21] have provided critical values for the beta statistic in relation to various sample sizes. These authors also show that the use of these critical values has considerably better power for detecting the presence of known DIF than the better-known

TABLE 1: Description of sample.

(a)

Gender	119 men, 88 women
Hispanic	22
Race	
Non-Hispanic White	9 (4.3%)
Hispanic	21 (10.1%)
Black	174 (83.7)
Native American	1 (0.5%)

(b)

Continuous variables			
Variable	Range	Mean	Standard deviation
Age	23–67	45.0	8.45
Education (years)	5–20	11.61	2.18
TOFHLA reading comprehension score	2–50	38.51	7.77

strategy of calculating Mantel-Haenszel chi-square values. We also used jMetrik, a freely available software package for item analysis (http://www.itemanalysis.com/), to estimate item difficulties, standard deviations, and discriminations (defined as the correlations of each item with the total scale score).

We divided our sample into two groups, those with ages less than and those with ages equal to or greater than 45 years. This cut point was chosen as it provided reasonably similar sample sizes for each group and lies in the age range related to both evidence of cognitive aging [22] and lower levels of health literacy [5]. Items that exceeded the critical value of beta for our sample size as reported by Zumbo and Witarsa [21] for a probability of less than 0.01 were flagged for examination of item plots and are marked in our results below.

3. Results

Statistics providing a characterization of the sample are presented in Table 1. The majority of participants were men and black, and there was a wide range of age and education in the sample.

Results of item analyses are presented in Table 2. Items with beta values greater than the $P < 0.01$ cut point provided by Zumbo and Witarsa are italicized [21]. It can be seen that 24 out of the 50 items show significant age-related DIF. The impact of age-related DIF on test performance is illustrated in Figure 1, based on analyses for item 40 in paragraph C of the TOFHLA reading comprehension test. It shows item curves for younger and older individuals; each plots the probability of someone obtaining a correct answer on question 40 (left axis, ranging from 0 to 1) and the participant's underlying general health literacy ability estimated as their total score on the measure. The plot includes lines for younger participants (marked with a 1) and older participants (marked with a 2). If an item does not present DIF, the lines should approximately coincide, and the beta value should be near 0. A consistent distance between the lines suggests that the item is more or less difficult for members of one group or another. As illustrated in Figure 1, older individuals must have a higher level of ability to obtain a correct answer than younger persons do. The impact of age-related DIF would thus cause older individuals to have lower overall scores because of the relatively greater difficulty of these items.

4. Discussion

Results of these analyses suggest the existence of substantial age-related DIF in the reading comprehension subtest of the TOFHLA. To the best of our knowledge, this is the first study to evaluate at an item level the influence of age on TOFHLA scores. Based on our observations of participants in an earlier study, we investigated the possibility that the response format of the TOHFLA might have an influence on older adults' performance independent of their actual levels of health literacy. Our results suggest that this may be the case. The implication of this finding is that at least a portion of the difference in health literacy associated with age on the TOFHLA may be the result of DIF rather than actual differences in health literacy.

It should be noted that some studies have not found age-related differences in health literacy when using a measure that does not use the cloze response format (Rapid Estimate of Health Literacy in Medicine or REALM [10]). One study, for example, administered both the S-TOFHLA and the short form of the REALM in adults with diabetes [23]. While the expected age-related differences emerged for the reading section of the S-TOFHLA, none were found for the REALM. Shigaki et al. [24] compared the REALM and another measure, the Newest Vital Sign (NVS) [12]. In this study, age differences emerged for the NVS (which requires that patients generate answers) but not for the REALM. In a large sample of persons with a wide range of educational and health backgrounds, Sudore et al. [25] also failed to find

TABLE 2: Item difficulties, discriminations, and betas.

Item	Difficulty	SD	Discrimination	Beta
A1[a]	0.880	0.326	0.398	***0.087***
A2	0.918	0.275	0.520	0.047
A3	0.809	0.394	0.504	***0.116***
A4	0.924	0.267	0.510	0.049
A5	0.940	0.238	0.499	0.032
A6	0.967	0.179	0.163	0.012
A7	0.874	0.332	0.549	0.025
A8	0.880	0.326	0.444	0.058
A9	0.858	0.350	0.386	***0.085***
A10	0.880	0.326	0.562	0.026
A11	0.902	0.299	0.472	0.063
A12	0.951	0.217	0.444	0.060
A13	0.902	0.299	0.417	0.052
A14	0.863	0.344	0.395	0.062
A15	0.842	0.366	0.391	***0.073***
B16	0.934	0.248	0.396	0.054
B17	0.924	0.267	0.473	0.044
B18	0.951	0.217	0.431	0.058
B19	0.645	0.480	0.393	***0.094***
B20	0.902	0.299	0.390	0.057
B21	0.721	0.450	0.504	***0.115***
B22	0.836	0.371	0.427	0.044
B23	0.934	0.248	0.369	0.036
B24	0.634	0.483	0.361	***0.170***
B25	0.809	0.394	0.464	***0.071***
B26	0.809	0.394	0.451	***0.099***
B27	0.863	0.344	0.601	***0.082***
B28	0.913	0.283	0.470	0.051
B29	0.820	0.386	0.543	0.034
B30	0.754	0.432	0.660	***0.109***
B31	0.798	0.403	0.520	***0.072***
B32	0.814	0.390	0.520	***0.118***
B33	0.869	0.339	0.526	0.054
B34	0.426	0.496	0.394	***0.151***
B35	0.874	0.332	0.666	0.062
B36	0.863	0.344	0.641	0.052
C37	0.863	0.344	0.570	***0.079***
C38	0.743	0.438	0.707	0.031
C39	0.579	0.495	0.512	***0.091***
C40	0.579	0.495	0.522	***0.146***
C41	0.448	0.499	0.529	0.050
C42	0.710	0.455	0.627	0.051
C43	0.628	0.485	0.633	***0.100***
C44	0.678	0.469	0.630	***0.074***
C45	0.251	0.435	0.346	***0.183***
C46	0.481	0.501	0.621	***0.110***
C47	0.197	0.399	0.244	***0.074***
C48	0.519	0.501	0.535	0.048
C49	0.568	0.497	0.564	***0.090***
C50	0.628	0.485	0.694	***0.070***

[a]Letter prefixes before items numbers denote from which of the three test paragraphs the item is drawn.

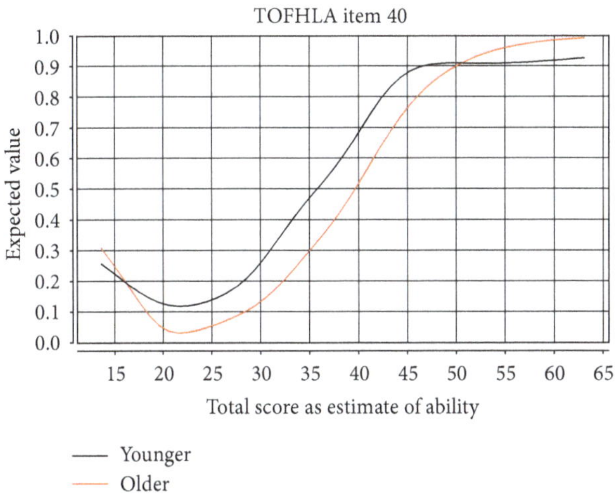

FIGURE 1: Item curve illustrating DIF between younger and older persons.

age-related differences in health literacy as assessed by the REALM.

Limitations of this study should be acknowledged. Our sample included only persons treated for HIV infection, potentially limiting the extent to which these findings can be generalized to other populations of older adults. Although our participants may have had HIV-related cognitive deficits that could have affected their performance on the S-TOFHLA, it is also likely that they would have had age-related changes in cognitive function. The dual effects of HIV infection and aging on cognitive function (presumably the basis for finding DIF on the S-TOFHLA) are difficult to distinguish; studies of the issue have suggested that both aging and HIV have an impact on cognition [26] while at least one study did not find a relation [27]. Older participants might be differentially more susceptible to fatigue during testing procedures. Since the TOFHLA questions were embedded in a larger battery of cognitive measures, this might have affected older persons' responses. We note that the entire battery is only required for at most 2 hours and that our participants were all community-dwelling and ambulatory, reducing the likelihood of serious fatigue affecting their responses. This possibility, however, cannot be ruled out.

While it thus might appear that age-related deficits in health literacy may be related to the response format of the measure used to assess it, it must be noted that other measures have found age-related differences in health literacy. Although (due to concerns for test security that prohibit revealing actual items) it is difficult to know the precise format of responses on the measure, the National Assessment of Adult Literacy found significant deficits in health literacy among older adults. Haun et al. found age-related differences in performance on the S-TOFHLA and a self-report measure of health literacy, the BRIEF [28], but not on the REALM. It may be reasonable to conclude, as have others, that it may be important to consider task demands and purpose when selecting a health literacy measure for a particular purpose [29]. These results thus further support others' observations of the variable relations of common measures of health literacy with age. Given the evidence of age-related DIF on a substantial number of items in the reading comprehension subtest of the TOFHLA, it would appear prudent to be cautious in interpreting the significance of age-related deficits in health literacy when it is assessed using the TOHFLA or S-TOFHLA.

Conflict of Interests

The authors have declared that they have no conflict of interests with any entity discussed in this paper.

References

[1] N. D. Berkman, S. L. Sheridan, K. E. Donahue, D. J. Halpern, and K. Crotty, "Low health literacy and health outcomes: an updated systematic review," *Annals of Internal Medicine*, vol. 155, no. 2, pp. 97–107, 2011.

[2] N. D. Berkman, D. A. Dewalt, M. P. Pignone et al., "Literacy and health outcomes," *Evidence Report/Technology Assessment*, no. 87, pp. 1–8, 2004.

[3] Department of Health and Human Services, "Healthy people 2020: topics and objectives," Tech. Rep., Department of Health and Human Services, Washington, DC, USA, http://healthypeople.gov/2020/topicsobjectives2020/pdfs/HP 2020objectives.pdf.

[4] D. A. Dewalt, N. D. Berkman, S. Sheridan, K. N. Lohr, and M. P. Pignone, "Literacy and health outcomes: a systematic review of the literature," *Journal of General Internal Medicine*, vol. 19, no. 12, pp. 1228–1239, 2004.

[5] S. White and S. Dillow, "Key concepts and features of the 2003 National Assessment of Adult Literacy," Tech. Rep. NCES 2006-471, US Department of Education, National Center for Educational Statistics, Washington, DC, USA, 2005.

[6] C. Y. Osborn, M. K. Paasche-Orlow, T. C. Davis, and M. S. Wolf, "Health literacy: an overlooked factor in understanding HIV health disparities," *American Journal of Preventive Medicine*, vol. 33, no. 5, pp. 374–378, 2007.

[7] R. M. Parker, D. W. Baker, M. V. Williams, and J. R. Nurss, "The test of functional health literacy in adults: a new instrument for measuring patients' literacy skills," *Journal of General Internal Medicine*, vol. 10, no. 10, pp. 537–541, 1995.

[8] P. L. Ackerman, M. E. Beier, and K. R. Bowen, "Explorations of crystallized intelligence: completion tests, cloze tests, and knowledge," *Learning and Individual Differences*, vol. 12, no. 1, pp. 105–121, 2000.

[9] D. C. Park and A. H. Gutchess, "Cognitive aging and everyday life," in *Aging and Communication*, N. A. Charness, D. C. Park, and B. Sabel, Eds., pp. 217–232, Springer, New York, NY, USA, 2000.

[10] P. W. Murphy, T. C. Davis, S. W. Long, R. H. Jackson, and B. C. Decker, "Rapid Estimate of Adult Literacy in Medicine (REALM): a quick reading test for patients," *Journal of Reading*, vol. 37, pp. 124–130, 1993.

[11] V. F. Reyna, W. L. Nelson, P. K. Han, and N. F. Dieckmann, "How numeracy influences risk comprehension and medical decision making," *Psychological Bulletin*, vol. 135, no. 6, pp. 943–973, 2009.

[12] B. D. Weiss, M. Z. Mays, W. Martz et al., "Quick assessment of literacy in primary care: the newest vital sign," *Annals of Family Medicine*, vol. 3, no. 6, pp. 514–522, 2005.

[13] J. E. Jordan, R. H. Osborne, and R. Buchbinder, "Critical appraisal of health literacy indices revealed variable underlying constructs, narrow content and psychometric weaknesses," *Journal of Clinical Epidemiology*, vol. 64, no. 4, pp. 366–379, 2011.

[14] A. Pleasant, J. McKinney, and R. V. Rikard, "Health literacy measurement: a proposed research agenda," *Journal of Health Communication*, vol. 16, 3, pp. 11–21, 2011.

[15] R. L. Ownby, C. Hertzog, and S. J. Czaja, "Tailored information and automated reminding to improve medication adherence in Spanish- and English-speaking elders treater for memory impairment," *Clinical Gerontologist*, vol. 35, no. 3, pp. 221–238, 2012.

[16] R. L. Ownby, C. Hertzog, and S. J. Czaja, "Relations between cognitive status and medication adherence in patients treated for memory disorders," *Ageing Research*, vol. 3, no. 1, 2012.

[17] P. L. Ackerman, M. E. Beier, and M. O. Boyle, "Individual differences in working memory within a nomological network of cognitive and perceptual speed abilities," *Journal of Experimental Psychology*, vol. 131, no. 4, pp. 567–589, 2002.

[18] S. E. Embretson and S. P. Reise, *Item Response Theory for Psychologists*, Lawrence Erlbaum, Mahwah, NJ, USA, 2000.

[19] D. Waldrop-Valverde, D. L. Jones, F. Gould, M. Kumar, and R. L. Ownby, "Neurocognition, health-related reading literacy, and numeracy in medication management for HIV infection," *AIDS Patient Care and STDs*, vol. 24, no. 8, pp. 477–484, 2010.

[20] J. O. Ramsay, *TestGraft98 Manual*, McGill University, Montreal, Canada, http://www.psych.mcgill.ca/faculty/ramsay/TestGraf.html.

[21] B. D. Zumbo and P. M. Witarsa, "Nonparametric IRT methodology for detecting DIF in moderate-to-small scale measurment: operating characteristics and a compartions with the Mantel Haenszel," in *Proceedings of the Annual Meeting of the American Educational Research Association*, 2004, http://educ.ubc.ca/faculty/zumbo/aera/papers/Zumbo_Witarsa_AERA.pdf.

[22] D. C. Park, G. Lautenschlager, T. Hedden, N. S. Davidson, A. D. Smith, and P. K. Smith, "Models of visuospatial and verbal memory across the adult life span," *Psychology and Aging*, vol. 17, no. 2, pp. 299–320, 2002.

[23] J. K. Kirk, J. G. Grzywacz, T. A. Arcury et al., "Performance of health literacy tests among older adults with diabetes," *Journal of General Internal Medicine*, vol. 27, pp. 534–540, 2012.

[24] C. L. Shigaki, R. L. Kruse, D. R. Mehr, and B. Ge, "The REALM vs. NVS: a comparison of health literacy measures in patients with diabetes," *Annals of Behavioral Science and Medical Education*, vol. 18, pp. 9–13, 2012.

[25] R. L. Sudore, K. M. Mehta, E. M. Simonsick et al., "Limited literacy in older people and disparities in health and healthcare access," *Journal of the American Geriatrics Society*, vol. 54, no. 5, pp. 770–776, 2006.

[26] D. E. Vance, V. G. Wadley, M. G. Crowe, J. L. Raper, and K. K. Ball, "Cognitive and everyday functioning in older and younger adults with and without HIV," *Clinical Gerontologist*, vol. 34, no. 5, pp. 413–426, 2011.

[27] L. A. Cysique, P. Maruff, M. P. Bain, E. Wright, and B. J. Brew, "HIV and age do not substantially interact in HIV-associated neurocognitive impairment," *Journal of Neuropsychiatry and Clinical Neurosciences*, vol. 23, no. 1, pp. 83–89, 2011.

[28] L. D. Chew, J. M. Griffin, M. R. Partin et al., "Validation of screening questions for limited health literacy in a large VA outpatient population," *Journal of General Internal Medicine*, vol. 23, no. 5, pp. 561–566, 2008.

[29] J. Haun, S. Luther, V. Dodd, and P. Donaldson, "Measurement variation across health literacy assessments: implications for assessment selection in research and practice," *Journal of Community Health*, vol. 17, supplement 3, pp. 141–159, 2012.

6

Universal Design: A Step toward Successful Aging

Kelly Carr,[1] Patricia L. Weir,[1] Dory Azar,[2] and Nadia R. Azar[1]

[1] *Department of Kinesiology, University of Windsor, 401 Sunset Avenue, Windsor, ON, Canada N9B 3P4*
[2] *Dory Azar Architect, 870 Revland Drive, Tecumseh, ON, Canada N8N 5B2*

Correspondence should be addressed to Nadia R. Azar; azar5@uwindsor.ca

Academic Editor: Ioannis Trougakos

The concept of aging successfully has become increasingly important as demographics shift towards an aging population. Successful aging has been defined to include (1) a low probability of disease and disease-related disability; (2) a high level of physical and cognitive functioning; and (3) an active engagement in life. The built environment can create opportunities or constraints for seniors to participate in social and productive activities. Universally designed spaces are more easily accessed and used by a spectrum of people without specialized adaptations. Thus, a universally designed environment creates opportunities for older adults to participate in these activities without the stigmatization associated with adapted or accessible designs. Providing older adults with specific universal design options (e.g., lever handle faucets) has the potential to increase the ease of completing activities of daily living, which promotes a continual engagement in life. Literature regarding universal design is promising; however, its theory requires further attention from professionals designing the built environment, evidence of the significance of its application from academics, and the embracement of its core principles from society. Overall, universal design has the potential to provide a stepping stone toward successful aging.

1. Introduction

A rise in life expectancy and a decline in fertility rates have created a shift in demographics leading to an aging population [1–4]. Currently, Canada's population of citizens 65 years of age and older is at a record high (14.8%; [3]). This older adult population has experienced a 14.1% growth in the past five years, with 60–64 year olds experiencing the greatest increase, followed by centenarians [3]. If this trend continues, seniors will account for nearly a quarter of the population by 2036 [4]. At that point, the number of older adults will surpass the number of children, a first in Canadian history [4]. These demographic trends span beyond Canadian borders and have been recognized globally [1]. As a result, successful aging has become an important concept worldwide [5].

Successful aging has been empirically defined to include (1) a low probability of disease and disease-related disability; (2) a high level of physical and cognitive functioning; and (3) an active engagement in life [6, 7]. To some extent, these components represent a hierarchical relationship, as it is suggested that the absence of disease and disability leads to a prolonged maintenance of physical and cognitive functioning, which enables a higher level of engagement defined as the combination of social activity and productive activity [7, 8], participation in leisure activities [9], and belonging to neighborhood groups [10] (see [11] for an extensive review). Individuals who meet these hierarchical components during the aging process maintain the capacity to adequately function during daily living, leading to greater independence [12]. Continued independence is suggested to be an important factor throughout the aging process as it facilitates control and autonomy, both of which increase well-being and life satisfaction [6, 13]. In addition to the psychosocial benefits associated with successful aging, the absence of chronic disease seen in older adults who have aged successfully has the potential to reduce the health care costs required for an aging population [14]. While there are older adults who are successfully aging, the majority of older adults are dealing with some kind of limitation. Putting these ideas into a practical setting, we need to consider older adults, living in the broader community who are active in their homes, church groups, recreation centers and are out and about in their community doing errands to manage their personal lives (e.g., shopping, banking, appointments, etc.). All of these represent forms of engagement. Though planning and design of the built environment has long been considered an influential factor on the aging process, only recently has the philosophy of universal design flourished [15, 16]. Universal design includes designing environments and products that are more easily accessed and used by a spectrum of people without specialized adaptations [16]. A key concept of universal design is to provide accessibility without stigmatization, by integrating accessibility features such that they benefit all users while going essentially unnoticed [16]. For example, automatic sliding doors are standard features at many shopping centers. These doors remove barriers to entry for individuals in a wheelchair, and for older adults or young children who have difficultly opening heavy doors. However, they also benefit all customers carrying purchased goods and are a convenience feature for the able-bodied individual with free hands. They provide accessibility without stigmatization, since everyone entering or exiting the store uses them, regardless of ability.

The concept of universal design proves to be timely, as it complements the implementation of the Accessibility for Ontarians with Disabilities Act (2005), which requires full accessibility of public and private buildings by the year 2025 [17]. While being mindful of complete accessibility, universal design aims to accommodate human diversity with a focus on inclusion and equality [18]. It is these aspects of universal design that set it apart from accessibility design and specialized adaptation and create the potential to further enhance well-being and quality of life [19]. Specific to older adults, implementing universal design could enable individuals to continue to complete activities of daily living independently while providing a safer environment for daily functioning and navigation, both of which can reduce the chances of an older adult entering a nursing home [19, 20]. These benefits are provided through the implementation of any of the seven structured universal design principles outlined in Table 1 [16]. For example, providing automatic sliding doors at the entrance of a public building meets at least 6 of these principles. As described in the previous paragraph, they provide equal access for individuals with diverse abilities and needs (Principles 1 and 2). They are very simple and intuitive to use (Principle 3), and since they open when sensors detect the presence of a person within range (as opposed to having to open the door manually or even by pushing a button), they require no physical effort to operate (Principle 6). These sensors also ensure that the sliding door will remain open for as long as the person remains within the sensor's range, minimizing the risk of injury due to the door shutting before they are able to walk all the way through (Principle 5). Finally, automatic sliding doors are frequently much wider than a typical swinging door, making it easier to maneuver through the door while using ambulatory aids (e.g., canes, walkers, scooters, wheelchairs, crutches, etc.) or while manipulating other large items (e.g., carrying large/irregular packages, pushing a stroller, or shopping cart) (Principle 7). For older adults who no longer have enough upper limb strength to open a heavy door, and/or who use a walker or a wheelchair, and/or may have age-related visual impairments, and/or move slowly; automatic sliding doors remove a significant barrier to entering public buildings independently and facilitate their ability to engage in the activities within.

As the population experiences a substantial increase in older adults it is imperative to understand the impact thoughtful design and planning has on the ability to age successfully [3, 4]. Specifically, universal design may have the potential to affect older adult's engagement with life, by providing accessible and accommodating environments in which this population can thrive without stigmatization. As Rowe and Kahn [6] proposed, it is the environment surrounding the older adults (i.e., residential and community environment) that is the primary factor that creates opportunities and constraints for the individual. Thus, modifications to the built environment can impact the engagement levels (i.e., interpersonal relations and involvement in productive activities) of older adults to promote successful aging [7]. This approach is favorable, as it increases an individual's functional abilities with the least amount of effort required from the individual when compared to approaches attempting to change the person (i.e., exercise to increase strength, to enable the individual to operate a regular door) or provide assistive tools (i.e., provide an electronic push button to open the door) [16]. Therefore, the aim of this review is to conceptualize the importance of older adults actively engaging in life, the roles the built environment and universal design play in maintaining engagement, and provide examples to implement this approach for optimal engagement in late adulthood. Through this review, we hope to bring attention to the potential for universal design to promote successful aging by facilitating active engagement in one's life.

2. Active Engagement in Life

2.1. Predictor of Successful Aging. While Rowe and Kahn's [7] definition of successful aging has been the most widely empirically tested, their description of active engagement is limited to the maintenance of interpersonal relationships and continued involvement in productive activities. Interpersonal relationships are connections and interactions with others, including the availability of emotional support and physical assistance, whereas productive activities are all activities that provide value regardless of compensation to the individual (i.e., volunteering, paid employment; [7]). Though Rowe and Kahn's definition of engagement in life is highly regarded in academia, it should be noted that there is little consensus regarding this concept [21]. As highlighted by Levasseur et al. [11], it might be thought of as a continuum ranging from social participation to social engagement, with activities being performed by oneself, with others, or for others.

Despite this inconsistency, continued engagement is commonly regarded as a significant predictor of successful aging [21]. Specifically, it is suggested that older adults perceive social and familial relationships as fundamental to aging successfully [22–24]. Older adults residing in nursing homes

Table 1: Seven principles of universal design (adapted from Story [16]).

Universal design principle	Description	Example
(1) Equitable use	Useful and marketable to people with diverse abilities	Doors that automatically open
(2) Flexibility of use	Accommodates a wide range of individual preferences and abilities	Automated teller machines' buttons far enough apart to be pressed accurately
(3) Simple and intuitive use	Easy to understand, regardless of user's experience, knowledge, language skills, or current concentration level	Providing furniture assembly instructions in a series of clear illustrations instead of text
(4) Perceptible information	Communicates necessary information effectively to the user, regardless of ambient conditions or the user's sensory abilities	Computer software that relays information visually through text and pictures, and audibly through speakers
(5) Tolerance for error	Minimizes hazards and the adverse consequences of accidental or unintended actions	Hallways that return to common areas rather than stop in dead ends
(6) Low physical effort	Can be used efficiently and comfortably with a minimum of fatigue	Bottle caps that are easy to grip and require only a small range of motion to open
(7) Size/space for approach/use	Appropriate size and space is provided for approach, reach, manipulation, and use regardless of the user's body size, posture, or mobility	Wall mounted components (i.e., toilet paper) that are visible, easy to reach, and easy for all hand sizes to use

also emphasize the importance of social interactions [25]. This view may be a product of the companionship and sustained connection to the broader community these contacts offer [26]. Complementing interpersonal relations with involvement in productive activities has also been perceived as beneficial; a sample of older adults reported participating in activities (i.e., gardening) to be among the most important factors required to age successfully [27]. Therefore, continued engagement in life is not only valued within empirical definitions of successful aging, it is perceived by older adults to be pertinent to the aging process as well.

2.2. Benefits of Engagement. Engagement in life has received the least research attention of the three components of successful aging described by Rowe and Kahn [7]; however, the benefits obtained through continued engagement have not gone unnoticed [21, 28]. Research suggests that a positive correlation exists between the number of activities older adults participate in and quality of life and well-being [29, 30]. This relationship is even more pronounced for individuals with minimal contact with family members, individuals suffering from functional loss, and during bereavement of loss of a spouse [30, 31]. These findings suggest continued engagement in life has a compensatory role for maintaining well-being and quality of life following adverse events during older adulthood [30]. Older adults residing in nursing homes also experience increases in quality of life from productive activities, such as perceiving oneself as being able to help others [25]. Furthermore, interpersonal relations (i.e., large social networks), as well as participation in activities, are suggested to increase the potential to age successfully by facilitating happiness, contentment, life satisfaction, and enjoyment [32, 33].

Increases in health have also been attributed to engagement in social, intellectual, cultural, leisure, and productive pursuits [29]. Individuals reporting higher levels of social engagement, irrespective of the activity, are significantly less likely to require health services and are prescribed less medication [34]. This finding is complemented by reports of increased objective and subjective health, reductions in all causes of mortality, and reductions in loneliness and depression through participation in social, productive, and physical activities [32, 35–37]. Taken together, these findings are highly suggestive that continued engagement in life provides an avenue to age successfully.

2.3. Engagement and the Built Environment. The usual aging process is associated with natural changes in health and functioning [6]. These changes include (but are not limited to) reductions in muscle mass, the development of osteoporosis, and declines in cognitive and sensory function [6, 38–41]. Although these natural age-related changes have the potential to impact the ability to maintain an active engagement in life, the built environment can influence engagement profiles of older adults as well, both positively and negatively [19]. For example, the characteristics of the home environment can increase or reduce functional limitations of older adults by creating or removing barriers to daily tasks [42]. Furthermore, both residential and community designs that enable older adults to satisfy individual needs, and to access services and resources, are necessary to promote successful aging [22, 26]. Ultimately, these accommodating environments can increase well-being, quality of life, and participation in activity, all of which can aid in successful aging [25, 37]. In order to implement such environments to optimize the aging process, a comprehensive understanding of the theories of universal design is warranted.

3. Universal Design

3.1. More than Accessibility. The built environment has also been proposed to negatively impact older adults by creating barriers to maintain a continued engagement with life [18]. In consequence, social bonds and community connections can be severed due to an environment that hinders the functioning of this population [18]. However, environments that are thoughtfully designed or modified to accommodate varying abilities have the potential to reduce disability and foster engagement in social and productive activities in later life [43, 44]. Due to the impact the built environment has on daily functioning in older adulthood, it is imperative for designers to take into consideration changes experienced during the aging process [45].

Research specific to older adults and the built environment suggests that adults have a strong preference for aging in a place of familiarity, in regards to the home and broader community [18, 58]. Specifically, 75% of middle aged and older adults report a strong desire to reside as long as possible in their current homes [58]. Keeping in mind the current shift in demographics, such a preference creates a high demand for built environments that are accommodating and accessible to older adults. A number of design theories have principles that accommodate the aging process in the design of the built environment. In addition to universal design, these theories include accessible design, adaptable design, and transgenerational design (Table 2; [46, 48]). Although accessible and adaptable design features provide accommodations that could be helpful for older adults, these features are often fixed in place and noticeable [59] and may promote a sense of segregation among end-users [16] and of stigmatization as being "seniors" or "disabled" [60]. Since these features require specialized adaptations or equipment, they may also come at a substantial financial cost, particularly if they are added as retrofits to existing spaces [16]. Transgenerational design seeks to create products and environments that are compatible with the physical and sensory impairments associated with aging, often from the initial planning stages [48]. There is some overlap between universal design and transgenerational design: Farage et al. [61] maintain that many of the design principles of transgenerational design are consistent with the principles of universal design, and that thoughtful application of the universal design principles will lead to design that is transgenerational. However, since the focus of transgenerational design is on accommodating the adaptations that arise as a result of aging [62], accommodations for other populations may be overlooked [16], and this approach may still be stigmatizing due to its emphasis on "age" [62].

Though all thoughtful design has the potential to reduce or remove barriers associated with aging and disability; universal design strives to provide accessible environments without stigmatization or ageism, as the design principles are not specialized and are incorporated into the environment in the initial stages of planning [16, 18, 44]. Universal design is founded on the premise that there is only one population with varying characteristics rather than a "normal" and "diverging from normal" population [63]. "Because all groups are placed within the context of normal expectations of the human condition, trying to justify the importance of each vulnerable population group becomes unnecessary." (Pastalan, as cited in [64], page 3). Thus, universal design removes segregation of the older population resulting in an ideal approach to increase successful aging throughout the lifespan.

Universal design, often used interchangeably with inclusive design and design for all, is a 21st century professional, academic, and social movement [65, 66]. If implemented properly, universal design creates safe, accessible, and usable environments for the broadest spectrum of people possible [67]. Empirical evidence of the success of the universal design philosophy on the professional (i.e., architecture) and academic (i.e., theoretical application) fronts has been reported. Danford [68] provided a tour of a universally designed and a non-universally designed building to 24 adults with either a visual, auditory, or mobility impairment and eight adults with no impairments. All people, with and without impairments, reported less difficulty and required less effort and assistance to complete standard tasks (i.e., finding a public washroom, entering the building) in the building constructed using the universal design principles.

The social movement of universal design has a theoretical foundation rather than an empirical framework. Currently, literature refers to universal design as a philosophy and a process, rather than a legal code and a result [63, 69]. While being mindful of this construct, universal design should be implemented as good practice as it not only incorporates building code requirements of design, it goes beyond the basic code requirements and provides equality regarding usability and accessibility among a wide spectrum of the population. Overall, this provides evidence that universal design is more than simply creating accessible environments; it encourages a shift in attitude toward democracy and equality for all citizens, including the continually growing older adult population [63]. With such an influence on society, it is plausible to propose universal design can facilitate continued engagement in life, and ultimately successful aging.

3.2. A Step toward Successful Aging. The built environment can impact the engagement profiles of older adults both positively and negatively [18, 43, 44]. Therefore, it is important to consider specific examples of universal design that can allow for positive changes to engagement levels and ultimately promote successful aging. The recommendations provided in Table 3 are based on three basic activities of daily living (BADLs) and three instrumental activities of daily living (IADLs) that are identified in the literature as pertinent to the independence of older adults and are directly related to the built environment [70–72]. BADLs refer to activities of personal care and physical self-maintenance, whereas IADLs include community and domestic activities that require an individual to adapt to the environment [70, 71]. The implementation of the universal design options described in Table 3 would provide a stepping stone toward successful aging: Older adults would be provided with an opportunity to more easily accomplish BADLS and IADLs, which would promote independence in both social and productive activities and ultimately foster active engagement in life.

3.3. Identifying and Overcoming Challenges. Despite the positive implications universal design offers to adults experiencing natural age-related declines, this design philosophy

TABLE 2: Additional theories of design.

Design theory	Definition	Example
Accessible design [46]	Provides separate design features for user groups with disabilities Usually permanent and noticeable Fulfills code requirements for use by individuals with disabilities	Provide the minimum level of accessibility required by the local building code. This can vary by region (e.g., province or state), and with different building types within the same region. For example, Ontario Building Code requires power door operators (e.g., push button, automatic sensor, etc.) on entrances to hotels, but not on entrances to stand-alone office spaces of less than 300 m^2 [47].
Adaptable design [46]	Provides design features that are usable by groups with disabilities, however remain concealed or omitted until needed Features are either adjustable or easily and quickly added or removed in order to "adapt" the environment for specific individuals	An electronic push button is provided to open the door, but the use of the push button is optional (i.e., door will open manually).
Transgenerational design [48]	Develops products and environments that are compatible with the natural physical and sensory declines experienced during the aging process	Provide a power assist door, which augments the force applied by the user to fully open the door [49].

TABLE 3: Examples of universal design techniques that will allow older adults to complete basic activities of daily living (BADLs) and instrumental activities of daily living (IADLs) with greater ease.

Activities of daily living	Examples of universal design
BADL	
Bathing	Make provisions during construction to reinforce walls in the shower area to facilitate future installation of grab bars [50] Bathtub/shower controls positioned to allow for operation outside the fixture [20] Lever handle faucets [20] No threshold walk-in shower [20]
Physical ambulation	No threshold, zero step entrances [50] Wider doorways and corridors [50] Open floor plan [20] Straight staircases with consistent risers and treads and a stopping place (landing) midway between levels [51]
Toileting	Make provisions during construction to reinforce bathroom walls to facilitate future installation of grab bars by the toilet [50] Installation of a downstairs bathroom [50] Adjustable toilet and sink for easy access, with a short reaching distance to paper dispenser and grab bars [20]
IADL	
Food preparation	Kitchen counter tops at varying levels to accommodate standing and seated users, and people of varying heights [52] Kitchen cabinets that accommodate limited reach ranges and allow various ways for approach and manipulation [53] Color contrasts, large-print readouts, audible and tactile feedback of controls [53] Close access to ovens with counter space directly next to the oven [53]
Shopping	Lowering or making height adjustable electronic devices used in typical purchasing transaction (i.e., credit card reader/swipe; [54]) Larger print on signs indicating aisle numbers and locations of goods, and on packaging of items [55] Larger aisle ways [55] Automatic powered doors at entrances and exits [56]
Transportation	Complement higher-order roads (i.e., interstates) with lower-speed, two lane through-routes [57] Connect local street networks within communities to create short drives and walking distances [57]

is not without challenges and limitations. Primarily, the implementation of universal design is challenged by the minimal education provided to engineers, architects, and environmental planners regarding the importance and use of this design theory [73]. Furthermore, the lack of a standard education regarding universal design may partially account for the little consensus and consistency surrounding the definitions pertaining to universal design [63]. Secondly, universal design is limited in its implementation as we are currently at a time when norms and codes of practice take precedence over theory for guiding decisions and actions [63]. Universal design has a theoretical foundation and has yet to be adopted as "best practice" that goes beyond mandated codes and guidelines, and thus its principles are often overlooked. Thirdly, incorporating designs that simultaneously meet the needs of multiple end-users with widely diverse abilities into the built environment is challenging [62], and achieving this level of accommodation may not be realized if the architects assume an understanding of the barriers that the end-users will experience [74]. Despite the knowledge the architect may have regarding accessible design, and the sincerity of the architect's intentions to understand the end-users' specific needs; such needs are often difficult to interpret by able-bodied persons who may not experience them as barriers, and decisions regarding the application of accessible design within the built environment are often made with little or no input from end-users [75]. With respect to aging, architects may not be aware of the barriers presented to older adults within the built environment and may not recognize these individuals as those who may benefit from various accommodations. A fourth challenge regards the discrepancy between professionals and academics concerning the cost associated with implementing universal design. Academics have often reported that universal design can be implemented at little or no additional cost [16]. However, accessible and universal designs require more square footage within buildings and homes (i.e., larger bathroom stalls or residential bathrooms to allow wheelchair access and/or a caregiver), which will increase construction costs [65]. Finally, the architect's primary objective in designing any building is to meet the needs of the client (i.e., the decision makers). As such, an architect can provide suggestions to clients and rationalize them accordingly; however, an architect cannot force their values into a design. Therefore, the incorporation of universal design is dependent on the client's perceived importance of its implementation. Ultimately, if the client does not desire universal design and local building code does not require it, the architect will be unable to implement it.

The aforementioned challenges to implementing universal design are obstacles that need to be overcome through a multidimensional approach. Future directions for professionals in architecture and environmental planning could include (1) increasing the incorporation of universal design into the educational curriculum while emphasizing the importance of applying the philosophy to the built environment; (2) communicating with older adults and persons with disabilities during the design process to ensure an understanding of the diversified needs of the population as a whole; (3) collaborating among one another to include universal design as a "best practice" guideline, making it a common implementation that exceeds minimal code requirements; and (4) develop more cost-effective ways to implement universal design in order to increase the affordability of such design, thereby increasing the client's willingness to include universal design principles in the design process [45]. The theory and literature surrounding universal design is very promising; however, many more randomized controlled trials testing the effectiveness of specific universal design options are needed. As a result of rigorous research and knowledge translation efforts, universally designed environments may become the norm and code of practice for architects and design professionals. As a society, the philosophy of universal design needs to be embraced with the aim of shifting individual attitudes towards perceiving the population as whole where individuals can equally thrive in the environment, regardless of ability or age.

4. Conclusion

The concept of successful aging has become increasingly important as senior citizens begin to dominate the population demographics [3, 5]. Maintaining an active engagement in life through participation in social and productive pursuits is one component of successful aging [6, 7]. Since the built environment directly impacts the engagement profiles of older adults, it is necessary to provide environments designed to suit the needs of older adults [18]. Of all the design theories that attempt to accommodate the aging process, the philosophy of universal design may be the most desirable option as it provides built environments that benefit everyone, prevent stigmatization, and increase the ease of engagement in activities of daily living [16]. Currently, universal design is a promising voluntary philosophy that requires increased attention from facility planners and coordinators, evidence of the significance of its application from academics, and the embracement of its core principles by society. Taken as a whole, it is evident that the application of universal design to the built environment is the step toward successful aging that the graying population needs.

Acknowledgments

Kelly Carr is supported by the Social Sciences and Humanities Research Council of Canada (SSHRC) Joseph-Armand Bombardier Canada Graduate Scholarships Program. Patricia Weir is supported by a SSHRC Standard Research Grant (no. 862-2010-0007).

References

[1] G. F. Anderson and P. S. Hussey, "Population aging: a comparison among industrialized countries," *Health Affairs*, vol. 19, no. 3, pp. 191–203, 2000.

[2] P. Lloyd-Sherlock, "Population ageing in developed and developing regions: implications for health policy," *Social Science and Medicine*, vol. 51, no. 6, pp. 887–895, 2000.

[3] Statistics Canada, "The Canadian population in 2011: age and sex," Catalogue 98-311-X2011001, Statistics Canada Minister of Industry, Ottawa, Canada, 2012.

[4] Statistics Canada, "Population projections: Canada, the provinces and territories," *The Daily*, pp. 6–7, 2010.

[5] K. A. Lowry, A. N. Vallejo, and S. A. Studenski, "Successful aging as a continuum of functional independence: lessons from physical disability models of aging," *Aging and Disease*, vol. 3, no. 1, pp. 5–15, 2012.

[6] J. W. Rowe and R. L. Kahn, "Human aging: usual and successful," *Science*, vol. 237, no. 4811, pp. 143–149, 1987.

[7] J. W. Rowe and R. L. Kahn, "Successful aging," *The Gerontologist*, vol. 37, no. 4, pp. 433–440, 1997.

[8] R. B. Tate, L. Lah, and T. E. Cuddy, "Definition of successful aging by elderly canadian males: the Manitoba Follow-Up Study," *The Gerontologist*, vol. 43, no. 5, pp. 735–744, 2003.

[9] E. Del Bono, E. Sala, R. Hancock, C. Gunnell, and L. Parisi, *Gender, Older People and Social Exclusion. A Gendered Review and Secondary Analysis of the Data*, Institute for Social and Economic Research, Essex, UK, 2007.

[10] M. V. Zunzunegui, A. Koné, M. Johri, F. Béland, C. Wolfson, and H. Bergman, "Social networks and self-rated health in two French-speaking Canadian community dwelling populations over 65," *Social Science and Medicine*, vol. 58, no. 10, pp. 2069–2081, 2004.

[11] M. Levasseur, L. Richard, L. Gauvin, and E. Raymond, "Inventory and analysis of definitions of social participation found in the aging literature: proposed taxonomy of social activities," *Social Science and Medicine*, vol. 71, no. 12, pp. 2141–2149, 2010.

[12] J. M. Guralnik, L. P. Fried, and M. E. Salive, "Disability as a public health outcome in the aging population," *Annual Review of Public Health*, vol. 17, pp. 25–46, 1996.

[13] J. E. Hertz and C. A. Anschutz, "Relationships among perceived enactment of autonomy, self-care, and holistic health in community-dwelling older adults," *Journal of Holistic Nursing*, vol. 20, no. 2, pp. 166–186, 2002.

[14] K. E. Thorpe and M. Philyaw, "The medicalization of chronic disease and costs," *Annual Review of Public Health*, vol. 33, pp. 409–423, 2012.

[15] M. P. Lawton, "Environment and other determinants of well-being in older people," *The Gerontologist*, vol. 23, no. 4, pp. 349–357, 1983.

[16] M. F. Story, "Maximizing usability: the principles of universal design," *Assistive Technology*, vol. 10, no. 1, pp. 4–12, 1998.

[17] Ontario Ministry of Community and Social Services, "About the Accessibility for Ontarians with Disabilities Act (AODA), 2005," Catalogue 7710-AODA-B01, Queen's Printer for Ontario, Toronto, Canada, 2008.

[18] H. Demirkan, "Housing for the aging population," *European Review of Aging and Physical Activity*, vol. 4, no. 1, pp. 33–38, 2007.

[19] D. E. Crews and S. Zavotka, "Aging, disability, and frailty: implications for universal design," *Journal of Physiological Anthropology*, vol. 25, no. 1, pp. 113–118, 2006.

[20] E. A. DeMerchant and J. O. Beamish, "Universal design in residential spaces," *Housing and Society*, vol. 22, no. 1-2, pp. 77–91, 1995.

[21] C. F. Mendes de Leon, "Social engagement and successful aging," *European Journal of Ageing*, vol. 2, no. 1, pp. 64–66, 2005.

[22] A. Bowling and P. Dieppe, "What is successful ageing and who should define it?" *British Medical Journal*, vol. 331, no. 7531, pp. 1548–1551, 2005.

[23] D. L. Charbonneau-Lyons, P. M. Mosher-Ashley, and M. Stanford-Pollock, "Opinions of college students and independent-living adults regarding successful aging," *Educational Gerontology*, vol. 28, no. 10, pp. 823–833, 2002.

[24] E. A. Phelan, L. A. Anderson, A. Z. LaCroix, and E. B. Larson, "Older adults' views of "successful aging"—how do they compare with researchers' definitions?" *Journal of the American Geriatrics Society*, vol. 52, no. 2, pp. 211–216, 2004.

[25] L. W. Guse and M. A. Masesar, "Quality of life and successful aging in long-term care: perceptions of residents," *Issues in Mental Health Nursing*, vol. 20, no. 6, pp. 527–539, 1999.

[26] B. J. Fisher and D. K. Specht, "Successful aging and creativity in later life," *Journal of Aging Studies*, vol. 13, no. 4, pp. 457–472, 1999.

[27] T. Knight and L. A. Ricciardelli, "Successful aging: perceptions of adults aged between 70 and 101 years," *International Journal of Aging and Human Development*, vol. 56, no. 3, pp. 223–245, 2003.

[28] J. A, Liffiton, S. Horton, J. Baker, and P. L. Weir, "Successful aging: how does physical activity influence engagement with life?" *European Review of Aging and Physical Activity*, vol. 9, no. 2, pp. 103–108, 2012.

[29] S. Fone and B. Lundgren-Lindquist, "Health status and functional capacity in a group of successfully ageing 65–85 years olds," *Disability and Rehabilitation*, vol. 25, no. 18, pp. 1044–1051, 2003.

[30] M. Silverstein and M. G. Parker, "Leisure activities and quality of life among the oldest old in Sweden," *Research on Aging*, vol. 24, no. 5, pp. 528–547, 2002.

[31] M. J. Bergstrom and M. E. Holmes, "Lay theories of successful aging after the death of a spouse: a network text analysis of bereavement advice," *Health Communication*, vol. 12, no. 4, pp. 377–406, 2000.

[32] C. A. Brown, F. A. McGuire, and J. Voelkl, "The link between successful aging and serious leisure," *International Journal of Aging and Human Development*, vol. 66, no. 1, pp. 73–95, 2008.

[33] W. J. Strawbridge, M. I. Wallhagen, and R. D. Cohen, "Successful aging and well-being: self-rated compared with Rowe and Kahn," *The Gerontologist*, vol. 42, no. 6, pp. 727–733, 2002.

[34] P. A. Bath and A. Gardiner, "Social engagement and health and social care use and medication use among older people," *European Journal of Ageing*, vol. 2, no. 1, pp. 56–63, 2005.

[35] K. M. Bennett, "Social engagement as a longitudinal predictor of objective and subjective health," *European Journal of Ageing*, vol. 2, no. 1, pp. 48–55, 2005.

[36] T. A. Glass, C. Mendes de Leon, R. A. Marottoli, and L. F. Berkman, "Population based study of social and productive activities as predictors of survival among elderly Americans," *British Medical Journal*, vol. 319, no. 7208, pp. 478–483, 1999.

[37] E. Grundy and A. Bowling, "Enhancing the quality of extended life years. Identification of the oldest old with a very good and very poor quality of life," *Aging and Mental Health*, vol. 3, no. 3, pp. 199–212, 1999.

[38] T. Hedden and J. D. E. Gabrieli, "Insights into the ageing mind: a view from cognitive neuroscience," *Nature Reviews Neuroscience*, vol. 5, no. 2, pp. 87–96, 2004.

[39] T. Lang, T. Streeper, P. Cawthon, K. Baldwin, D. R. Taaffe, and T. B. Harris, "Sarcopenia: etiology, clinical consequences, intervention, and assessment," *Osteoporosis International*, vol. 21, no. 4, pp. 543–559, 2010.

[40] U. Lindenberger and P. Ghisletta, "Cognitive and sensory declines in old age: gauging the evidence for a common cause," *Psychology and Aging*, vol. 24, no. 1, pp. 1–16, 2009.

[41] D. C. Park and P. Reuter-Lorenz, "The adaptive brain: aging and neurocognitive scaffolding," *Annual Review of Psychology*, vol. 60, pp. 173–196, 2009.

[42] H. W. Wahl, A. Fänge, F. Oswald, L. N. Gitlin, and S. Iwarsson, "The home environment and disability-related outcomes in aging individuals: what is the empirical evidence?" *The Gerontologist*, vol. 49, no. 3, pp. 355–367, 2009.

[43] S. Y. Liu and K. L. Lapane, "Residential modifications and decline in physical function among community-dwelling older adults," *The Gerontologist*, vol. 49, no. 3, pp. 344–354, 2009.

[44] L. M. Verbrugge and A. M. Jette, "The disablement process," *Social Science and Medicine*, vol. 38, no. 1, pp. 1–14, 1994.

[45] O. Demirbilek and H. Demirkan, "Universal product design involving elderly users: a participatory design model," *Applied Ergonomics*, vol. 35, no. 4, pp. 361–370, 2004.

[46] Centre for Universal Design, "Definitions: Accessible, Adaptable, and Universal Design," 2006, http://www.ncsu.edu/www/ncsu/design/sod5/cud/pubs_p/phousing.htm.

[47] Building Code Act, "Ontario Regulation 350/06, Sentence 3. 8. 3. 3.(4)," 1992, http://www.search.e-laws.gov.on.ca/en/isysquery/cbd0d22c-40df-4754-b58e-e261ddd42ecb/4/doc/?search=browseStatutes&context=#hit1.

[48] J. J. Pirkl, "Transgenerational design: prolonging the American dream," *Generations*, vol. 19, no. 1, pp. 32–36, 1995.

[49] E. Steinfeld and G. S. Danford, "Automated Doors: Towards Universal Design," Buffalo, The Center for Inclusive Design and Environmental Access, School of Architecture and Planning SUNY/Buffalo, 1993, http://www.ap.buffalo.edu/idea/publications/automateddoors.htm.

[50] L. K. Weisman, "Creating the universal designed city: prospects for the new century," *Architectural Theory Review*, vol. 5, no. 2, pp. 156–173, 2000.

[51] C. Leibrock and S. Behar, *Beautiful Barrier-Free: A Visual Guide to Accessibility*, Van Nostrand Reinhold, New York, NY, USA, 1993.

[52] J. P. Marsden, R. A. Meehan, and M. P. Calkins, "Therapeutic kitchens for residents with dementia," *American Journal of Alzheimer's Disease and other Dementias*, vol. 16, no. 5, pp. 303–311, 2001.

[53] Y. Afacan and H. Demirkan, "A priority-based approach for satisfying the diverse users' needs, capabilities and expectations: a universal kitchen design case," *Journal of Engineering Design*, vol. 21, no. 2-3, pp. 315–343, 2010.

[54] K. Bajaj, G. A. Mirka, C. M. Sommerich, and H. Khachatoorian, "Evaluation of a redesigned self-checkout station for wheelchair users," *Assistive Technology*, vol. 18, no. 1, pp. 15–24, 2006.

[55] C. F. Kaufman, "Shop 'til you drop: tales from a physically challenged shopper," *Journal of Consumer Marketing*, vol. 12, no. 3, pp. 39–55, 1995.

[56] M. F. Story, J. L. Mueller, and R. L. Mace, "The universal design file: designing for people of all ages andabilities," 1998, http://design-dev.ncsu.edu/openjournal/index.php/redlab/article/view/102.

[57] E. Dumbaugh, "Designing communities to enhance the safety and mobility of older adults: a universal approach," *Journal of Planning Literature*, vol. 23, no. 1, pp. 17–36, 2008.

[58] American Association of Retired Persons, *Home and Community Preferences of the 45+ Population*, Keenan, T. A, Washington, DC, USA, 2010.

[59] C. J. Deardorff and C. Birdsong, "Universal design: clarifying a common vocabulary," *Housing and Society*, vol. 30, no. 2, pp. 119–138, 2003.

[60] I. Audirac, "Accessing transit as universal design," *Journal of Planning Literature*, vol. 23, no. 1, pp. 4–16, 2008.

[61] M. A. Farage, K. W. Miller, F. Ajayi, and D. Hutchins, "Design principles to accommodate older adults," *Global Journal of Health Science*, vol. 4, no. 2, pp. 2–25, 2012.

[62] S. Keates, P. J. Clarkson, L. A. Harrison, and P. Robinson, "Towards a practical inclusive design approach," in *Proceedings of the Conference on Universal Usability*, pp. 45–52, New York, NY, USA, November 2000.

[63] S. Iwarsson and A. Ståhl, "Accessibility, usability and universal design—positioning and definition of concepts describing person-environment relationships," *Disability and Rehabilitation*, vol. 25, no. 2, pp. 57–66, 2003.

[64] Center for Universal Design, "Universal design. Housing for the lifespan of all people," 2000, http://design-dev.ncsu.edu/openjournal/index.php/redlab/article/view/101.

[65] Commission for Architecture and the Built Environment, *Inclusion By Design: Equality, Diversity and the Built Environment*, Seacout, London, UK, 2008.

[66] H. Froyen, E. Verdonck, D. De Meester, and A. Heylighen, "Documenting handicap situations and eliminations through universal design patterns," *Australasian Medical Journal*, vol. 1, no. 12, pp. 199–203, 2009.

[67] S. Kose, "From barrier-free to universal design: an international perspective," *Assistive Technology*, vol. 10, no. 1, pp. 44–50, 1998.

[68] G. S. Danford, "Universal design people with vision, hearing, and mobility impairments evaluate a model building," *Generations*, vol. 27, no. 1, pp. 91–94, 2003.

[69] G. Trost, "State of affairs in universal design in Europe," *Fujitsu Scientific and Technical Journal*, vol. 41, no. 1, pp. 19–25, 2005.

[70] J. Fricke, "Activities of Daily Living," International Encyclopedia of Rehabilitation, 2010, http://hdl.handle.net/1959.9/160364 .

[71] S. Katz, "Assessing self-maintenance: activities of daily living, mobility, and instrumental activities of daily living," *Journal of the American Geriatrics Society*, vol. 31, no. 12, pp. 721–727, 1983.

[72] M. P. Lawton and E. M. Brody, "Assessment of older people: self-maintaining and instrumental activities of daily living," *The Gerontologist*, vol. 9, no. 3, pp. 179–186, 1969.

[73] F. Aslaksen, S. Bergh, O. R. Bringa, and E. K. Heggem, *Universal Design: Planning and Design for All*, Norwegian State Council on Disability, Oslo, Norway, 1997.

[74] P. Hall and R. Imrie, "Architectural practices and disabling design in the built environment," *Environment and Planning B*, vol. 26, no. 3, pp. 409–425, 1999.

[75] R. Luck, H. Haenlein, and K. Bright, "Project briefing for accessible design," *Design Studies*, vol. 22, no. 3, pp. 297–315, 2001.

7

Home-Living Elderly People's Views on Food and Meals

Ellinor Edfors and Albert Westergren

The PRO-CARE Group, School of Health and Society, Kristianstad University, 291 88 Kristianstad, Sweden

Correspondence should be addressed to Albert Westergren, albert.westergren@hkr.se

Academic Editor: Joseph R. Sharkey

Background. The aim of the study was to describe home-living elderly people's views on the importance of food and meals. *Methods.* Semistructured interviews with twelve elderly people. The interviews were analysed using qualitative content analysis. *Results.* Respondents described how their past influenced their present experiences and views on food and meals. Increased reliance on and need of support with food and meals frequently arose in connection with major changes in their life situations. Sudden events meant a breaking point with a transition from independence to dependence and a need for assistance from relatives and/or the community. With the perspective from the past and in the context of dependency, respondents described meals during the day, quality of food, buying, transporting, cooking, and eating food. *Conclusions.* Meeting the need for optimal nutritional status for older people living at home requires knowledge of individual preferences and habits, from both their earlier and current lives. It is important to pay attention to risk factors that could compromise an individual's ability to independently manage their diet, such as major life events and hospitalisation. Individual needs for self-determination and involvement should be considered in planning and development efforts for elderly people related to food and meals.

1. Introduction

Malnutrition, which includes undernutrition as well as overweight/obesity, is a common problem among the elderly. The prevalence of undernutrition among home-living elderly people was found to be 14.5% according to the Mini Nutritional Assessment (MNA) [1]. Among elderly people who had recently moved to a residential home, 33–37% were malnourished according to the MNA [2]. The higher prevalence of undernutrition among elderly people admitted to residential homes highlights the importance of identifying elderly people who live at home and are at risk of malnutrition, to prevent the development and aggravation of undernutrition, followed by increased dependency on and need for institutional care [1]. In addition, among 70-year-old Swedes, 20% of the men and 24% of the women were obese (BMI > 30) [3]. In Swedish nursing homes the prevalence of overweight was 22% and another 8% were obese [4]. Thus, obesity is also a frequent problem among the elderly.

The consequences of undernutrition in elderly people include functional decline or frailty [5–7], decreased quality of life [8], increased health care utilisation and costs [9, 10], higher rates of adverse complications from other health conditions [11], and increased mortality [6, 7, 12]. The consequences of obesity include negative impact on physical functions and quality of life, decreased survival rates, metabolic syndromes, arthritis, pulmonary abnormalities, urinary incontinence, cataracts, and cancer [13]. Thus, from a nutritional perspective, obesity as well as undernutrition are a concern among elderly people as they exacerbate age-related decline in physical functioning and can cause frailty [13].

Myriad risk factors are associated with inadequate caloric intake and malnutrition. Risk factors for undernutrition have been identified as higher age, lower self-perceived health, low functional status, diseases, taking several medicines, and symptoms of depression [1, 14–18]. It was also found that people who were hospitalised prior to receiving home health services were more likely to undereat than those not hospitalised [19]. Eating with others increases caloric intake [20]. Aging is associated with a decrease in total energy expenditure, and if this coincides with a maintained or increased energy intake, overweight/obesity may develop [13].

Currently in Sweden, fewer elderly people with functional impairment move to nursing homes, and more choose or have to remain in their own homes. Many of these people are disabled and dependent on others for acquiring, preparing and/or consuming their food. The need for help with acquiring food typically occurs before the need for assistance with meal preparation arises [21]. Some elderly people get help with these activities from informal providers. Previous research has shown that living with others or receiving help from informal providers is beneficial for dietary intake [22, 23], and that frequent provision of meals from a formal agency can improve food intake [24] and decrease undernutrition risk [21]. Furthermore, by getting meals from a formal agency, those who would otherwise not be able to obtain or prepare food without assistance are able to keep living in their own homes [25].

Considering all the negative effects of malnutrition, it seems of utmost importance to identify elderly people living at home at risk of developing malnutrition, or who have already developed it, so that suitable preventive actions and/or treatment can be provided. To do so we need a deeper understanding of the circumstances of older people living at home, with respect to nutrition, from their perspectives. The aim of the study was to describe home-living elderly people's views on circumstances that are of importance regarding food and meals.

2. Methodology

The study was carried out in a small community in southern Sweden (approximately 12500 inhabitants), containing two smaller towns. Elderly care interventions, such as getting meals from a formal agency (food distribution/meals on wheels), were provided from two different kitchens, one localised in the towns. The meals were distributed to the elderly by home care staff. The elderly person had to pay a subsidised fee for the meal and meal delivery. Even though respondents lived independently they could have access to elderly centres for social activities and restaurants.

This study was a descriptive qualitative study based on semistructured interviews with twelve elderly people living in their own homes in a small municipality in southern Sweden. Criteria for inclusion in the study were elderly people over age 65 living in their own homes (with or without home help service and/or meals from a formal agency) and able to communicate in Swedish. Respondents were recruited by the nutritionally responsible nurse and the unit managers in the municipality. Written information about the aim of the study, that participation was voluntary and who to contact for further information, was distributed to potential respondents by home care staff. It is unknown how many people received this information. Those who agreed to participate were contacted by phone by the first author (E. Edfors); further information about the study was given and the time and place for the interview were set.

Twelve people were interested and actually participated in the study, seven men and five women, aged 82 to 94 (average 87.7 years). Four of them lived as couples and both partners were included in the study. Six of the respondents had no home help service and out of these three had food distribution from a formal agency. Three of the respondents had no food distribution while nine had food distribution that varied from three to seven days a week. Half of the respondents rated their severity of disease as moderate and only one as severe (Table 1).

The interviews were conducted by the first author (EE) in the respondents' homes. Before the interview started, the respondent was given clarifying information about the aim of the study, their right to withdraw at any time with no personal consequences, and that participation was voluntary. Written informed consent was obtained. As there could be a risk that the interviews were perceived as an invasion of privacy and cause emotional strain, respondents were offered the opportunity to contact the authors afterwards. All collected materials and personal data relating to respondents were treated confidentially. The study was performed in accordance with the Helsinki declaration of ethical principles [26]. Formal approval was not needed for this type of study, in accordance with Swedish law [27].

The interviews were conducted as semistructured interviews [28] based on the aim of the study. The interview started with an open-ended question and the respondent was asked to talk freely about an ordinary day, focusing on food and meals, "describe an ordinary day and try to focus on the food and meals during the day." Thereafter the questions were about food preferences and intake, physiological difficulties (swallowing, chewing), and functional difficulties (cooking, shopping), and on social dimensions of eating. These questions were inspired from themes in "Seniors in the Community: Risk Evaluation for Eating and Nutrition, Version II" (SCREEN II) that measures the risk of malnutrition among elderly people living in their own home [29]. Throughout the interview, the author, using follow-up questions, tried to capture the importance of circumstances and factors affecting food and meals. The interviews lasted 40–90 minutes and were recorded with digital equipment and transcribed verbatim.

The interview texts were inductively analysed by using qualitative content analysis [30]. Content analysis is described on two levels: the manifest content analysis that focuses on the content of the texts from a superficial perspective based on the written word, and latent content analysis that goes in-depth on content and interprets the underlying meaning conveyed by the text [30]. In this study the analysis was mainly based on manifest content analysis. The analysis was conducted in all stages by the two authors and work continuously alternated between the whole and parts of the collected material. In step one, texts were read and reread as a whole, a so-called naive reading. Statements were then made based on the impressions of and reflections about the wholeness and important elements in the text that had emerged during the naive reading. Then all parts of the text relating to the aim of the study were divided into meaning units that seemed to be about the same thing. In next step the meaning units were coded. The codes were critically discussed and a number of categories with subcategories emerged. Finally, all texts were re-read and compared with the outcome of the analysis to ensure that

Table 1: Characteristics of the respondents.

Interview number	Gender	Age	Cohabitation	Living in town (T) Countryside (CS)	Home help service	Food distribution, days/week	Severity of disease(1)
1	Male	84	Alone	CS	No	7	Moderate
2	Male	90	Together	T	Yes	7	Mild
3	Female	87	Together	T	Yes	7	Severe
4	Female	94	Alone	T	Yes	7	Moderate
5	Male	82	Alone	T	No	7	None
6	Male	89	Alone	CS	Yes	3	Moderate
7	Female	84	Alone	T	Yes	5	Mild
8	Female	85	Alone	T	No	0	Moderate
9	Male	89	Alone	T	Yes	7	Mild
10	Female	88	Together	CS	No	0	Moderate
11	Male	94	Together	CS	No	0	Moderate
12	Male	86	Alone	T	No	7	Mild

(1) Self-perceived severity of disease graded as none, mild, moderate, or severe.

Table 2: Categories and subcategories regarding home-living elderly people's views of food and meals.

Categories	Subcategories
Habits founded in the past affect the present	Food and meals
	Roles
To get help from others with food and meals	The breaking point
	Transition from independence to dependence
	Meals during the day
	Quality of food
Food and meals in present life	Buying and transporting food
	Cooking
	Eating

the categories covered the contents of the texts and codes. "Open Code" (freeware) software was used for the qualitative analysis (UMDAC and Epidemiology, University of Umeå).

3. Results

Three categories, with two-to-five subcategories each, were developed based on the text analysis: habits developed in the past affect the present; getting help from others with food and meals; current food and meals (Table 2).

3.1. Habits Founded in Past Life Affect Present Life

3.1.1. Food and Meals. The interviews showed that experiences in childhood and earlier adulthood had a great impact on the respondent's current feelings and views concerning food and meals. It was evident that the foundations of norms and values regarding food culture, traditions and eating habits were laid early and did not change to any great extent throughout life.

> *As children we were never allowed to say "I do not want that, I won't eat it." No, that was just not possible (no. 4, female, age 94).*

> *I eat the same type of food and about the same time as I always have done, as I did when my wife lived and when I worked (no. 9, male, age 89).*

The majority of the respondents had lived their lives in an environment where they were used to cooking for themselves and there was a difference between everyday meals and special occasions. Food and meals had also played an important social role. It was, for instance, important to be generous to the "outside world".

> *There were people in the whole house, and there were a lot of rooms, and there was food, a lot of food, yes really (no. 4, female, age 94).*

> *I feel that when you are out, or come someplace, you should be offered a cup of coffee, that's what I'm used to. Back home in the country, the coffee would be on as soon as someone walked in the door (no. 4, female, age 94).*

The respondents had grown up on a diet of home-cooked dishes made from locally produced ingredients. Meals consisted of, for example, porridge, wholemeal bread, potatoes, pork, and fresh fish. At ceremonies and celebrations one might be offered freshly slaughtered meat and more luxurious food.

> *I am used to home-cooked dishes since I was a child, not macaroni and spaghetti (no. 7, female, age 84).*

> *"When I grew up, pigs were supposed to weigh 125 kg when they were slaughtered. There was a thick layer of fat on their backs" (no. 11, male, age 94).*

The diet was based on what the season had to offer and it was vital to "make do with what the house could offer" and seize every opportunity to increase the food supply, for instance, by hunting, fishing, and picking berries.

> *I still pick berries and make syrup. I grew vegetables before (no. 10, female, age 88).*

> *I grew up by the sea and do not know anything else. I have been fishing myself, and everything (no. 6, male, age 89).*

3.1.2. Roles. The interviews showed a division in gender roles regarding the responsibility for the diet. Usually, the woman in the family had the main responsibility for food and meals. *"My wife was a very good cook"* (no. 5, male, age 82). The majority said that they had always been served homemade and carefully cooked food and that they knew how good and nutritious food should taste.

> *I worked as a cook; I used to do the cooking at home before I got my heart attack (no. 1, male, age 84).*

> *I've always been a good cook, and have always appreciated good food. My husband always said, "you cook such good food, I get way too fat". But I so appreciated good things.... I wanted... if you are going to eat, you might as well have good food (no. 4, female, age 94).*

3.2. To Get Help from Others with Food and Meals

3.2.1. The Breaking Point. The interviews revealed that in several cases, major changes in the ability to be independently responsible for food and meals were linked to some form of sudden event. It could be that the female partner who was responsible for meals passed away. Other causes could be falls, infections, and other diseases, such as myocardial infarction, conditions that in many cases had led to a hospitalisation. Other factors that affected independence were general frailty and an inability *"to use one's old body,"* that is, factors linked to "normal ageing."

> *About five years ago my wife had an accident, and she could no longer do the cooking. We had to get food from the service house (no. 1, male, age 84).*

3.2.2. Transition from Independence to Dependence. Becoming dependent on others on a daily basis can be difficult to deal with. One man had a strong desire to get well and return to independence.

> *I believe that everything changes. I dream of being able to buy myself a car in the spring so that I can go shopping (no. 6, male, age 89).*

Other respondents felt that they had no choice but get used to it and accept the situation.

> *I have become so used to it that I do not even think about whether it is difficult or not, it is just something you have to put up with (no. 4, female, age 94).*

One man seemed pleased to be dependent and he had strongly questioned the community's decision to discontinue his food distribution.

> *Well now that it has been so long, you might consider cooking again (note, said aid assessors)... Oh, said I, aren't you being a bit too hard now... It's quite expensive, she said... will they lose five crowns? Ten crowns? I can pay the difference because I've never been a burden for the community. (no. 12, male, age 86).*

3.3. Food and Meals in Present Life

3.3.1. Meals during the Day. Currently, and in the past, respondents' daily meals were distributed as breakfast, dinner and supper, usually served at the same time every day. The majority had their principal meal at noon, while supper mostly consisted of lighter food, such as tea and sandwiches. However, one male respondent preferred to have a proper cooked meal also for supper. From the interviews it could be discerned that the majority of respondents distributed their meals so that at night there was a long period without eating.

> *All my life I've had lunch at twelve o clock. So I usually eat at noon, and then I eat once in the evening, usually very light food (no. 6, male, age 89).*

Regular snacks were not common, except when someone occasionally felt hungry and had, for example, a piece of fruit, a cookie, or a sandwich. On the other hand, snacks in the form of coffee breaks were considered a natural and important element in social gatherings with other people, such as when friends came for a visit or when the respondents participated in social activities.

> *I do not eat snacks unless there is a study circle, like today, where we get served nice little cookie (no. 8, female, age 85).*

The four respondents who lived as couples ate their meals together, while single respondents mostly ate their meals alone. Two women felt lonesome with no companion at mealtimes. Four men, on the other hand, preferred to eat alone. They found it easier to be able to sit comfortably and eat at any time they wanted at their own pace, without having to consider other people.

> *I think it's great, I have no major, no problems at all. I think it's nice to sit quietly and eat my meal (no. 1, male, age 84).*

Even though respondents lived independently they could have access to elderly centres for social activities and restaurants.

> *I generally eat by myself. I have thought many times that I should go to the restaurant, because*

> *they do have a separate dining room at XXX (note, elderly centre). But I end up feeling more comfortable eating at home (no. 5, male, age 82).*

One woman said that eating at the elderly centre demanded suitable clothing, social behaviour and sociability. The noisy environment, caused by young people from a nearby school who also had their lunch there, could be another reason for eating alone at home instead.

> *... And then the young people from the school there, they also eat there, and when they're there, it is not easy for the older people to be among them, since they are noisy and do not behave (no. 7, female, age 84).*

Overall, the interviews revealed that the respondents usually did not skip a meal. Their appetite was normally good. Poor appetite and weight loss could be caused by psychological malaise, other illnesses, grief, lack of outdoor activities and bad temper.

> *Yes, it's psychological and that eliminates a lot of things. Very, very sensitive... when these problems occur (note, depression)... the food does not taste good, no. Then I ended up skipping meals and eating only two or three crackers a day (no. 11, male, age 94).*

Other reasons for a poor appetite or skipping a meal were related to the content of the distributed food, such as food having an unappealing appearance, not tasting good or containing ingredients that the older person did not like or tolerate, such as hot spices, or being difficult to chew and digest.

> *And it is served in such an unappealing way in these trays, it's not exactly exciting. There is one container for the sauce and one for the potatoes and the pieces of meat just lying there... it's not, it does not give you an appetite... and you feel like, oh, that does not look good at all... (no. 4, female, age 94).*

3.3.2. Quality of Food. The interviews revealed different perceptions of the quality of food among respondents who had food distribution. Respondents who got their food from a separate kitchen were very satisfied with the food content and quality. They understood that they would not always be served their favourite dishes. This group of respondents felt that the food consisted of varied and tasty dishes and appreciated the variation in content between weekday and weekend.

> *Wonderful, yes... It is very, very, very good. I cannot complain... It's varied and that's good. There are some things I do not like so much, but I still do not cancel. I could... (no. 12, male, age 86).*

Other respondents, who got their food from another kitchen, felt that the food was poor, tasteless, and badly cooked. They also said the food looked unappetising, contained spices that they were not familiar with, and was too influenced by modern food trends, such as pizza. They requested more varied old fashioned food, cooked in the traditional way with well-known spices such as salt, pepper, dill, and bay leaves.

> *It varies, it does, I'm being frank now... food for us elderly people is probably supposed to be cooked with care, but it happens that some food is not properly cooked" and "... It should be properly boiled or fried, depending on the dish. Very important. It happens that this is overcooked (no. 5, male, age 82).*

They also wanted certain ingredients in their food, such as fresh fish, veal, lamb, vegetables, fat, and cream. One respondent preferred the restaurant service and seemed to get much better food there than in food distribution. One woman chose to throw away food when it did not taste good or looked unappetising.

> *Now that I have reached this age, I should be allowed to... have things I like, and not... food that makes me think: Ugh, what is that, that's no good. What do I need that for? I do not want that... straight into the rubbish... I've thrown out a lot of money there (no. 4, female, age 94).*

Usually it was the home care staff who received the complaints about the food, even though the respondents knew that they not could influence the food content to any significant degree. Several interviews revealed that respondents perceived shortcomings in the municipality's interest in listening to their views about the food distribution.

> *I have talked to these girls. I feel sorry for the girls. They're the only ones I've talked to. The others, the people at the top, yes, well, I do not have time to talk to you right now, maybe I can call you some other time or something (no. 6, male, age 89).*

3.3.3. Buying and Transporting Food. The interviews showed that those who lived in urban areas were satisfied with the availability of well-stocked supermarkets. Having more than one shop in the community was believed to promote choice, quality and good prices. The majority of the respondents emphasised the importance of having access to an open-air market that was open one day a week, which gave them the opportunity to buy local products and good quality fresh fish. An important service to one couple that lived outside the urban area was the regular visits of a fish van and a private supplier of food.

One man and one woman, who arranged their shopping independently, said that the premise for this was that they could drive their car to the store themselves. Respondents who were no longer able to buy their food themselves stated different reasons for this, such as the inability to drive and difficulties in mobility. Five of the respondents, who got no help with shopping from the community, got help from children, other relatives and/or friends, usually once a week.

> *I always keep a list. When I know that something is missing, I write it down, and then when he*

comes (note, the son) it's ready (no. 9, male, age 89).

Before we had four shops, now there is none. Now my daughter helps me with shopping (no. 12, male, age 86).

One respondent, who had access to transport service (subsidised transport by taxi) for purchases, did not use this help because he tended to need more than one ride to and between the shops.

I get transport service, but it's so complicated and difficult... I do not know quite how long I have, and sometimes I need to go to the pharmacy, and then I have to go all the way from the supermarket to the pharmacy, and then I get a pain in my chest and have to order an extra trip... (no. 1, male, age 84).

Five of the respondents got community assistance with buying and transporting food, usually once a week. They had a strong desire to have control of food planning, such as shopping lists and purchases. Most of them wrote their own shopping list, and the shopping was carried out by the home care staff. Sometimes the respondent would forget to write things down on the list, or the wrong things were purchased by the home care staff. When this happened, the respondent usually had to wait until the next week's shopping.

They bought the wrong things... That's why it's important that when I order something there are people who know what it is all about, especially those who have their own household. And then they send a girl working temporarily... Here I am ... and sometimes when they are gone.. oh goodness, I forgot... (no. 6, male, age 89).

One woman requested more than one hour for shopping, since the staff's short allotment of time for this purpose made it impossible for her to come along to the shop. She wanted to be able to compare what different shops had to offer and make her own decisions.

One hour is too short. I want to spend some time in the shop. Two hours would give enough time to go to both XXX and YYY without hurry (note, two shops). See for yourself and not just request something. I do not know what they have and what's good. (no. 4, female, age 94).

3.3.4. Cooking. Cooking was sometimes seen as a meaningful and enjoyable thing to do. One woman liked to cook all the food, both for herself and for others. Four male respondents with food distribution appreciated it and felt it was easier to prepare the morning and evening meals, when they did not have to be responsible for the main meal. Several respondents chose to buy precooked frozen dishes and full meals for the main meal. One reason for this could be that they were frail and did not have enough strength to cook the main meal themselves. Another reason could be that it was boring to cook just for themselves. Prepared dishes were also considered easier to cook, for example, in a microwave, a cheap alternative and sometimes better tasting than the food that was served at the municipality's elderly centre.

It is not fun to cook anymore, now when I'm alone, therefore I buy pre-cooked food (no. 7, female, age 84).

I buy pre-cooked food at the shop. I think it is better than the XXX (note, elderly centre restaurant)... (no. 7, female, age 84).

I do not miss cooking; it is enough with managing morning and evening meals (no. 9, male, age 89).

3.3.5. Eating. The issues that respondents raised about eating were, in most cases, related to their oral health and dental status. Broken teeth and poorly adapted prostheses could be the causes of difficulties with chewing. Some respondents thought the meat from food distribution was leathery and difficult to chew.

Things that are hard to digest, such as brown beans, pea soup and stuff, I do not eat that, and whole meat, I cannot chew (no. 2, male, age 90).

Problems with eating were also linked to the presence of other symptoms, such as fungal infection in the mouth and nausea caused by problems from the oesophagus and stomach. Difficulties in swallowing food were also connected to oral health, dental status, food content, and the cooking method. The respondents emphasised the importance of caring for their teeth and regular dental visits to maintain optimal dental and oral health.

... It's worse now with the teeth. I can usually chew the food I get from... Yet, some of it is tough (no. 2, male, age 90).

Most respondents had, at some time, choked on something. In two cases the situation had developed to a life-threatening condition. Items the respondents mentioned having choked on included tablets, crumbly bread, large pieces of food, and tough meat.

... I'm a bit narrow in the throat... I choke... bread crumbs and things (no. 10, female, age 88).

4. Discussion

The aim of the study was to describe home-living elderly people's views on important circumstances regarding food and meals. The analysis of the interviews showed that respondents' earlier life had a strong influence on current views of food and meals. Souter and Keller [31] presented similar results in a study describing how what older people ate depended on past life experiences and their approach to old age [31]. Other studies concerning food and meals showed that habits and preferences that are formed during childhood and youth are difficult to change in adult life [32] and that dietary intake was often similar to what the elderly people grew up with [33]. This has also been documented in other cultures. Interviews with elderly Taiwanese people showed only small changes in eating patterns, and how preferences for traditional habits from earlier generations influenced their food and meals [34]. Developing assistance regarding food and meals for elderly people requires knowledge about the individual's current needs, but habits founded in earlier life must also be taken into consideration.

The results of the study showed that the respondents' needs for help to manage their daily food and meals often arose in relation to a sudden life event. Stressful life events also contribute to an increased risk of developing malnutrition. Examples include being widowed or falling ill and requiring hospitalisation. They perceived their dependence on others both positively and negatively. Most respondents stated that the woman in the family had had the main responsibility for meals. Several men in the study reported that their wife's death had been the breaking point for becoming dependent on food distribution and they thought the food distribution was a good alternative to get nourishing food. However, women who previously had cooked all their food mentioned difficulties in accepting the situation and in reconciling themselves with the conditions of food distribution. This is consistent with a study that showed that being dependent on others was difficult to accept, but dependence on meals from food distribution could also mean better quality of life [35]. Another study showed that elderly women living alone tended to simplify cooking and eating and had fewer cooked meals and events with coffee with cakes [36], and that poor cooking skills among elderly men was a barrier to improving energy intake, healthy eating and appetite [37]. Sudden life events often change habits relating to food and meals, and men and women seem to adapt to the new circumstances in different ways depending on earlier roles and experiences. These events are important to capture in order to highlight the need for assistance so that necessary actions can be taken.

In this study habits founded in past life, and negative life events affected the food and meals in present life. It might be that also the view of the future influences current food intake. Shifflet has studied food habit changes in a couple of studies including elderly patients visiting nutrition sites [38, 39]. Even though the focus for these studies was on food habit changes there are some interesting implications for the understanding of the findings in the present study. In one of the studies [38], the temporal frameworks within which food habit changes are negotiated were explored. Food habit changes were found to be externally motivated (following physician-prescribed diets, altering food intake due to taste changes, social isolation, and reduced income) or internally motivated (self-prescribed diets, maintenance of lifelong food habits, reduction of food intake due to being less active). In addition, past experiences in conjunction with a negative or positive view of the future resulted in varying levels of compliance with special diets [38]. The respondents in the present study expressed a wish to maintain their lifelong food habits and it is likely that such a wish would negatively affect eventual efforts to achieve positive food habit changes, if that would be necessary. However, the respondents did not express any concerns about the future affecting their food habits to any great extent. This might be due to that they already had made some food habit changes in connection with previous negative life events. In another study by Shifflett and McIntosh [39] it was found that among people with a positive future time perspective 9.7% of respondents had made negative food habit changes. However, among those with a negative future time perspective 32.4% had made negative food habit changes. Some types of disruptions and concerns that may be associated with a negative view of the future and possible changes in food habits were identified—females, loss of spouse, living alone, perception of declining health, and low income [39]. Also in the present study especially loss of spouse, living alone, and declining health seemed to negatively influence the ability to acquire, prepare and/or consume food. Considering the findings from Shifflet's studies [38, 39] together with the findings from this study it seems important not only to consider the past experiences and negative life events but also the elderly persons future time perspective in the negotiation of appropriate food use patterns.

The results of the study are guided by the respondents' desires to choose and make decisions about shopping, cooking and eating. This could mean access to fresh food of good quality, sitting by yourself and eating in peace or the opportunity to go to the shop with the home care staff. Similar findings are also highlighted in a study by Pajalic et al. [35], where elderly people with food distribution wanted good food from natural products and tasting "home-cooked food" [35]. The findings showed that the quality of assistance offered to older people living in their own home is dependent on the ability to be involved in decisions about food and meals, and on whether the help is given on the individual's own terms and is designed based on personal preferences and habits [40]. Swedish health care laws [41] and social services [42] make it clear that care and help must be based on respect for individual autonomy and integrity. Ageing and disease can cause physical and mental decline, which may result in the individual no longer being able to make the choices he or she wishes, but having to adapt to the new situation. There is self-determination as long as the person can freely choose between offered options, even if it is not always the most wanted option [43]. For those with formal home help service, all care staff can help the older person to maintain their independence and autonomy by building trusting relationships, being aware of needs and offering necessary help. The older people's autonomy can be promoted and affirmed through empowerment and opportunities to influence their own situation. Writing shopping lists, having access to flyers, going shopping, cooking with staff, having more than one dish to choose from, and being able to influence the content of menus and dishes are factors that can affirm participation and empowerment.

In planning and implementing qualitative studies, it is important to consider factors such as trustworthiness and transferability. A prerequisite for forming an opinion on trustworthiness is that all steps in the research process are well described [30]. Data were collected through semistructured interviews with older people living in their own home. The respondents were recruited by the community unit heads and there is a risk that only those elderly who had positive feelings agreed to participate. We had no way of knowing how many declined to participate or why. The results of the study, however, reveal both positive and negative aspects, and despite a low number of respondents, the results can be considered to provide valuable insight into what is important to consider regarding food and meals for older people living in their own home. The interview texts were analysed using content analysis [30]. To minimise the risk of researcher influence, the two authors read the texts several times independently and then discussed their interpretation during each step of the analysis. To ensure that no data relating to the aim were excluded, the results were finally tested against the original texts [30]. The contents of the results are also supported by illustrative quotations that show extractions from the study interview texts [44].

5. Conclusions

Meeting the need for optimal nutritional status for older people living at home requires knowledge of individual preferences and habits, from both their earlier and current lives. It is important to pay attention to risk factors that could compromise an individual's ability to independently manage their diet, such as major life events and hospitalisation. Individual needs of self-determination and involvement should be considered in planning and development efforts for elderly people related to food and meals. Preventive home visits to elderly people, without home help service and/or meals from a formal agency, can be one way to capture difficulties with acquiring, preparing and/or consuming food. This can be done in order to give advice and/or suggest provision of formal help. Another intervention could be to develop a program, promoting eating with other seniors. Elderly people can be picked up at home and driven to an elderly centre restaurant at which they receive nutritious meals and opportunities to socialise with others.

Conflict of Interests

The authors declare that they have no Conflict of interests.

Authors' Contribution

E. Edfors and A. Westergren have contributed equally to this work, that is, to designing and conceiving the study, analysis, coordinating, and drafting the paper. Data collection was made by E. Edfors. Both authors have read and approved the final paper.

Acknowledgments

The authors wish to thank all the respondents for their participation. They also thank Kerstin Ulander (deceased) for her initial involvement in the study. The study was supported by the Swedish Research Council and the Skåne County Council's Research and Development Foundation. The study was conducted within the Patient-Reported Outcomes-Clinical Assessment, Research, and Education (PRO-CARE) Group, Kristianstad University.

References

[1] Y. Johansson, M. Bachrach-Lindström, J. Carstensen, and A. C. Ek, "Malnutrition in a home-living older population: prevalence, incidence and risk factors. a prospective study," *Journal of Clinical Nursing*, vol. 18, no. 9, pp. 1354–1364, 2009.

[2] K. Wikby, A. C. Ek, and L. Christensson, "Nutritional status in elderly people admitted to community residential homes: comparisons between two cohorts," *Journal of Nutrition, Health and Aging*, vol. 10, no. 3, pp. 232–238, 2006.

[3] G. Eiben, D. K. Dey, E. Rothenberg et al., "Obesity in 70-year-old Swedes: secular changes over 30 years," *International Journal of Obesity*, vol. 29, no. 7, pp. 810–817, 2005.

[4] A. Westergren, C. Lindholm, C. Axelsson, and K. Ulander, "Prevalence of eating difficulties and malnutrition among persons within hospital care and special accommodations," *Journal of Nutrition, Health and Aging*, vol. 12, no. 1, pp. 39–43, 2008.

[5] B. Bartali, E. A. Frongillo, S. Bandinelli et al., "Low nutrient intake is an essential component of frailty in older persons," *Journals of Gerontology A*, vol. 61, no. 6, pp. 589–593, 2006.

[6] J. L. Locher, D. L. Roth, C. S. Ritchie et al., "Body mass index, weight loss, and mortality in community-dwelling older adults," *Journals of Gerontology A*, vol. 62, no. 12, pp. 1389–1392, 2007.

[7] C. S. Ritchie, J. L. Locher, D. L. Roth, T. McVie, P. Sawyer, and R. Allman, "Unintentional weight loss predicts decline in activities of daily living function and life-space mobility over 4 years among community-dwelling older adults," *Journals of Gerontology A*, vol. 63, no. 1, pp. 67–75, 2008.

[8] L. I. Vailas, S. A. Nitzke, M. Becker, and J. Gast, "Risk indicators for malnutrition are associated inversely with quality of life for participants in meal programs for older adults," *Journal of the American Dietetic Association*, vol. 98, no. 5, pp. 548–553, 1998.

[9] I. Janssen, D. S. Shepard, P. T. Katzmarzyk, and R. Roubenoff, "The healthcare costs of sarcopenia in the United States," *Journal of the American Geriatrics Society*, vol. 52, no. 1, pp. 80–85, 2004.

[10] H. Payette, C. Coulombe, V. Boutier, and K. Gray-Donald, "Nutrition risk factors for institutionalization in a free-living functionally dependent elderly population," *Journal of Clinical Epidemiology*, vol. 53, no. 6, pp. 579–587, 2000.

[11] C. MacIntosh, J. E. Morley, and I. M. Chapman, "The anorexia of aging," *Nutrition*, vol. 16, no. 10, pp. 983–995, 2000.

[12] H. Payette, C. Coulombe, V. Boutier, and K. Gray-Donald, "Weight loss and mortality among free-living frail elders: a prospective study," *Journals of Gerontology A*, vol. 54, no. 9, pp. M440–M445, 1999.

[13] D. T. Villareal, C. M. Apovian, R. F. Kushner, and S. Klein, "Obesity in older adults: technical review and position statement of the American society for nutrition and NAASO, the obesity society," *American Journal of Clinical Nutrition*, vol. 82, no. 5, pp. 923–934, 2005.

[14] A. M. Beck, L. Ovesen, and M. Osler, "The "mini nutritional assessment" (MNA) and the "determine your nutritional health" checklist (NSI checklist) as predictors of morbidity and mortality in an elderly Danish population," *British Journal of Nutrition*, vol. 81, no. 1, pp. 31–36, 1999.

[15] H. Payette, "Nutrition as a determinant of functional autonomy and quality of life in aging: a research program," *Canadian Journal of Physiology and Pharmacology*, vol. 83, no. 11, pp. 1061–1070, 2005.

[16] C. Alberda, A. Graf, and L. McCargar, "Malnutrition: etiology, consequences, and assessment of a patient at risk," *Best Practice and Research: Clinical Gastroenterology*, vol. 20, no. 3, pp. 419–439, 2006.

[17] C. C. H. Chen, Y. Y. Bai, G. H. Huang, and S. T. Tang, "Revisiting the concept of malnutrition in older people," *Journal of Clinical Nursing*, vol. 16, no. 11, pp. 2015–2026, 2007.

[18] B. L. Callen and T. J. Wells, "Screening for nutritional risk in community-dwelling old-old," *Public Health Nursing*, vol. 22, no. 2, pp. 138–146, 2005.

[19] J. L. Locher, C. S. Ritchie, C. O. Robinson, D. L. Roth, D. S. West, and K. L. Burgio, "A multidimensional approach to understanding under-eating in homebound older adults: the importance of social factors," *Gerontologist*, vol. 48, no. 2, pp. 223–234, 2008.

[20] J. L. Locher, C. O. Robinson, D. L. Roth, C. S. Ritchie, and K. L. Burgio, "The effect of the presence of others on caloric intake in homebound older adults," *Journals of Gerontology A*, vol. 60, no. 11, pp. 1475–1478, 2005.

[21] H. H. Keller, "Meal programs improve nutritional risk: a longitudinal analysis of community-living seniors," *Journal of the American Dietetic Association*, vol. 106, no. 7, pp. 1042–1048, 2006.

[22] J. V. White, "Risk factors for poor nutritional status," *Primary Care*, vol. 21, no. 1, pp. 19–31, 1994.

[23] C. P. G. M. de Groot, W. A. van Staveren, and C. de Graaf, "Determinants of macronutrient intake in elderly people," *European Journal of Clinical Nutrition*, vol. 54, supplement 3, pp. S70–S76, 2000.

[24] E. A. Gollub and D. O. Weddle, "Improvements in nutritional intake and quality of life among frail homebound older adults receiving home-delivered breakfast and lunch," *Journal of the American Dietetic Association*, vol. 104, no. 8, pp. 1227–1235, 2004.

[25] J. L. Locher, K. L. Burgio, W. C. Yoels, and C. S. Ritchie, "The social significance of food and eating in the lives of older recipients of meals on wheels," *Journal of Nutrition For the Elderly*, vol. 17, no. 2, pp. 15–33, 1998.

[26] Medical Association Declaration of Helsinki, "Ethical principles for medical research involving human subject," http://www.wma.net/en/30publications/10policies/b3/.

[27] SFS 2003:460, "Lag om etikprövning av forskning som avser människor (The act concerning the ethical review of research involving humans)," http://www.riksdagen.se/sv/Dokument-Lagar/Lagar/Svenskforfattningssamling/Lag-2003460-om-etikprovning_sfs-2003-460/.

[28] S. Kvale and S. Brinkman, *Interviews: Learning the Craft of Qualitative Research Interviewing*, Sage, Los Angeles, Calif, USA, 2nd edition, 2009.

[29] H. H. Keller, R. Goy, and S. L. Kane, "Validity and reliability of SCREEN II (seniors in the community: risk evaluation for eating and nutrition, version II)," *European Journal of Clinical Nutrition*, vol. 59, no. 10, pp. 1149–1157, 2005.

[30] U. H. Graneheim and B. Lundman, "Qualitative content analysis in nursing research: concepts, procedures and measures to achieve trustworthiness," *Nurse Education Today*, vol. 24, no. 2, pp. 105–112, 2004.

[31] S. Souter and C. Keller, "Food choice in the rural dwelling older adult," *Southern Online Journal of Nursing Research*, vol. 3, no. 5, pp. 1–18, 2002.

[32] C. Fjellström, B. Sidenvall, and M. Nydahl, "Foodintake and the elderly: social aspects," in *Food, People and Society: A European Perspective of Consumers' Food Choices*, L. Frewer, E. Risvik, and H. Schifferstein, Eds., pp. 197–209, Springer, Berlin, Germany, 2001.

[33] C. Banwell, J. Dixon, D. Broom, and A. Davies, "Habits of a lifetime: family dining patterns over the lifecourse of older Australians," *Health Sociology Review*, vol. 19, no. 3, pp. 343–355, 2010.

[34] C. H. Chen and J. H. Shao, "Have you had your bowl of rice?': a qualitative study of eating patterns in older Taiwanese adults," *Journal of Clinical Nursing*, vol. 21, no. 1-2, pp. 2–10, 2012.

[35] Z. Pajalic, L. Persson, A. Westergren, B. Vanja, and K. Skovdahl, "The experiences of elderly people living at home related to their receiving meals distributed by a municipality in sweden," *Journal of Food Research*, vol. 1, no. 1, article 68, 2012.

[36] K. Gustafsson and B. Sidenvall, "Food-related health perceptions and food habits among older women," *Journal of Advanced Nursing*, vol. 39, no. 2, pp. 164–173, 2002.

[37] G. Hughes, K. M. Bennett, and M. M. Hetherington, "Old and alone: barriers to healthy eating in older men living on their own," *Appetite*, vol. 43, no. 3, pp. 269–276, 2004.

[38] P. A. Shifflett, "Future time perspective, past experiences, and negotiation of food use patterns among the aged," *Gerontologist*, vol. 27, no. 5, pp. 611–615, 1987.

[39] P. A. Shifflett and W. A. McIntosh, "Food habits and future time: an exploratory study of age-appropriate food habits among the elderly," *International Journal of Aging and Human Development*, vol. 24, no. 1, pp. 1–17, 1986.

[40] K. Östman, "Erfarenhet av arbete med mat för äldre i eget boende," in *Mat för äldre inom vård och omsorg nr 16*, Socialstyrelsen, Stockholm, Sweden, 2007.

[41] Hälso-och sjukvårdslag SFS 1982:763 (Health and medical services act), http://www.riksdagen.se/sv/Dokument-Lagar/Lagar/Svenskforfattningssamling/Halso–och-sjukvardslag-1982_sfs-1982-763/.

[42] Socialtjänslag SFS 2001:453 (Social services act), http://www.riksdagen.se/sv/Dokument-Lagar/Lagar/Svenskforfattningssamling/Socialtjanstlag-2001453_sfs-2001-453/.

[43] L. Sandman, "On the autonomy turf. Assessing the value of autonomy to patients," *Medicine, Health Care, and Philosophy*, vol. 7, no. 3, pp. 261–268, 2004.

[44] P. Burnard, "Writing a qualitative research report," *Accident and Emergency Nursing*, vol. 12, no. 3, pp. 176–181, 2004.

8

The Relationship between Health and Community across Aging Cohorts

Julie Norstrand[1] and Keith T. Chan[2]

[1] *Boston College Graduate School of Social Work, McGuinn Hall, Chestnut Hill, MA 02467, USA*
[2] *School of Social Welfare, University at Albany, State University of New York, 135 Western Avenue, Richardson 277, Albany, NY 12222, USA*

Correspondence should be addressed to Julie Norstrand; norstraj@bc.edu

Academic Editor: Barbara Shukitt-Hale

Research is needed to examine the connection between older adults and their community as they age. This is important as increasing numbers of older adults wish to age in place. Regression models were examined across 3 cohorts testing relationships among social capital indicators (neighborhood trust, neighborhood support, neighborhood cohesion, neighborhood participation, and telephone interaction) with health outcomes (self-rated health, activities of daily living (ADL), and instrumental activities of daily living (IADL)). Results showed that most social capital indicators remained significant for all health outcomes into very old age. Development of tools for individual and community interventions to ensure optimal fit between the aging individual and their environment is discussed, along with recommendations for enhancing social work theory and practice.

1. Introduction

Interest in age-friendly community and aging-in-place concepts has grown over recent years as the majority of older adults wish to remain within the neighborhood in which they have become familiar and emotionally attached to. Social capital has previously been used to capture community connectedness or social glue [1]. Social capital is relevant to aging-in-place as it provides a framework to examine neighborhoods' fit for older adults; this has important implications for adapting neighborhoods to become more age-friendly and ensure opportunity to aging-in-place. Hence, social capital has gained increased attention from both practice and policy makers [2]. The research has demonstrated a positive relationship between social capital and wide range of health outcomes [3]. In other words, individuals with high social capital are more likely to experience good health. However, most of the research to date has been done on middle-aged adults. It is still not clearly understood how social capital functions in relation to health as adults reach very old age. The goal of this paper was to elucidate this relationship by examining the association between five indicators of social capital with three physical health outcomes among adults aged 65 years and older.

1.1. Social Capital. The use of social capital is increasingly recognized as a means for adapting environments for aging-in-place. As Emlet and Moceri argue, an elder friendly community captures the core features of social capital including "civic participation, and the nature of social networks and mutuality/reciprocity" [4, p. 2]. Despite the growing interest in social capital, it remains controversial due to its conceptual polysemy. Therefore, it is important to fully clarify how social capital was conceptualized in this study. Four out of the five social capital indicators used in this study focused on neighborhood (neighborhood trust, neighborhood support, neighborhood cohesion, and neighborhood participation), while the fifth measure (telephone interaction) captured community connections beyond the neighborhood. Therefore, social capital in this study should be considered to be primarily a measure of the neighborhood, with the understanding that social connections can stretch beyond physical borders.

Putnam's definition was used for this study: "features of social organization such as networks, norms, and social trust that facilitate coordination and cooperation for mutual benefit" [5]. There were several reasons for using Putnam's definition; primarily Putnam's conceptualization of social capital has a communitarian focus [6]. A fundamental aspect to communitarianism is the establishment and maintenance of social norms that are fundamental to making communities stronger [7]. Strong communities enable healthier populations; and so Putnam's definition has been widely applied in the health related literature [8]. Since health was the key focus of this study, Putnam's definition of social capital was considered appropriate here. Finally, many of the indicators of social capital available in the dataset used for this study mirror those used to measure social capital as conceptualized by Putnam. Previous research has used a number of these same indicators to reflect social capital [1, 9]. The five indicators used in this study (namely, neighborhood trust, neighborhood support, neighborhood cohesion, neighborhood participation, and telephone interaction) have been used widely in the social capital and health literature [3].

1.2. Social Capital and Health among Older Adults. Social capital has been shown to have significant positive associations with a vast array of health outcomes for all ages, including older adults [3, 10]. Kawachi and colleagues [3] found in a number of studies that indicators of social capital are linked to a wide range of health conditions, such as mortality, life-expectancy, self-rated health, cancer, cardiovascular disease, obesity, diabetes, and functional limitations.

Social capital may be particularly important for older adults because this group is "more tethered to their immediate surroundings (and so) the impact of the environment is likely greater" [11, p. 253]. There is growing support for the positive impact of social capital on the health of older adults, even among the oldest-old [12]. In their study, Nyqvist and colleagues found that the *structural* dimension of social capital (i.e., social networks, social integration, and attachment) was important for depressive symptoms among the oldest-old aged 85 and older. The authors argued that this dimension of social capital might be particularly important for this cohort due to their increasing physical frailty and reduced social networks. Therefore, the examination of the relationship between structural dimensions of social capital and health, when conducted across cohorts that represent the changing lifespan of elders (young-old (65–74 years), the middle-old (75–84 years), and the oldest-old (85+ years)), can shed new light on how networks grow, develop, and adapt for this population.

1.3. Influence of Age on Social Capital and Health Relationship. Research on whether there are changes in the level of social capital over the lifespan is limited. Research by Axler and colleagues suggested that social capital was the lowest among older adults (aged 60 years and over) compared to younger cohorts [9]. In terms of varying dimensions of social capital, some research has found a decrease as people live into very old age, such as size of social networks and frequency of contacts [13], and civic participation as older adults become less physically active [14]. It is not clear what occurs with other aspects of social capital such as sense of belonging and trust as older adults age. Place attachment, a concept closely related to sense of belonging, does seem to increase with age [15]. However, important physical environmental factors, such as crime, may diminish the sense of belonging [16]. Furthermore, the impact of age on the relationship between social capital and health remains poorly understood. As Cagney and Wen point out: "models of the social capital-health relationship must be attentive to age" [11, p. 239]. Considering the increase in population longevity, the effect of age on the relationship between social capital and health is an important public health query. By understanding the role of age in the relationship between social capital and health, interventions can be developed to optimize the fit between older adults and their community as they age in place.

By partitioning social capital into five indicators, this study was focused on examining how separate dimensions of the social environment can act as determinants of health for older adults, particularly during the latter part of their lifespan. By examining these indicators separately, it is hoped that this will provide a more multifaceted understanding of how elders may feel about their sense of belonging in their neighborhoods and beyond.

1.4. Purpose of Study. The relationship among five indicators of social capital (neighborhood trust, neighborhood support, neighborhood cohesion, neighborhood participation, and telephone interaction) which were examined with three health outcomes: self-rated health, activities of daily living (ADL), and instrumental activities of daily living (IADL). Analyses were conducted to examine differences across three cohorts, the young-old (65–74 years), the middle-old (75–84 years), and the oldest-old (85+ years). In order to understand the relationship between social capital and health by age, this study was designed to investigate two questions: (1) does the level of social capital change with age? And (2) does the relationship between social capital and health outcomes change with increasing age? For the first research question we hypothesized that older adults will possess lower levels of certain indicators of social capital (specifically, participation and telephone interaction) while other indicators will increase (specifically, trust, cohesion, and support). As some components of social capital are lost or gained with increasing age, we hypothesized that certain indicators of social capital will have an increased or decreased association with health as individuals progress to a later stage in their lifespan. Specifically, social capital indicators, neighborhood trust, neighborhood cohesion, and neighborhood support, which mirror cognitive dimensions of social capital, will more likely be significantly associated with health among the very old (i.e., oldest-old cohort) compared to younger cohorts. This assumption is based on previous research carried out with the oldest-old, where cognitive dimensions of social capital were found to become increasingly important [12]. The other social capital indicators, neighborhood participation and telephone interaction, will be less likely associated with

TABLE 1: Socioeconomic characteristics by cohort.

	65–74 yrs (N = 1233) (%)	75–84 yrs (N = 845) (%)	85+ yrs (N = 266) (%)	χ^2 (df)	P
Gender (female)	67	69	69	1.12 (2)	0.60
Race (nonwhite)	26	20	17	17.33 (2)	0.001
Education (<HS)	10	13	15	26.66 (8)	0.001
Poverty (200% FPL)	28	34	41	22.46 (2)	0.001
Marital status				268.21 (6)	0.001
Married/living with someone	51	36	25		
Widowed	20	47	61		
Divorced/separated	16	8	4		
Single	13	10	10		
Living arrangements (alone)	37	48	66	86.16 (2)	0.001

health outcomes into late adulthood compared to younger cohorts. As described previously, neighborhood participation and telephone interaction have been found to decrease with increased frailty in old age [13, 14].

2. Methods

This study used cross-sectional data from the 2010 Community Health Data Base (CHDB) managed by Philadelphia Health Management Corporation. The survey has been conducted biennially since 1994 in five urban and suburban counties of southeastern Pennsylvania (Bucks, Chester, Delaware, Montgomery, and Philadelphia). Random digit dialing (RDD) was used to survey approximately 10,000 households. Persons aged 60 and older were oversampled for the analysis, representing over 700,000 older adults in the area. If a randomly selected adult respondent was unable to be interviewed because of health impairments or language barriers, the interview was conducted with an adult proxy. All respondents who had an adult proxy (N = 14, <1%) respond for them were removed from the sample as it was considered important to gain first-hand information from respondents themselves.

3. Sample

The sample consisted of 2,344 adults (65 years and older) from a five-county southeastern Pennsylvania region. Just over half (53%) belonged to the young-old cohort, 36% belonged to the middle-old cohort, and 11% belonged to the oldest-old cohort. There were significant differences across the three cohorts across all socioeconomic indicators except by gender. The oldest-old cohort was significantly more likely to be white, have a lower level of education, be poor, and live alone. Marital status varied across cohorts, where older cohorts reported higher percentages of widowed status (Table 1). When comparing this complete sample of older adults to peers nationwide, the percent of older adults (14.5%) was slightly higher than national figures (13%) [17]. However, it should be noted that Pennsylvania (15.4%) had the fourth largest proportion of older adults in 2010 [17]. The complete sample was similar to elders nationwide in terms of age (74.8 years and 74.0 years, resp.). However, generally there were fewer females, minority, and lower level of educational attainment among elders nationwide [18] compared to the sample examined in this study. Poverty (@ 100% FPL) among elders nationwide (9.0%) was higher than the complete sample (7.6%) [18]. However, there was considerable variation in poverty level in the complete sample by county. For example, 13.6% older Philadelphians were poor [19].

4. Measures

4.1. Physical Health Outcomes

Self-Rated Health. This was measured by a single item that asked to rate health on a 5-point Likert scale, with a high number indicating better self-rated health.

ADL and IADL. ADL reflected eight basic activities that generally occur within the home (i.e., eating, dressing, grooming, walking, transferring, bathing, continence, and soiling). IADL measured more complex tasks needed for the ADLs that generally require interaction with the surrounding environment (i.e., talking on the phone, walking, shopping, meal preparation, housework, taking medicine, and handling money). For this study, ADL and IADL scales were dichotomized with 0 representing no ADL/IADL limitations and 1 representing 1 or more ADL/IADL limitations. In this study, only 10.7% had 1 or more ADL and 25.4% had 1 or more IADL, similar to national statistics from other large-scale studies from the CDC and the US Census. Conceptually, having 1 or more limitations with ADLs or IADLs can have a direct impact on an older person's ability to age in place.

4.2. Social Capital Indicators. The five social capital indicators were originally derived from the Social Capital Community Benchmark Survey [20]. The items were as follows.

Neighborhood Support. This was assessed by "please rate how likely people in your neighborhood are willing to help their neighbors with routine activities such as picking up their trash cans, or helping to shovel snow. Would you say that most people in your neighborhood are always, often, sometimes, rarely, or never willing to help their neighbors?" Response categories were recoded from 1 to 4, with 1 being rarely/never, 2 being sometimes, 3 being often, and 4 being always.

Neighborhood Participation. This was assessed by "How many local groups or organizations in your neighborhood do you currently participate in such as social, political, religious, school-related, or athletic organizations?" Responses categories ranged from 0 to 12 groups. Due to very small number of cases in category responses 6 and higher, this variable was top-coded so response categories ranged from 0 to 6.

Neighborhood Cohesion. This was assessed by "Please tell me if you strongly agree, agree, disagree, or strongly disagree with the following statement: I feel that I belong and am a part of my neighborhood." Responses categories were coded from 1 to 4 with 1 being strongly disagree, 2 being disagree, 3 being agree, and 4 being strongly agree.

Neighborhood Trust. This was assessed by "Please tell me if you strongly agree, agree, disagree, or strongly disagree with the following statement: Most people in my neighborhood can be trusted." Response categories were also coded from 1 to 4 with 1 being strongly disagree, 2 being disagree, 3 being agree, and 4 being strongly agree.

Telephone Interaction. This was assessed by "About how often do you talk with friends or relatives on the telephone?" Response categories included several times a day, once a day, a few times a week, once a week, less often than once a week, and never. Responses categories were recoded from 1 to 4, with 1 being once a week or less, 2 being few times a week, 3 being once a day, and 4 being several times a day.

4.3. Demographic and Socioeconomic Covariates. Demographic and socioeconomic variables entered into the analyses were *age* in years ranging from 65 and higher; *sex*, 0 representing female and 1 representing male; *race*, a dichotomized variable with 0 representing white and 1 representing minority, (minority includes all nonwhite plus all Hispanics of any race); *education*, coded along 5 response categories: less than high school graduate (0–11 years), high school graduate (12 years), some college (13–15 years), and postcollege (more than 16 years) with high school (16 years) as comparison group; *poverty* at 200% of the federal poverty line dichotomized into poor (coded 1) and nonpoor (coded 0); *marital status*, recoded into 4 dummy variables (single, divorced, and widowed with married as comparison group); and *living arrangements*, a dichotomized variable representing living alone (coded 0) versus living with others (coded 1). Poverty at 200% was used because it represented a more reasonable cut-off for poverty than 100% [21].

5. Data Analysis

The first research question was tested using Kruskal-Wallis rank sum tests on the five social capital indicators (neighborhood trust, neighborhood support, neighborhood cohesion, neighborhood participation, and telephone interaction) with the sample (>65 yrs) split along by three cohorts (65–74, 75–84, and 85 and older). Cohort analysis was used to examine differences across the lifespan of older adults, where important differences may emerge for the oldest-old (85 and older), who are the most at risk. The second research question was tested using binary logistic (ADL and IADL) and ordinal logistic regression (self-rated health), analyses for each of the health outcomes as separate dependent variables for each of the three cohorts. Standard socioeconomic indicators were accounted for as covariates in the analyses.

6. Results

6.1. Research Question 1. Findings suggest that age did not play a role in terms of possession of social capital except for neighborhood support (Table 1). Results from Kruskal-Wallis rank sum tests showed significant differences across cohorts for the indicator neighborhood support. The rank sum was the highest for the youngest group and became gradually lower as respondents aged (65–74: 1,240,000; 75–84: 887,372; 85+: 251,588), suggesting that support from neighbors as an indicator of social capital deteriorates as participants progressed to a later lifespan.

Differences across the three cohorts were more notable for health (Table 2). Significant differences were found on all four health outcomes across the three groups, with worsening health profiles as age increased. Post hoc tests showed significant differences between all groups for ADL and IADL. Significant differences were found between the young-old and oldest-old for self-rated health. Significant differences in terms of sociodemographic characteristics were also found across groups (Table 3). As age increased, the sociodemographic profile was more likely to be white, less educated, poor, and living alone.

6.2. Research Question 2. Tables 4, 5, and 6 showed the results of the logistic regressions carried out for each of the health outcomes across the three cohorts. Generally the fit of these regression models was significant for health outcomes across all three groups, except for self-rated health and ADL among the oldest-old. Despite the limited variance explained by the models, the results showed a complex set of associations between social capital indicators and health outcomes that changed with age. All of the social capital indicators, except telephone interaction, were significantly associated with all of the health outcomes. Interestingly, these social capital indicators were relevant at different stages of the lifespan. Specifically, for the health outcome self-rated health (Table 4) neighborhood cohesion improved health among the young-old (OR = 1.31, $P < 0.05$), while neighborhood trust (OR = 1.87, $P < 0.001$) and neighborhood participation (OR = 1.14, $P < 0.05$) improved health among the middle-old. For the middle-old, respondents who reported greater neighborhood trust (OR = 0.63, $P < 0.05$) and neighborhood participation (OR = 0.74, $P < 0.05$) were around 30% less likely to have an ADL limitation (Table 5). No significant associations were observed for social capital indicators among the young-old

TABLE 2: Social capital characteristics by cohort.

	65–74 yrs (N = 1233) (%)	75–84 yrs (N = 845) (%)	85+ yrs (N = 266) (%)	χ^2 (df)[a]	P
SC: cohesion				16.97 (6)	0.009
Strongly disagree	1	0	2		
Disagree	6	4	9		
Agree	60	64	58		
Strongly agree	34	31	31		
SC: support				15.84 (6)	0.015
Never/rarely	11	11	15		
Sometimes	26	22	22		
Often	32	28	27		
Always	31	38	36		
SC: Trust				5.32	0.503
Strongly disagree	2	2	1		
Disagree	10	9	8		
Agree	62	66	62		
Strongly agree	26	23	29		
SC: participation				25.67	0.177
0	44	45	49		
1	26	26	27		
2	15	13	14		
3+	15	16	10		
SC: telephone interaction				5.87	0.438
Once a week	10	12	10		
Few times a week	25	28	27		
Once a day	23	22	25		
Several times a day	42	38	38		

[a]The Kruskal-Wallis statistic, a test of rank for nonparametric samples, was also conducted for all social capital items to examine differences in the 3 groups. Results indicated statistical differences for support (KW = 6.59, df = 2, and P = 0.04), but no differences for cohesion, trust, and participation (cohesion: KW = 1.58, df = 2, and P = 0.46; trust: KW = 1.66, df = 2, and P = 0.44; telephone interaction: KW = 3.71, df = 2, and P = 0.16). In the case of support, the cohort of 65 to 74 was ranked the highest for support (rank sum = 1,240,000), followed by those who are 75 to 84 (rank sum = 887,372), and last for those who are 85 and older (rank sum = 251,588).

TABLE 3: Health outcomes by cohort.

	65–74 yrs (N = 1233) (%)	75–84 yrs (N = 845) (%)	85+ yrs (N = 266) (%)	χ^2 (df)	P
Self-rated health[a]				33.03	0.000
Poor	4.07	7.13	7.52		
Fair	16.12	17.34	24.81		
Good	33.96	36.82	32.33		
Very good	30.37	27.43	24.81		
Excellent	15.47	11.28	10.53		
No ADL	92.94	88.17	77.82	55.81 (2)	0.000
No IADL	83.94	69.47	51.13	147.22 (2)	0.000

[a]The Kruskal-Wallis statistic, a test of rank for nonparametric samples, was also conducted for each self-rated health to examine differences in the 3 groups. Results for the KW indicated significant differences in self-rated health between groups (KW = 23.194, df = 2, and $P < 0.0001$), with those who are 65 to 74 having the highest health (rank sum = 1,510,000), followed by those who are 75 to 84 (rank sum = 943,626), and those who are 85 and older having the lowest health (rank sum = 277,376).

for ADL. In terms of IADL limitations (Table 6), the oldest-old group with more neighborhood cohesion were 50% less likely to have an IADL limitation (OR = 0.45, $P < 0.05$). On the other hand, those who were 85 and older who reported higher levels of neighborhood trust were twice as likely to report an IADL limitation (OR = 2.00, $P < 0.05$). Social capital indicators were not observed to be significant with IADL limitations for the two other cohorts.

7. Discussion

We hypothesized that certain indicators of social capital would increase (namely, neighborhood trust, neighborhood cohesion, and neighborhood support) or decrease (namely, neighborhood participation and telephone interaction) with increasing age. The trends in the percentage breakdowns did show some support for this (Table 2). For example, the oldest-old reported lower levels of both neighborhood participation

TABLE 4: Self-rated health with all predictors (odds ratios with 95% interval confidence).

Age category	65–74 yrs		75–84 yrs		85+ yrs	
Predictor	OR	95% C.I.	OR	95% C.I.	OR	95% C.I.
Age	1.00	0.96; 1.04	0.92***	0.87; 0.97	1.06	0.96; 1.17
Sex (male)	0.81	0.62; 1.04	0.76	0.56; 1.05	0.72	0.37; 1.38
Race (minority)	0.57***	0.43; 0.76	0.59**	0.41; 0.87	0.69	0.31; 1.55
Education	1.34***	1.20; 1.49	1.17*	1.02; 1.35	1.19	0.89; 1.58
Poverty @ 200% (poor)	0.49***	0.37; 0.66	0.61**	0.44; 0.87	1.40	0.75; 2.62
Marital status (married)						
Widowed	0.59*	0.40; 0.87	0.91	0.59; 1.41	1.25	0.55; 2.86
Divorced/separated	0.48**	0.32; 0.74	1.18	0.59; 2.38	0.56	0.12; 2.55
Single	0.50*	0.32; 0.77	1.07	0.58; 1.94	0.98	0.34; 2.83
Living arrangement (with others)	0.76	0.54; 1.06	0.66*	0.44; 0.99	1.59	0.78; 3.24
SC: neighborhood cohesion	1.31*	1.04; 1.65	1.10	0.82; 1.48	1.15	0.71; 1.89
SC: neighborhood support	1.05	0.92; 1.19	1.11	0.95; 1.30	1.35*	1.01; 1.80
SC: neighborhood trust	1.06	0.87; 1.31	1.87***	1.42; 2.46	1.23	0.76; 1.97
SC: neighborhood participation	1.05	0.96; 1.14	1.14*	1.02; 1.26	1.09	0.94; 1.26
SC: telephone interaction	1.02	0.91; 1.14	0.90	0.79; 1.04	0.93	0.71; 1.23
Model fit						
R^2	0.07		0.05		0.04	
F(df)	$F(14{,}997) = 194.82$**		$F(14{,}641) = 94.13$*		$F(14{,}186) = 20.94$	

***$P \leq 0.001$; **$P \leq 0.01$; *$P \leq 0.05$.

TABLE 5: ADL with all predictors (odds ratios with 95% interval confidence).

Age category	65–74 yrs		75–84 yrs		85+ yrs	
Predictor	OR	95% C.I.	OR	95% C.I.	OR	95% C.I.
Age	0.97	0.89; 1.07	1.20***	1.09; 1.31	1.08	0.95; 1.23
Sex (male)	0.66	0.35; 1.24	0.81	0.46; 1.43	0.78	0.31; 1.95
Race (minority)	1.90*	1.08; 3.31	2.13**	1.20; 3.78	0.30	0.07; 1.18
Education	1.06	0.82; 1.37	1.07	0.84; 1.37	1.16	0.78; 1.73
Poverty @ 200% (poor)	3.64***	1.98; 6.71	2.08*	1.17; 3.69	1.89	0.76; 4.68
Marital status (married)						
Widowed	0.94	0.41; 2.17	1.61	0.79; 3.28	0.73	0.21; 2.48
Divorced/separated	1.20	0.50; 2.86	3.12*	1.08; 9.05	1.67	0.27; 10.44
Single	1.45	0.61; 3.46	1.70	0.59; 4.85	1.26	0.31; 5.21
Living arrangement (with others)	0.87	0.45; 1.69	2.07*	1.08; 3.95	1.13	0.38; 3.43
SC: neighborhood cohesion	0.97	0.57; 1.64	1.33	0.80; 2.21	0.74	0.38; 1.46
SC: neighborhood support	1.08	0.81; 1.43	0.90	0.69; 1.17	0.95	0.63; 1.43
SC: neighborhood trust	0.85	0.55; 1.30	0.63*	0.41; 0.98	0.89	0.47; 1.70
SC: neighborhood participation	1.03	0.84; 1.26	0.74*	0.58; 0.94	1.05	0.85; 1.30
SC: telephone interaction	0.94	0.73; 1.20	1.06	0.83; 1.36	0.96	0.66; 1.39
Model fit						
R^2	0.09		0.11		0.06	
F(df)	$F(14{,}999) = 44.65$***		$F(14{,}644) = 50.05$***		$F(14{,}186) = 11.83$	

***$P \leq 0.001$; **$P \leq 0.01$; *$P \leq 0.05$.

and telephone interaction than their younger cohorts. Also, the oldest-old also reported higher levels of trust than younger cohorts. Neighborhood cohesion did not follow the expected trend as it decreased with age. These findings add to the limited literature on the change in social capital over the lifespan. In terms of support, our findings found the perception that neighbors are willing to help did increase to a certain age. According to our study, middle-old cohort reported the highest level of neighborhood support. What is interesting to note about this cohort is that they possessed high (or higher) levels of neighborhood support, neighborhood cohesion, and neighborhood trust compared to the other two cohorts. This could suggest that the neighborhood, in terms of support, cohesion, and trust, may be particularly

TABLE 6: IADL with all predictors (odds ratios with 95% interval confidence).

Age category	65–74 yrs		75–84 yrs		85+ yrs	
Predictor	OR	95% C.I.	OR	95% C.I.	OR	95% C.I.
Age	1.00	0.94; 1.06	1.15***	1.08; 1.22	1.12	0.99; 1.27
Sex (male)	0.75	0.48; 1.15	0.80	0.54; 1.20	0.45*	0.20; 0.99
Race (minority)	1.74**	1.17; 2.59	1.71*	1.09; 2.69	0.92	0.37; 2.32
Education	0.88	0.74; 1.06	1.03	0.87; 1.23	1.01	0.71; 1.44
Poverty @ 200% (poor)	2.15***	1.42; 3.26	1.74**	1.15; 2.64	1.48	0.68; 3.22
Marital status (married)						
Widowed	1.79*	1.02; 3.14	1.79*	1.06; 3.02	1.83	0.65; 5.16
Divorced/separated	1.51	0.81; 2.82	1.98	0.86; 4.55	2.80	0.53; 14.96
Single	1.99*	1.07; 2.73	1.50	0.70; 3.24	4.41*	1.13; 17.24
Living arrangement (with others)	1.25	0.78; 2.00	1.79*	1.10; 2.92	1.22	0.50; 2.98
SC: neighborhood cohesion	0.79	0.55; 1.14	1.17	0.81; 1.68	0.45*	0.23; 0.85
SC: neighborhood support	1.13	0.92; 1.37	0.83	0.69; 1.00	0.70	0.49; 1.01
SC: neighborhood trust	0.87	0.64; 1.18	0.94	0.68; 1.31	2.00*	1.08; 3.70
SC: neighborhood participation	0.97	0.83; 1.11	0.89	0.77; 1.02	0.94	0.76; 1.17
SC: telephone interaction	0.99	0.83; 1.19	1.08	0.91; 1.29	1.06	0.76; 1.46
Model fit						
R^2	0.09		0.06		0.14	
F(df)	$F(14,999) = 77.37^{***}$		$F(14,644) = 50.38^{***}$		$F(14,186) = 35.75^{***}$	

$^{***}P \leq 0.001$; $^{**}P \leq 0.01$; $^{*}P \leq 0.05$.

meaningful for this cohort. Other indicators of social capital examined in this study (i.e., neighborhood participation and telephone interaction) did not follow this trend. For example, the middle-old cohort reported the lowest frequency of telephone interactions with friends, relatives, and neighbors, although this difference was not significant. The variation in possession of different indicators of social capital by cohort could be used in terms of developing communities that maximize the potential for successful aging-in-place; such policy implications are described further below.

Logistic regressions for each of the four health outcomes showed that different indicators of social capital continued to be significant predictors of health outcomes even when accounting for standard sociodemographic predictors; however, the nature of these associations changed with increasing age. With respect to the second hypothesis, our expectation was supported in the fact that different indicators of social capital were relevant to health as age increased. We had specifically predicted that the social capital indicators, neighborhood trust, neighborhood cohesion, and neighborhood support, would more likely be associated with improved health among those of advanced age (i.e., the oldest-old cohort) compared with the younger cohorts (i.e., young-old). This prediction did bear out for IADL with respect to neighborhood trust and neighborhood cohesion for the oldest-old. However, the relationship was in the opposite direction with neighborhood trust. It is likely that this finding reflects endogeneity in the relationship of neighborhood trust and reporting an IADL limitation; elders who are among the oldest and most vulnerable must trust the people around them to even be able to seek out help for complex tasks with negotiating the outside world. We also predicted that the social capital indicators, neighborhood participation and telephone interaction, would be less likely to be significant with increasing age. The results indicated that there was no relationship to health for these variables.

Albeit the fact that social capital explained a very small part of the overall variance of each of the health outcomes, what is important to derive from these findings is how different aspects of the social environment matter for different health outcome at different stages of life. Specifically, neighborhood trust was only significant among the middle-old cohort for self-rated health and ADL, whereas neighborhood trust had an unexpected relationship with IADL limitations for the oldest-old. Neighborhood cohesion was significant for the young-old for self-rated health whereas neighborhood cohesion was significant for the oldest-old in terms of IADL. Neighborhood support was significant for the oldest-old in terms of self-rated health. Finally, neighborhood participation was only significant for the middle-old for self-rated health and ADL. This mixed pattern of associations suggests that all parts of the social environment play a role across the aging lifespan and for different indicators of health. This is a significant finding suggesting that the social environment is a critical factor to be considered when adapting settings for aging-in-place. This also highlights the importance of looking at social capital in terms of multiple indicators rather than creating a single factor. Furthermore, these findings also suggest that the "age structure of the community" also needs to be taken into account [11, p. 251]; in other words, the social environment must fit the needs of the age demographics.

The nature of the relationship between the five social capital indicators and the three health outcomes may provide some interesting insight into the meaning of these health outcomes in relation to the social environment. Compared to ADL and IADL, the relationship between social capital and self-rated health was noted across all three age groups. Both self-rated health and social capital are highly subjective concepts; and it is possible that subjective processes applied to each of these domains (i.e., self-rated health and social capital) influence one another. In terms of functional health, social capital was significant only among the oldest-old for IADL whereas it was significant only among the middle-old for ADL. It is important to pay attention to which dimensions of the social environment mattered: among the oldest-old, neighborhood support and neighborhood trust were critical for IADL. Among the middle-old, neighborhood trust and neighborhood participation were significant. Although these patterns of relationships do make sense, it is difficult to explain why social capital did not matter for either ADL or IADL for the youngest-old. Perhaps grandparent/family responsibilities diminish as people move from young-old to middle-old age. This may give them more time to engage with neighbors; and this builds familiarity (experienced as trust and sense of belonging) with the neighborhood. As Kahn and Antonucci [22] Convoy model explicates, relationships change over the lifespan that can impact health and well-being. More research is needed to better understand what and how older adults interact with their neighborhoods.

The associations between social capital indicators and health outcomes were in the expected direction; in other words, high levels of social capital indicators were associated with better health outcomes. There was one exception though, and that was with the relationship between neighborhood trust and IADL limitation among the oldest-old. Among this cohort, higher neighborhood trust was associated with higher IADL limitations. This was an unexpected finding. It may be that individuals who experienced high levels of IADL limitations required help from neighbors and thus develop higher levels of trust through this interaction. This interpretation does bring up an important point regarding the need for caution when making assumptions about the direction of the relationship between social capital and health.

The one indicator of social capital that was not significant for any of the four health outcomes examined in this study was telephone interaction. The principal author also found similar findings in a previous study; in that study it was noted that it may be not the frequency of contact (as was measured in this study) but rather the level of support provided by the network that was the critical factor for physical and mental health [10]. Lack of significant association for telephone interaction with any of the three health outcomes in this study may provide some insight into social capital: it is quality of connection rather than quantity of connections within the neighborhood that is important for social capital to capture. This finding may also pertain to other dimensions of social capital, such as neighborhood participation. In other words, the quality of neighborhood participation (i.e., measuring the type of activity) rather than the number of organizations that the individual is participating with might better capture the benefits of social capital. Ultimately, the findings in this study suggest that more attention needs to be paid to the perception of community and the people living in these communities. Indeed, the role of neighbors is likely to increase in the future as the availability of spouses or children to provide care for aging parents is expected to diminish. This is due to reduction in fertility rates, increased divorces rates, and low rates of remarriage [23, 24].

8. Conclusions

It is hoped that the findings of this research may build on optimal environments for aging-in-place and elder-friendly communities by furthering our understanding of what dimensions of the social environment matter for health. As Emlet and Moceri have argued, there is a need "to further elucidate the importance of social relationships and social connectedness with aging in place and in developing elder friendly communities" ([4, p. 3]). It was the aim of this research to provide a comprehensive empirical examination of the fit between the aging individual and their surrounding environment in relation to health.

The dynamic between the aging individual and the community in which they live is a complex one. Although previous research has described an important role of the environment in which older adults live, this study has provided rich empirical evidence for this by examining relationships between *multiple* indicators of social capital and health across three cohorts. It is hoped that these findings will encourage the development of programs and interventions that allow for greater exposure to these important indicators of the social environment among older adults. Indeed, the results suggest that there is opportunity for intervention at numerous points throughout the end of the lifespan, and different dimensions of the social environment may be more critical at different points of the lifespan. For example, this study showed that neighborhood support was important for self-rated health among the oldest-old. A possible means of building support could be through programs that help establish connections between neighbors who have volunteered to assist with those who need assistance. Although this type of intervention may appear intrusive, the need for assistance among elders is increasingly recognized and accepted by elders themselves, as well as by family who live at a distance. Additionally, neighbors may not mind helping others if they understand that there is a need, and this is part of the problem they can help to address in their proverbial backyards. Such awareness has grown after infamous events such as the heat waves in Chicago in 1995 [25] and in Paris in 2003 [26] where rates of death were particularly high among the frail elderly. These events highlighted the need for greater awareness of and reaching out to frail neighbors. Neighbors providing assistance present as an alternative to cost-prohibitive home care. Interventions directed at the oldest-old could also incorporate neighborhood trust and neighborhood cohesion, as these were indicators of social capital found to be critical for IADL of the oldest-old. Interventions focused on the oldest-old are mentioned here, yet it is important to point out that each of the indicators of social capital (except telephone interaction) could be incorporated into interventions directed at the young-old and middle-old as well.

From a lifespan perspective, an important question to ask here is when should interventions aimed at increasing social capital be made? For example, should an effort be made to intervene during the middle-old aged years or earlier? Ideally interventions aimed at augmenting an individual's social capital should be implemented early in life, during youth as research has shown that children that volunteer are more likely to volunteer in adulthood and later in life (Oesterle, Johnson, and Mortimer, 2004). Perhaps interventions aimed at building social capital specifically among older adults should be done at or before the point when retirement is being considered. It is possible to conceive of a program, which at the exit job interview puts the individual, who is soon to retire, in connection with volunteer organizations in the community. In this way, the program helps build a bridge between the individual and their community, and so the older adult can start to build social capital through volunteering in the community.

When considering interventions aimed at building social capital, the geographic context should also be taken into account. The sample of older adults in this study resided is urban and suburban settings of five counties of southeastern Pennsylvania. Philadelphia, the county with the highest proportion of older adults (namely, 39% of sample), represented a highly urbanized context while the other four counties reflected mostly suburban settings. Pathways that link social capital and health may differ according to geographic context [27]. These authors describe characteristics of urbanization such as crime, minority, inequality, and population stability that may influence social capital and health. Specifically, Pridmore and colleagues write, "Poor urban settlements require special interventions to address social exclusion, disruption of social networks and trust, insecurity and violence, and high mortality and morbidity" [27, p. i138]. Ultimately, the context in which the individual lives requires consideration when developing interventions aimed at building social capital. Furthermore, the level at which the intervention is to be provided must also be taken into account. For example, the approach will be different if the intervention is to occur at the individual or microlevel, city or mesolevel, or the macrolevel.

8.1. Limitations of the Study. An important limitation of this study is that the data is based on a cross-sectional design. This means that definitive statements about causality cannot be made. Most likely the association between social capital and health is bidirectional, as has been demonstrated in previous research [28]. Some additional limitations to be considered when interpreting the findings: first and foremost, size of the sample for the oldest-old was fairly small ($N = 266$) compared to the young-old ($N = 1233$) and the middle-old ($N = 845$). These sample sizes were further reduced in the regression models. Small sample size of the oldest-old cohort may have limited the power of the statistical significance tests. This may explain the nonsignificant models for self-rated health and ADL for oldest-old. This also brings up the important consideration regarding survival. In other words, those examined in this study represented those who were by default healthier and had chosen to stay aging in place. Another limitation was that the definition and measurement of social capital remain elusive. As was found in this study, not all the measures used were associated with health, specifically telephone interaction. We continue to need a better understanding of how to best measure social capital. Furthermore, as Nyqvist and colleagues have stated:, "It is generally assumed that social capital indicators measure the same thing in different groups and places" [12, p. 105]. However, research has demonstrated that there are marked differences in the questions about social capital that are considered appropriate for various groups depending, for instance, on the subjects' age [29].

It is also important to note that the effect sizes for the analyses were somewhat low, given the small R^2 findings. However, because this study employed nonparametric techniques for estimation, it can be problematic to rely too heavily on these measures of linear fit. Despite these concerns, the results do clearly indicate that community-level neighborhood social capital does have a relationship to health for elders, even when including important individual-level factors. This speaks to the mezzo- and macrolevel implications of these findings and warrants further investigation in research.

8.2. Considerations for Future Research. This research clearly calls for use of longitudinal data as this could provide answers regarding causality as age increases, in the hope of developing age-sensitive interventions across the lifespan. These findings also need to be replicated with larger sample sizes, especially for the oldest-old group. Furthermore, as highlighted above, the geographic context needs to be given greater focus in future research. Also, in response to Nyqvist and colleagues' concerns, there is a need for social capital scale development that reflects the specific characteristics of older persons. Furthermore, questions asking whether residents plan to move in the near future and why should be included in order to get a better understanding of how the social environment might impact decisions leading to moving away from one's neighborhood. Finally, based on the findings of this study certain dimensions of the social environment (namely, trust, cohesion, support, and participation) were found to be associated with health at different parts of the aging lifespan. However, the question still remains as how does one build, for example, trust and cohesion? Successful implementation of programs that build social capital should also take into consideration individual characteristics, such as gender, race, and economic status that may influence the relationship between social capital and health. Finally, impact of social capital on the individual needs to be examined in the light of Lawton's environmental docility and environmental proactivity distinction. In other words, as age progresses how do different dimensions of the social environment either benefit or impede functioning? Ultimately, there continues to be a need to refine the person-environment fit model over the lifespan [30].

Conflict of Interests

The authors declare that there is no conflict of interests regarding the publication of this paper.

References

[1] PHMC, "CHDB report: measuring the correlation between social connectedness and health," in *Directions Winter 2010-2011*, 2010, http://www.phmc.org/site/index.php?option=com_content&view=category&layout=blog&id=62&Itemid=1623.

[2] J. Lomas, "Social capital and health: implications for public health and epidemiology," *Social Science and Medicine*, vol. 47, no. 9, pp. 1181–1188, 1998.

[3] I. Kawachi, S. V. Subramanian, and D. Kim, *Social Capital and Health*, Springer Science + Business Media, New York, NY, USA, 2008.

[4] C. A. Emlet and J. T. Moceri, "The importance of social connectedness in building age-friendly communities," *Journal of Aging Research*, vol. 2012, Article ID 173247, 9 pages, 2012.

[5] R. Putnam, "Bowling alone: America's declining social capital," *Journal of Democracy*, vol. 6, no. 1, pp. 65–78, 1995.

[6] M. T. Hyyppa, "Definitions and forms of social capital," in *Healthy Ties: Social Capital, Population Health and Survival*, T. M. Hyyppa, Ed., pp. 9–17, Springer, London, UK, 2010.

[7] G. Gwyther, *Social Capital and Communitarianism*, Sociological Sites/Sights, Finders University, Adelaide, Australia, 2000, http://www.tasa.org.au/docs/conferences/2000_10/171100%20Gwyther.pdf.

[8] C. Stephens, "Social capital in its place: using social theory to understand social capital and inequalities in health," *Social Science and Medicine*, vol. 66, no. 5, pp. 1174–1184, 2008.

[9] F. Axler, L. Kotranski, G. Klein, D. Levengood, I. Stalberg, and R. Wilcox, *Social Capital and Health: Does a Relationship Exist?* PHMC, Philadelphia, Pa, USA, 2002, http://www.chdbdata.org/uploads/datareports/APHA%20Presentation.pdf.

[10] J. A. Norstrand, A. Glicksman, J. Lubben, and M. Kleban, "The role of the social environment on physical and mental health of older adults," *Journal of Housing for the Elderly*, vol. 26, no. 1–3, pp. 290–307, 2012.

[11] K. A. Cagney and M. Wen, "Social capital and aging-related outcomes," in *Social Capital and Health*, I. Kawachi, S. V. Subramanian, and D. Kim, Eds., pp. 239–258, Springer Science + Business Media, New York, NY, USA, 2008.

[12] F. Nyqvist, J. Gustavsson, and Y. Gustafson, "Social capital and health in the oldest old: the Umeå 85+ study," *International Journal of Ageing and Later Life*, vol. 1, no. 1, pp. 91–114, 2006.

[13] T. C. Antonucci, K. S. Birditt, and H. Akiyama, "Convoys of social relations: an interdisciplinary approach," in *Handbook of Theories of Aging*, V. L. Bengston, D. Gans, N. M. Putney, and M. Silverstein, Eds., pp. 247–259, Springer, New York, NY, USA, 2nd edition, 2009.

[14] J. A. Burr, F. G. Caro, and J. Moorhead, "Productive aging and civic participation," *Journal of Aging Studies*, vol. 16, no. 1, pp. 87–105, 2002.

[15] C. Gilleard, M. Hyde, and P. Higgs, "The impact of age, place, aging in place, and attachment to place on the well-being of the over 50s in England," *Research on Aging*, vol. 29, no. 6, pp. 590–605, 2007.

[16] L. de Donder, N. de Witte, T. Buffel, S. Dury, and D. Verté, "Social capital and feelings of unsafety in later life: a study of the influence of social networks, place attachment, and civic participation on perceived safety in Belgium," *Research on Aging*, vol. 34, no. 4, pp. 425–448, 2012.

[17] Census Bureau, *The Older Population: 2010*, 2010 Census Briefs, 2011, http://www.census.gov/prod/cen2010/briefs/c2010br-09.pdf.

[18] Census Bureau, "Table S0103: population 65 years and over in the United States," 2010 American Community Survey 1-Year Estimates, 2010, http://factfinder2.census.gov/faces/tableservices/jsf/pages/productview.xhtml?pid=ACS_10_1YR_S0103&prodType=table.

[19] PHMC, *Community Health Data Base*, PHMC, Philadelphia, Pa, USA, 2010, http://www.chdbdata.org/.

[20] Kennedy School of Government, *Social Capital Community Benchmark Survey*, Kennedy School of Government, Cambridge, UK, 2000, http://www.hks.harvard.edu/saguaro/communitysurvey/.

[21] Elder Economic Security Initiative, "The elder economic security standard Index for Pennsylvania," 2008, http://www.wow-online.org/pdf/WOW_PA_Index_FINAL.pdf.

[22] R. L. Kahn and T. C. Antonucci, "Convoys over the life course: attachment, roles and social support," in *Life-Span Development and Behavior*, P. B. Baltes and O. Brim, Eds., vol. 3, pp. 253–286, Academic Press, New York, NY, USA, 1980.

[23] J. E. Lubben and M. W. Gironda, "Centrality of social ties to the health and well-being of older adults," in *Social Work and Health Care in an Aging World*, B. Berkman and L. K. Harooytan, Eds., pp. 319–350, Springer, New York, NY, USA, 2003.

[24] J. Karuza, "Social support," in *Practice of Geriatrics*, E. H. Duthie, P. R. Katz, and M. L. Malone, Eds., pp. 53–59, Saunders Elsevier, Philadelphia, Pa, USA, 2007.

[25] E. Klinenberg, *Heat Wave: A Social Autopsy of Disaster in Chicago*, University of Chicago Press, Chicago, Ill, USA, 2002.

[26] J.-F. Dhainaut, Y.-E. Claessens, C. Ginsburg, and B. Riou, "Unprecedented heat-related deaths during the 2003 heat wave in Paris: consequences on emergency departments," *Critical Care*, vol. 8, no. 1, pp. 1–2, 2004.

[27] P. Pridmore, L. Thomas, K. Havemann, J. Sapag, and L. Wood, "Social capital and healthy urbanization in a globalized world," *Journal of Urban Health*, vol. 84, no. 1, pp. i130–i143, 2007.

[28] N. Sirven and T. Debrand, "Social capital and health of older Europeans: causal pathways and health inequalities," *Social Science and Medicine*, vol. 75, no. 7, pp. 1288–1295, 2012.

[29] V. Cattell and R. Herring, "Social capital, generations and health in East London," in *Social Capital for Health: Insights from Qualitative Research*, C. Swann and A. Morgan, Eds., Health Development Agency, London, UK, 2002.

[30] W. A. Satariano, "Aging, health, and the environment: an ecological model," in *Epidemiology of Aging: An Ecological Approach*, W. A. Satariano, Ed., pp. 39–84, Jones & Bartlett Learning, 2006.

9

A Brief Report on the Factor Structure of the Cognitive Measures in the HRS/AHEAD Studies

A. Nayena Blankson[1] and John J. McArdle[2]

[1] *Department of Psychology, Spelman College, 350 Spelman Lane S. W., Box 259, Atlanta, GA 30314, USA*
[2] *Department of Psychology, University of Southern California, 711 Seeley G. Mudd Building, Los Angeles, CA 90089, USA*

Correspondence should be addressed to A. Nayena Blankson; ablanksl@spelman.edu

Academic Editor: F. R. Ferraro

Using cognitive data from the Health and Retirement Study and Asset Health Dynamics Among the Oldest Old studies that were collected between 1992 and 2004, McArdle and colleagues (2007) found that a two-factor model (episodic memory and mental status) fit better than a one-factor model. The question that was addressed in the present study was whether these results would replicate in newer cohorts of data, collected between 2006 and 2010. We also tested age, education, and gender as predictors of the identified factors. Results confirm that a two-factor structure fits better than the single-factor model in the newer cohorts. Differential predictors were also observed.

1. Introduction

The measurement of intelligence is an important area of research in psychology and, with the increased longevity among Americans, cognitive aging has become a pertinent issue. Studies of cognition in older individuals can lead to increased understanding of the role of cognitive decline in everyday functioning among an increasingly aging population. However, in most investigations, the measurement of cognitive abilities is often treated as a unitary construct—usually referred to as general intelligence or general cognitive functioning. There is now considerable evidence to challenge that simplified view: a one-factor theory of intelligence does not explain many important observed relationships between intelligence and other variables (see [1], for a review). This finding has been observed in many previous investigations. In particular, recent research by McArdle et al. [2] examined the factor structure underlying the cognitive measures in the Health and Retirement Study (HRS) and Asset Health Dynamics Among the Oldest Old (AHEAD) studies. Results provided support for a two-factor model, one factor representing mental status and the second factor representing episodic memory. The purpose of the present study was to determine whether results obtained by McArdle et al. [2] would replicate to a new cohort of data. Additionally, we examined several demographic variables as predictors of the identified factors.

2. Literature Review

For over 100 years, researchers have investigated the measurement of cognitive abilities, from populations ranging from infancy to older ages. With increased longevity of individuals, strengthening our ability to measure cognitive skills of older individuals will help to facilitate research on predictors and outcomes associated with cognitive aging at older ages. The HRS and AHEAD studies have been one of the most widely used data sets in addressing research questions associated with cognition in the older ages. For example, Suthers et al. [3] investigated the link between life expectancy and cognitive impairment. Moody-Ayers et al. [4] examined the effect of cognitive functioning on functional decline. Not often considered in past research was the factor structure underlying the cognitive measures. Yet, more recent research on intelligence and cognition has shown that there is added value in determining whether we are measuring one and only one factor or multiple factors. Such arguments have at their roots the work of Spearman [5], which suggested that all human abilities can primarily be classified under one factor, and the work of Cattell [6] and Horn [1], which suggested that multiple intelligences better represent human cognition. The accumulated evidence to date supports a multiple-factor theory. Thus, it is important to consider whether a multiple-factor theory will also obtain in measures of cognition in the older ages.

Using cognitive data from the HRS and AHEAD studies, McArdle et al. [2] found that a two-factor model (episodic memory and mental status) fit better than a one-factor model. Since the publication of that paper, three new cohorts have been added to the data. Thus, a question remains as to whether conclusions reached by McArdle et al. that were based on data collected between 1992 and 2004 are generalizable to the newer cognitive data set, collected between 2006 and 2010. According to Lykken [7], constructive replication is when original hypotheses are tested with new methodology. Constructive replication helps to provide stronger support for a theory by demonstrating that conclusions are not restricted to a specific method. The present analyses serve as a replication of the research conducted by McArdle et al. That is, in the present investigation we test hypotheses tested by McArdle et al. [2] using more recent data. Specifically, we tested (1) whether a 2-factor model fits better than a 1-factor model and (2) age, education, and gender as the predictors of the identified factors. These variables have been extensively studied in past research as predictors of cognition. Therefore, inclusion of these same predictors in the present analyses is of scientific import.

The Health and Retirement Study (HRS) and Asset Health Dynamics Among the Oldest Old (AHEAD) studies began in 1992 and 1993, respectively, and in 1998 were combined into one study that attempts to be nationally representative of Americans over 50 years of age. The studies use a panel design in which the same respondents are interviewed every two years, and new respondents are added to the sample every six years to replenish the sample to adjust for aging and attrition (see [8, 9]; http://hrsonline.isr.umich.edu/).

The cognitive performance tests in the HRS/AHEAD studies measuring episodic memory and mental status were used in the present study. Specifically, the immediate and delayed free recall tasks have been found to measure an episodic memory factor while a mental status factor is comprised of the serial 7s, counting backward from 20, naming, and dates tasks. For the immediate and delayed recall tasks, respondents are asked to recall a list of nouns read by an interviewer immediately and after a 5-minute delay [10]. Random assignment was used within time points to assign the list of words for recall. For the serial 7s task, participants are asked to subtract 7 from 100 across 5 trials. On the counting backward task, individuals count backward from 20 for 10 continuous numbers. For the names task, respondents state the US president and vice president by last name and name two objects (scissors and cactus). Finally, for the dates task, respondents provide the current date (month, day, year, and day of week). These tests were adapted from the Telephone Interview of Cognitive Status (TICS; [11]), which itself was adapted for telephone administration from the Mini-Mental State Exam (MMSE; [12]). Though the MMSE is one of the most widely used quick screen measures of cognition for diagnosing cognitive impairment, the HRS cognitive measures can be argued to be among the most widely used measures for assessing cognition in older individuals for research purposes, given the sample size of the HRS data. Thus, the HRS data provide a rich source of information on cognitive aging in the US. The data have been used extensively in the past, and it is anticipated that the data will continue to be used to study cognitive declines and their correlates among older individuals in the US. The present research will therefore inform researchers on the best practices for use of these data in addressing questions regarding cognitive functioning among older Americans.

3. Method

3.1. Participants. The HRS is a nationally representative longitudinal study sponsored by the National Institute on Aging and conducted by the University of Michigan. The HRS researchers targeted community-dwelling adults in the contiguous United States who were 51 to 61 years old in 1992, when the baseline interview was conducted. Blacks, Hispanics, and Florida residents were oversampled (for details, see [8]). In 1993 and 1995, the AHEAD study was conducted among a national sample of adults aged 70 or older. In 1998, the HRS and AHEAD studies merged, both assuming the name HRS, and two new cohorts were added to the HRS sampling frame. New cohorts are added every two years.

For the present study, we used data collected from Waves 8 (2006) through 10 (2010). More specifically, as part of the data cleaning process, previous researchers (i.e., [13]) imputed missing cognitive data for participants using a multivariate, regression-based procedure using Imputation and Variance Estimation (IVEware) software. Our initial sample ($N = 361$) is compromised of those participants from the 2006 to 2010 waves who had data (imputed or self-respondent) available on the cognitive variables of interest. We then eliminated any person who had a sampling weight of zero ($n = 133$) or missing data on the cognitive variables at the first occasion of testing ($n = 11$), resulting in the subsample of 217 respondents described in Table 1. The demographic variables presented in this table include (a) chronological age at baseline testing, (b) years of formal education, and (c) gender.

3.2. Measures. The cognitive performance tests in the HRS/AHEAD included immediate and delayed free recall, serial 7s, counting backwards from 20, naming the US president and vice president by last name, naming two objects (scissors and cactus), and providing the date (month, day, year, and day of week). For the recall tasks, participants recalled a list of 10 words. Individuals received a score of 1 point for each word recalled correctly. Regarding the serial 7s task, the respondents were asked to start from the number 100 and subtract 7 continuously, for up to 5 trials. Participants received 1 point for each correct subtraction among the 5 trials, with each subtraction scored independently. For the

TABLE 1: Sample demographics at initial testing.

	Age in years	Years of education	Female (%)
M	66.63	13.12	47
SD	9.25	2.88	0.50
Minimum	52.00	0.00	0 = male
Maximum	93.00	17.00	1 = female

counting backward task, participants received two trials, in which they were required to count backward from 20 for 10 continuous numbers. If participants responded correctly on the first trial, they received 2 points. If participants were correct on the second try, they received 1 point. Individuals who failed on both opportunities received 0 points. For the names task, respondents had to name the current US president and vice president by last name and name two objects. Each of the 4 names was scored independently, with 1 point for correct responses and 0 points for incorrect responses, and a total score was computed across the 4. Finally, for the dates task, respondents had to provide the current date (month, day, year, and day of week). Similar to the scoring of the names task, each of the 4 aspects of the date received 1 point for a correct answer and 0 points for an incorrect answer, and a total score was computed across the 4 dates.

To provide comparability across all scales and to simplify measurement for further statistical analysis, we scaled each variable into percent correct scores (i.e., based on division by the maximum score and multiplication by 100). The serial 7s, backward counting, dates, and names tasks were all skewed and therefore treated as categorical variables in the analyses.

3.3. Data Analyses. Substantive analyses included confirmatory factor analyses conducted to test the 1- and the 2-factor models and latent factor path modeling, to examine age, education, and gender as predictors of cognition. For the 2-factor model, the first factor was marked by two continuous variables (immediate recall and delayed recall), while the second factor was marked by four categorical variables (serial 7s, backward counting, dates, and names). Weighted least squares with mean and variance adjusted (WLSMV) estimation was used to account for the skewed categorical variables. Use of WLSMV estimation has been found to perform better than maximum likelihood estimation when data are categorical [14]. Delta parameterization was employed so that scale factors could be modeled for the categorical variables. Factors were identified by fixing the loadings for immediate recall and serial 7s at unity. Analyses were conducted using Mplus 7.0 [15]. In all analyses, goodness-of-fit indices were used to make decisions about the accuracy of the models. More specifically, overall χ^2 is presented and we also rely on the root-mean square error of approximation (RMSEA; [16, 17]) and comparative fit index (CFI; [18]) for the assessment of good fit. As a rule of thumb, RMSEA values smaller than 0.10 [16] and CFI values above 0.95 [19] were considered favorable although CFI values above 0.90 are tenable [18] and are still a widely used cut-off [20].

TABLE 2: Descriptive statistics for cognitive measures at initial testing.

Statistic	IR	DR	S7	BC	DA	NA
M	53.96	42.49	70.69	96.77	94.35	91.71
SD	16.58	19.56	31.39	17.71	11.78	14.84
Min	10	0	0	0	50	25
Max	100	100	100	100	100	100
Skewness	0.27	0.10	−0.74	−5.33	−1.97	−1.75
Kurtosis	0.22	0.14	−0.69	27.67	3.14	2.60

Note: IR: immediate recall; DR: delayed recall; S7: serial 7s; BC: backward counting; DA: dates; NA: names.

TABLE 3: Correlations among cognitive measures.

Variable	1	2	3	4	5
(1) Immediate recall	—				
(2) Delayed recall	0.76**	—			
(3) Serial 7s	0.27**	0.27**	—		
(4) Backward counting	0.08	0.09	0.06	—	
(5) Dates	0.26**	0.33**	0.26**	0.13*	—
(6) Names	0.20**	0.27**	0.36**	0.21**	0.33**

** $P < 0.01$.
* $P < 0.05$.

Once we establish the underlying factor structure among the cognitive variables, then we can begin to address questions regarding predictors of cognition in older ages. To address this question, the latent factors were regressed on age, education, and gender.

4. Results

Summary statistics on all cognitive data are presented in Table 2 and in Table 3 are the correlations among the cognitive variables. This information is based on the cognitive variables at the first time of testing for all participants. Immediate recall (IR) had an average near 50% but the delayed recall (DR) scale was somewhat harder. Backward counting (BC), dates (DA), and names (NA) had over 90% correct response rate and were negatively skewed.

Next, confirmatory factor modeling was applied to test the 1-factor versus 2-factor hypothesis. The 2-factor model fit better. The fit of the 1-factor model was chi-square = 53 (df = 9); CFI = 0.79; RMSEA = 0.15 (95% CI = 0.19; 0.19). The fit of the 2-factor model was chi-square = 20 (df = 8); CFI = 0.94; RMSEA = 0.08 (95% CI = 0.04; 0.13). Standardized factor loadings for the 1- and 2-factor models are displayed in Table 4.

Results of the latent factor path model predicting the two factors are shown in Table 5. Results revealed significant age and education effects for episodic memory. However, gender differences were observed only for episodic memory but not mental status.

5. Discussion

Recent research in cognitive aging has focused on determining the factor structure underlying cognitive tests. More

TABLE 4: Standardized loadings from confirmatory factor analyses.

	Memory			Mental status[a]		
	IR	DR	S7	BC	DA	NA
One-factor model						
Loading	0.78	0.84	0.49	0.20	0.72	0.62
Uniqueness	0.40	0.30	0.76	0.96	0.49	0.62
Two-factor model						
Loading	0.90	0.90	0.57	0.28	0.86	0.72
Uniqueness	0.19	0.19	0.67	0.91	0.27	0.48

[a]Uniqueness parameters estimated from thresholds.

TABLE 5: Parameter estimates for prediction of two factors (standardized estimates in parentheses).

Factor predictor	Episodic memory	Mental status
Age	−0.44 (−0.24)**	−0.02 (−0.22)*
Education	1.96 (0.34)**	0.11 (0.47)**
Female	8.58 (0.28)**	−0.19 (−0.15)

$^{**}P < 0.01$.
$^{*}P < 0.05$.

specifically, research by McArdle et al. [2] suggested that a 2-factor structure was a better fit to the cognitive tests in the HRS/AHEAD study than a 1-factor structure. The present study served as a replication of the McArdle et al. analyses by testing the factor structure in data collected between 2006 and 2010. Additionally, we tested age, education, and gender as predictors of the obtained factors. Results provided support for the 2-factor model, consistent with McArdle et al. [2].

The primary question that was addressed in the present investigation was whether the 2-factor structure would hold up in the new cohorts, and results indicate that this is indeed the case. Moreover, examination of the predictors of the factors indicates that while age and education predict both factors, gender predicted only the episodic memory factor. Younger individuals were found to perform better than the older participants, as did those with higher levels of education. Thus, in using these cognitive tests for research or clinical purposes, it is important to take these variables into consideration. Females were also found to perform better on the test of episodic memory than were males, but this same gender difference was not observed for mental status. The differential effects of gender on the two factors highlight the importance of considering the cognitive tests using a multiple-factor framework rather than a single-factor framework in future research.

Rarely are results replicated and published in research. Often, the argument is made that the replicated results do not add new information to the literature and, therefore, most replication studies go unpublished. Yet, it is through replication that we can enhance our understanding regarding various psychological phenomena, particularly because most of the research conducted in the fields of psychology and gerontology is correlational in nature. Thus, the primary aim of the present research presents an inherent strength of the study. Despite this strength, however, there is the limitation of the small sample size of the current data, precluding such tests such as invariance of measurement across groups. Nevertheless, the results indicate that researchers should use a 2-factor representation of the cognitive data rather than the 1-factor representation in future research. Moreover, because the tests that were examined in the present research are an adaptation of the Mini-Mental State Exam, these results also suggest that it may be of benefit to consider the 2 components as separate aspects of cognitive functioning in clinical screening of patients.

Conflict of Interests

The authors declare that there is no conflict of interests regarding the publication of this paper.

Acknowledgment

The authors thank the National Institute on Aging for a MERIT award to the second author (Grant no. AG-007137-21) for the support of this research.

References

[1] J. L. Horn and A. N. Blankson, "Foundations for better understanding of cognitive abilities," in *Contemporary Intellectual Assessment: Theories, Tests, and Issues*, D. P. Flanagan and P. L. Harrison, Eds., The Guilford Press, New York, NY, USA, 3rd edition, 2012.

[2] J. J. McArdle, G. G. Fisher, and K. M. Kadlec, "Latent variable analyses of age trends of cognition in the health and retirement Study, 1992–2004," *Psychology and Aging*, vol. 22, no. 3, pp. 525–545, 2007.

[3] K. Suthers, J. K. Kim, and E. Crimmins, "Life expectancy with cognitive impairment in the older population of the United States," *Journals of Gerontology B: Psychological Sciences and Social Sciences*, vol. 58, no. 3, pp. S179–S186, 2003.

[4] S. Y. Moody-Ayers, K. M. Mehta, K. Lindquist, L. Sands, and K. E. Covinsky, "Black-white disparities in functional decline in older persons: the role of cognitive function," *Journals of Gerontology A: Biological Sciences and Medical Sciences*, vol. 60, no. 7, pp. 933–939, 2005.

[5] C. Spearman, "General intelligence: objectively determined and measured," *The American Journal of Psychology*, vol. 15, pp. 201–292, 1904.

[6] R. B. Cattell, "Some theoretical issues in adult intelligence testing," *Psychological Bulletin*, vol. 38, article 592, 1941.

[7] D. T. Lykken, "Statistical significance in psychological research," *Psychological Bulletin*, vol. 70, no. 3, pp. 151–159, 1968.

[8] S. G. Heeringa and J. H. Connor, *Technical Description of the Health and Retirement Study Sample Design*, Institute for Social Research Pub. DR-002, University of Michigan, Ann Arbor, Mich, USA, 1996.

[9] C. Leacock, Ed., *Getting Started with the Health and Retirement Study, Version 1. 0*, Survey Research Center, Institute of Social Research, University of Michigan, Ann Arbor, Mich, USA, 2006.

[10] M. B. Ofstedal, G. G. Fisher, and A. R. Herzog, "Documentation of cognitive functioning measures in the Health and Retirement

Study," HRS/AHEAD Documentation Report DR-006, University of Michigan, Ann Arbor, Mich, USA, 2005.

[11] J. Brandt, M. Spencer, and M. Folstein, "The telephone interview for cognitive status," *Neuropsychiatry, Neuropsychology and Behavioral Neurology*, vol. 1, no. 2, pp. 111–117, 1988.

[12] M. F. Folstein, S. E. Folstein, and P. R. McHugh, "Mini-Mental State: a practical method for grading the cognitive state of patients for the clinician," *Journal of Psychiatric Research*, vol. 12, pp. 189–198, 1975.

[13] G. G. Fisher, H. Hassan, W. L. Rodgers, and D. R. Weir, *Health and Retirement Study Imputation of Cognitive Functioning Measures: 1992–2010 Early Release*, University of Michigan, Ann Arbor, Mich, USA, 2012.

[14] A. Beauducel and P. Y. Herzberg, "On the performance of maximum likelihood versus means and variance adjusted weighted least squares estimation in CFA," *Structural Equation Modeling*, vol. 13, no. 2, pp. 186–203, 2006.

[15] L. K. Muthén and B. O. Muthén, *Mplus User's Guide*, Muthén & Muthén, Los Angeles, Calif, USA, 1998–2012.

[16] M. A. Browne and R. Cudeck, "Alternative ways of assessing model fit," in *Testing Structural Equation Models*, K. A. Bollen and J. S. Long, Eds., Chapter 6, pp. 136–162, Sage, Newbury Park, Calif, USA, 1993.

[17] J. H. Steiger and J. C. Lind, "Statistically-based tests for the number of common factors," in *Proceedings of the Annual Spring Meeting of the Psychometric Society*, Iowa City, Iowa, USA, 1980.

[18] P. M. Bentler, "Comparative fit indexes in structural models," *Psychological Bulletin*, vol. 107, no. 2, pp. 238–246, 1990.

[19] L.-T. Hu and P. M. Bentler, "Cutoff criteria for fit indexes in covariance structure analysis: conventional criteria versus new alternatives," *Structural Equation Modeling*, vol. 6, no. 1, pp. 1–55, 1999.

[20] R. J. Van Lieshout, K. Cleverley, J. M. Jenkins, and K. Georgiades, "Assessing the measurement invariance of the Center for Epidemiologic Studies Depression Scale across immigrant and non-immigrant women in the postpartum period," *Archives of Women's Mental Health*, vol. 14, no. 5, pp. 413–423, 2011.

10

Robotics to Enable Older Adults to Remain Living at Home

Alan J. Pearce,[1,2] Brooke Adair,[2] Kimberly Miller,[2] Elizabeth Ozanne,[3] Catherine Said,[2] Nick Santamaria,[4] and Meg E. Morris[2,5]

[1] *Cognitive and Exercise Neuroscience Unit, School of Psychology, Deakin University, Melbourne, VIC, Australia*
[2] *Department of Physiotherapy, The University of Melbourne, Melbourne, VIC, Australia*
[3] *Department of Social Work, The University of Melbourne, Melbourne, VIC, Australia*
[4] *Department of Nursing, The University of Melbourne and Royal Melbourne Hospital, Melbourne, VIC, Australia*
[5] *School of Allied Health, La Trobe University, Melbourne, VIC, Australia*

Correspondence should be addressed to Meg E. Morris, m.morris@latrobe.edu.au

Academic Editor: Roger A. Fielding

Given the rapidly ageing population, interest is growing in robots to enable older people to remain living at home. We conducted a systematic review and critical evaluation of the scientific literature, from 1990 to the present, on the use of robots in aged care. The key research questions were as follows: (1) what is the range of robotic devices available to enable older people to remain mobile, independent, and safe? and, (2) what is the evidence demonstrating that robotic devices are effective in enabling independent living in community dwelling older people? Following database searches for relevant literature an initial yield of 161 articles was obtained. Titles and abstracts of articles were then reviewed by 2 independent people to determine suitability for inclusion. Forty-two articles met the criteria for question 1. Of these, 4 articles met the criteria for question 2. Results showed that robotics is currently available to assist older healthy people and people with disabilities to remain independent and to monitor their safety and social connectedness. Most studies were conducted in laboratories and hospital clinics. Currently limited evidence demonstrates that robots can be used to enable people to remain living at home, although this is an emerging smart technology that is rapidly evolving.

1. Introduction

Throughout the world rapid population ageing is occurring, with a large proportion of older adults preferring to stay living at home [1]. Most older people experience one to three chronic diseases [2] and, in very advanced age, frailty, disability, and social isolation are common. At the same time there are increasing demands on health service providers due to the low availability of home and community services, low uptake of e-health and smart technologies by healthcare professionals, and an ageing health workforce [3]. Although many older people express their desire to stay in the familiar social environment of their own home [4], many cannot do so due to impairments, immobility and social isolation. Many older people who live at home are at high risk of falls and injuries and report difficulty accessing health care services when they need them [5].

As previously discussed by Rowe and Kahn [6] the definition of successful aging requires three pillars. Firstly, there is a low probably of disease and/or disability from disease; secondly a high cognitive and physical functioning capacity; and three, the combination of the first two with an active engagement in life. In affecting successful aging, particularly with the nexus to an active engagement in life, there is a need for development of, and access to, smart technologies to monitor and maintain health and wellbeing, as well as to link older people with communities and health-care professionals. One area where technology is rapidly advancing is robotics. Robots are now available that provide services such as home cleaning, appliance operation, and safety monitoring. These "service robots" can be excellent for monitoring, surveillance, and basic tasks of everyday living yet they lack artificial intelligence. Morris et al. [3] argued the need for "smart" robotic technologies that not only respond to an individual's needs, but can also learn and modify their behaviour based upon their owner's requirements. This is particularly the case for older individuals who would need to interact with their robot to maintain mobility, health, safety, and social connectedness.

Service robots currently include commercialised domestic robots, such as self-navigating vacuum cleaners and mops, known as Roomba and Scooba respectively [7]. Service robots also include "pet" or sociable robots, such as the Aibo robotic pet dog, Paro the robotic pet seal, and similar robotic animals that use "pet therapy" to assist older people to maintain mobility, and to keep active [8]. Service robots have also been developed for hospital settings. One example of this is the iWARD project in Germany [9] where modular designed robots have been adapted for different roles for independent living, health, and safety. They can also act in a team to service the needs of medical and other health professional staff such as for remote consultations and communication between staff in different wards.

The literature reveals some misconceptions about the potential for robotic interaction with humans. For example, popular opinion holds that robotic technologies are only applied to individuals when they are disabled [10]. However, there is a small yet increasing awareness that robotic technologies can also complement current health care service provision by monitoring older people within their home environment [11] and assisting them to mobilise safely and prevent falls [12]. Narrative literature reviews on the role of robotics in health care [8, 11–13] or social assistance robots [14] have previously been completed mainly speculating about the future of robotics in health. The aim of this systematic review was to identify specific evidence-based research answering questions to address the potential of robotic technologies to monitor older individuals' health and wellbeing and to assist with activities of daily living. Another aim was to review the extent of robotic technologies currently tested and used in the home environment for older individuals.

2. Methods

We identified two key questions for the systematic review of the literature addressing robotics and ageing in the home environment.

(1) What is the range of robotic devices available to enable older people to remain mobile, independent and safe?

(2) What is the evidence demonstrating that robotic devices are effective in enabling independent living in community dwelling older people?

Where possible, in each database, searches for all topics were limited to peer-reviewed publications between January 1990–February 2012, published in English. We included human participants aged 45 years and older, as it is generally accepted that many chronic conditions may have their onset from approximately this age onwards. This broader definition of older individuals' was adopted by the authors, defined by MESH heading definitions of "middle-aged" 45–64 years, "aged" (65–79 years) and "aged 80+ years" with the understanding that "older individuals" were a heterogeneous group. The authors also accepted the definition of a "home" setting as the individual's place of residence [15]. This included establishments providing residence and care for special needs, such as retirement villages and aged care facilities providing low care services, service integrated housing, and supported accommodation.

To answer question 1, randomised controlled studies, quasi-experimental studies, and comparative studies with and without concurrent controls, case-series and feasibility studies, systematic and general review articles, and government reports (where relevant to topic area) were included to identify available technologies. The following publications were excluded from the paper: narrative reviews, descriptive or narrative papers without presentation of data, limited-review conference proceedings and abstracts, higher degree research theses (PhD/Masters), undergraduate research theses (Honours) and books.

To answer question 2, data extraction and quality assessments were predominantly performed on studies that met the criteria for question 1, however these studies were required to demonstrate that testing and/or data collection had been completed in a home (or simulated) environment.

Data base searches were limited to studies assessing humans and those published in English and included: Web of Science, Science Direct, MEDLINE, PSYCHINFO, SCOPUS, CINAHL, expanded version of the cumulative index to nursing and allied health by *EBSCO*, Australasian Medical Index, National Library for Health, Rehabilitation Research (USA), and TROVE.

Two independent, trained reviewers evaluated the title and abstracts of the yield articles against the decision rules inclusion criteria. The title of each article was scanned and the two reviewers independently excluded articles not related to the topic. The full texts of the articles were then obtained for data extraction, categorized according to National Health and Medical Research Council (NHMRC) guidelines on levels of evidence [16], and the quality of each article was assessed using the Downs and Black [52] quality appraisal tool. Downs and Black was specifically selected to assess the articles as it can be used for both experimental and quasi-experimental research designs. Two independent reviewers conducted data extraction and quality assessment for each article. Lack of agreement about inclusion of articles, data extracted, or grading against quality criteria was reconciled by mutual agreement.

3. Results

Figure 1 illustrates the breakdown of articles following the predetermined inclusion and exclusion criteria. The major reason for exclusion was that articles were descriptive and did not contain data providing evidence of effectiveness, feasibility, or validity. Table 1 shows the studies that have provided evidence of technologies assisting older people.

The yield of articles in response to question 1 showed that robotic technology is currently available to assist older

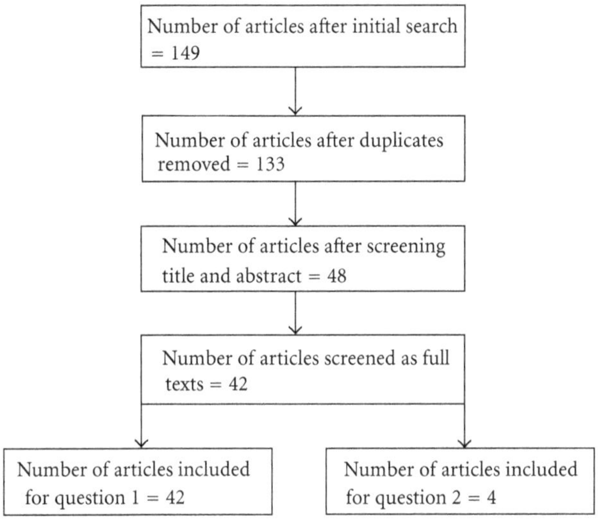

Figure 1: Yield of articles for the robotics literature.

people and people with physical disabilities. These were not "smart" robots per se, with no artificial intelligence interface, and the majority of these articles were lower limb "exoskeleton" technologies. Robotic exoskeletons are fitted to the outside of the limbs, rather than being internally fixed using surgical methods and supplies at the energy (or part of the energy) for limb movement. The "Lokomat" was the most widely tested robotic exoskeleton for the lower limbs [25, 27, 29, 33, 37, 48, 49] to trial its suitability as a supportive structure for walking. Other technologies to assist with walking and mobility included robotic walkers and robotic guidance systems [30, 38]. These systems, such as the "Guido", are extensions on the non-motorised walker frames, where the individual can control the speed of locomotion but also obtain environmental feedback, via sensors, to assist in obstacle avoidance and in navigating through doorways.

Upper limb technologies included both upper limb exoskeleton systems to guide arm movements and haptic visuomotor feedback systems to assist in compensation for disorders of sensation and visual impairment. The "MIT-MANUS", a visuomotor guidance system, was the most utilised of the upper limb robotic systems, particularly for people who were recovering from stroke [17, 19, 21, 24, 35]

Table 2 shows the articles that met the inclusion criteria for question 2. To date, four investigations have tested robots within a home, residential care setting, or simulated home environment. Generally, these studies demonstrated that robots are able to help older people with mobility issues around the home environment. However, this data presented was only low to moderate in terms of their level of evidence and research quality [52]. Shimada et al. [40] investigated the effectiveness of a lower limb exoskeleton device using a pre-post single group design in older healthy females within an independent home living facility. Unlike other lower limb robots, such as the Lokomat which is a relatively large driven gait orthosis that automates locomotion therapy, the exoskeleton technology in this study was smaller and more compact. This study reported improvements in walking speed and reduced energy expenditure (due to fitness gains) following 3 months of 2 sessions (90 minutes duration) per week of assisted walking using the exoskeleton technology with elderly females. Spenko et al. [28] investigated the effectiveness of a robotic personal mobility aid with sensors to guide elderly ambulatory individuals away from obstacles. Analysis of the effectiveness of the technology was difficult to interpret as only descriptive data were presented in the paper. Saeki et al. [32] presented a case study describing the use of an upper limb robotic trainer in an elderly woman two years post hemiparesis. Improvements in motor function were reported in musculature of the proximal arm compared to the distal hand and alterations in cortical representation maps of the affected area were suggestive of plastic adaptations. However, these cortical representation changes were not correlated with changes in movement performance of the hemi paretic upper limb. Finally, a recent study by Carlson and Demiris [51] demonstrated improvements in wheelchair mobility when combined with a robotic interface (collaborative control) compared to when participants had to control the wheelchair manually without robotic assistance. Moreover these authors showed, via self-reported questionnaire, that participants found manoeuvering the wheelchair less mentally demanding during collaborative control.

4. Discussion

This systematic review has highlighted that robotics is still an emerging field in terms of its application to health and rehabilitation for community dwelling older people. Despite these studies being of a lower design quality, the evidence to date shows that robotics research is used widely in engineering laboratories and, to a lesser extent, in clinical settings. Only a very small number of controlled clinical trials evaluated the effects of implementing robotic technology in the home for the purposes of potentially assisting with daily living activities, home care, home maintenance and housework, security, safety, falls detection, or social interaction. Moreover, none of the studies on robotics presented costing of the devices, discussed safety concerns to the user, whether the devices could be mass produced, or social issues such as acceptance by older people in their home environment.

It was also notable that the studies in this paper focussed on application of robotic technologies for purposes of movement rehabilitation in people who had impairments and disabilities arising from conditions such as arthritis, back pain, balance impairment, stroke, or spinal cord injury. To date no studies have objectively measured the potential application of robotic technologies as monitoring devices in the home setting. Potentially artificial intelligence could be used to measure the health status of their "owner," provide reminders for specific medications to be taken; or provide contingency procedures in the case of an adverse event such as a slip, trip, or fall.

One study in this paper demonstrated an increased exercise capacity when healthy older participants utilised a robotic exoskeleton for walking training in a "home" setting [40]; however as the study was limited to only

Table 1: Studies for question 1.

First Author/year	Study Design	Evidence Level [16]	Duration	Setting	Country	Sample size	Age mean	Age range	Characteristics	Gender M	Gender F	Sampling	Technology	Description
Aisen [17] 1997	Intervention study	III-1	Overall duration not stated. Robot trained 4-5 hrs/wk on top of conventional training. Sham trained 1-2 sessions/wk	Hospital rehabilitation clinic	USA	20	§	Robot trained—45–68; Sham trained—38–72	Post-stroke, hemiplegia	11	9	Pseudorandomised	"MIT-MANUS"	Robotic upper limb exoskeleton.
Morvan [18] 1997	Qualitative study	IV	<1 mnth	§	France	28	§	§	Young with either tetraplegia, myopathies or spasticity	#		Not stated	"MASTER" robotic arm system	Psychological preparedness by older people for robots.
Krebs [19] 1998	Intervention study	III-1	Overall duration not stated. Robot trained 4-5 hrs/wk on top of conventional training. Sham trained 1 sessions/wk	Hospital rehabilitation clinic	USA	20	Robot trained—58.5; Sham trained—63	§	§	#		Pseudorandomised	"MIT-MANUS"	Robotic upper limb exoskeleton.
Cozens [20] 1999	Intervention study	III-3	<1 d	Laboratory	England	10	§	47–69	Stroke or MS with upper limb weakness	#		Pseudorandomised	No name provided	Robotic upper limb apparatus.
Volpe [21] 1999	Intervention study	III-1	1 wk treatment, 3 yr follow-up	Hospital rehabilitation clinic	USA	20 total, 12 of 20 mea-sureat 3 yrs	Robot trained—54 ± 3 Sham trained—66 ± 2	§	Post-stroke	7	5	Pseudorandomised	"MIT-MANUS"	Robotic upper limb exoskeleton.
Reinkensmeyer [22] 1999	Intervention study	III-3	<1 d	§	USA	5	§	24–79	Brain injury (TBA/ABI)	#		Convenience	Robotic arm	Arm guidance system.
Burgar [23] 2000	Intervention study (x3)	III-2	1 wk–2 mnths	Laboratory	USA	24	§	21–80	Post-stroke hemiplegia	#		Convenience	MIME	Mirror Image Motion Enabler (MIME).
Volpe [24] 2000	Intervention study	III-1	25 × 1 hr sessions 5 d/wk	Hospital rehabilitation clinic	USA	56	64.5	27–83	Post-stroke hemiplegia	30	26	Randomised control	"MIT-MANUS"	Robotic upper limb exoskeleton.
Jezernik [25] 2003	Intervention study	III-3	2 × 1 hr sessions	Spinal cord injury clinic	Switzerland	6	§	38–73	Spinal cord	#		§	"Lokomat"	Robotic gait exoskeleton.
Loureiro [26] 2003	Intervention study	III-3	9 sessions over 3 wks	Hospital	England	30	§	§	Stroke hemiplegia	#		Randomised control	"GENTLE/S"	Haptic upper limb system.
Rentschler [13] 2003	Technical report	IV	<1 d	Laboratory	USA	1	29	29	Healthy	1	—	Case study	PAMA	Personal adaptive mobility aid (PAMA).
Winchester [27] 2005	Other	III-3	12 wks	Laboratory	USA	4	§	20–49	Spinal cord injury	4	—	Convenience	"Lokomat"	Robotic gait exoskeleton.
Spenko [28] 2006	Other	III-3	<1 d	Laboratory	USA	6	§	85–95	Healthy older	1	5	Convenience	"Smartcane" and "Smart walker"	Walking aid for mobility and monitoring.
Isreal [29] 2006	Other	III-3	5 sessions	Laboratory	USA	12	§	15–59	Spinal cord injury	#		Convenience	"Lokomat"	Robotic gait exoskeleton.

Table 1: Continued.

First Author/year	Study Design	Evidence Level	Duration	Setting	Country	Sample size	Age mean	Age range	Characteristics	Gender M	Gender F	Sampling	Technology	Description
Mehrholz [30] 2007	Systematic review	I [16]	n/a	n/a	n/a	n/a	n/a	n/a	n/a	n/a		n/a	Assisted gait device	Robotic-assisted gait training.
Rocon [31] 2007	Other	III-3	<1 d	Laboratory	Spain	10	52.3	§	Tremor	7	3	Convenience	"WOTAS"	Robotic exoskeleton to reduce arm tremor.
Saeki [32] 2008	Other	IV	6 mnths	Laboratory	Japan	1	48	n/a	Neuro-logical	—	1	N/a	"Bi-Manu-Track"	Robotic arm trainer.
Hidler [33] 2008	Intervention study	III-2	6 mnths	Laboratory	USA	5	44.1	24–59	Spinal cord injury	#		Randomised control	"Lokomat"	Robotic gait exoskeleton.
Janssen and Pringle [34] 2008	Intervention study	III-3	6 wks	Laboratory	USA	12	36	20–70	Spinal cord injury	12	—	Convenience	"ERGYS 1"	Functional electrical stimulator leg ergometry.
Krebs [35] 2008	Intervention study	III-2	6 wks	Rehabilitation clinic	USA	47	57.5	27–79	Stroke	#		Pre-post single group	"MIT-MANUS"	Robotic hand visuomotorguidance system.
Patton [36] 2008	Other	n/a	n/a	n/a	USA	n/a	n/a	n/a	n/a	n/a		n/a	"KineAssist"	Discussion paper on robot to improve balance and gait.
Querry [37] 2008	Intervention study	III-2	<1 d	Laboratory	USA	26	35.5	§	Spinal cord injury	17	9	Non-randomised control	"Lokomat"	Robotic gait exoskeleton.
Rentschler [38] 2008	Intervention study	III-2	1 d	Laboratory	USA	17	85.3	§	Healthy	#		Pseudorandomised	"GUIDO"	Robotic walker.
Galluppi [39] 2009	Intervention study	IV	§	Hospital	Italy	§	§	§	§	#		§	Robotic wheelchair	Collaborative control robotic wheelchair.
Shimada [40] 2009	Intervention study	III-2	<6 mths	Retirement village	Japan	15	78.3	72–85	Healthy	0	15	Convenience	Stride assistance system	Robotic exoskeleton stride assistance system to assist with walking but provide resistance for physical improvement.
Flinn [41] 2009	Case study	IV	6 wks	Hospital	USA	1	48	n/a	Post-stroke	n/a		n/a	"InMotion2"	Upper limb visuomotor guidance system.
Zeng [42] 2009	Intervention study	IV	§	Hospital rehabilitation clinic	Singapore	3	§	16–48	Cerebral palsy/TBI	#		Convenience	Robotic wheelchair	Collaborative control robotic wheelchair.
Lo [43] 2010	Intervention study	II	12 weeks (total of 36 hours training)	Multi-rehabilitation centres	USA	127	64.6	§	>6 months post-stroke	122	5	Random control trial	Modular robotic system (no name) for upper arm guidance.	Modular robotic upper arm guidance system for shoulder, forearm, wrist, and grasping movements.
Frizera Neto [44] 2010	Intervention study	III-3	<1 d	Indoor installation	Spain	5	§	§	Healthy	#		Convenience	"SIMBIOSIS"	Robotic walker—upper body force interaction.
Sharma [45] 2010	Intervention study	III-3	<1 d	Laboratory	USA	19	38.5	§	Healthy	13	6	Convenience	"Drive Safe" smart wheelchairs	Joystick driven, sensor controlled wheelchairs.
Wolpaw [46] 2010	Expert opinion	n/a	n/a	n/a	n/a	n/a	n/a	n/a	n/a	n/a		n/a	Brain-computer interfaces	Opinion based article on the progression in brain-computer interfaces and suggestions on where the technology paradigm should progress.
Galvez [47] 2011	Intervention study	III-3	n/a	Laboratory	USA	4	§	24–62	Spinal cord injury	#		Convenience	Sensor orthoses	Robotic body-weight support treadmill.
Turiel [48] 2011	Intervention study	III-3	1 hr/d, 5 d/wk, 30–45 mins/session	Laboratory	Italy	14	50.6	n/a	Spinal cord injury	10	4	Pre-post single group	"Lokomat"	Robotic gait exoskeleton.

Table 1: Continued.

First Author/year	Study Design	Evidence Level	Duration	Setting	Country	Sample size	Age mean	Age range	Character-istics	Gender M	Gender F	Sampling	Technology	Description
Schwartz [49] 2011	Intervention study	[16] III-3	2-3 times/wk, 30–45 mins/session	Rehabilitaion clinic	Israel	28	42	n/a	Spinal cord injury	18	10	Single group, matched historical control	"Lokomat"	Robotic gait exoskeleton.
Conroy [50] 2011	Intervention study	II	60 mins, 3 times/wk for 6 wks	Laboratory	USA	62	57.8	n/a	Stroke, hemiplegia upper limb	34	28	Random control trial	"InMotion2"	Upper limb visuomotor guidance system. 2D versus 3D including antigravity training, comparing the combination of vertical and planar robot with planar alone.
Carlson and Demiris [51] 2012	Intervention study	III-2	<1 d, 2 × 40 min sessions	Simulated home	England	21	§	17–47	Healthy	#		Convenience	No name	Collaborative controlled robotic wheelchair.

#No gender given, §Not given.

Table 2: Quality evaluation of data driven studies for question 2.

First Author/year	Design	Evidence Level [16]	Duration	Dosage	Setting	Country	Sample size	Age mean	Age range	Character-istics	Gender M	Gender F	Sampling	Key DV	Key measure	Results	Score (max27)* [15]
Spenko [28] 2006	Pilot Interven-tion study	IV	§	§	Residential care	USA	"several"	§	§	§	§	§	§	Distance from wall in meters before the smart-walker changed direction	Motor performance	Good performance outcome using both PAMM technologies. Subjective measures gave less confidence in robotic-controlled walkers to manually controlled walkers.	4
Saeki [32] 2008	Case study	IV	<6 mths	20 mins 2 d/wk for 4 mths	Home	Japan	1	48	§	Neurological	0	1	§	Oxygenated/ deoxygenated/ total haemoglobin level in motor cortex assessed by fMRI technique	Motor assessment scale (modified Ashworth Scale)	Improvement in modified Ashworth motor assessment scale (2 to 5); reduced score on modified Ashworth scale (3 to 2); no change in wrist and fine motor tasks; direct activation of motor area in affected hemisphere.	4
Shimada [40] 2009	Intervention study	III-2	<6 mths	2 × 90 mins/wk for 3 mths	Retirement village	Japan	15	78.3	72–85	Healthy	0	15	Conven-ience	Walking speed	5 m walk test	Increase in walking speed; reduction in energy consumption (lower glucose metabolism)	12
Carlson and Demiris [51] 2012	Intervention study	III-2	<1 d	2 × 40 mins	Simulated "home" environment	England	21	§	17–47	Healthy	§	§	Conven-ience	Wheel-chair control around a simulated home environment	Collision and cognitive perception	Less collisions with robotic assistance and lower scores on perceptions of concentration	13

§ Not given.

*The last question of the Downs and Black assessment tool was excluded due to ambiguity of the question. This meant that the maximum score possible was 27.

one group, with no direct comparison to an age-matched control group who participated in the walking program without the exoskeleton, it is difficult to rigorously evaluate the effectiveness of the use of the robotic exoskeleton in this study. Moreover, follow-up data measures were not taken, therefore it is not possible to ascertain the long-term effectiveness of the technology in assisting in maintaining independence.

However, this paper has demonstrated that applications of robotic technologies have progressed much further than what the general public perceive robots are capable of undertaking. Robotic technology studies, despite being methodologically weak [52], have demonstrated capability of functional improvements following loss of function in upper and lower limbs, or to assist with mobility in indoor environments. The range of the robotic technologies presented in in Table 2 show that the technology is now progressing to the point that that home trials of these different robotic technologies will be undertaken in the near future.

A limitation of this review was that non-English language studies were excluded. Therefore it is possible that studies of testing robotics in the home environment have been completed, but were not included in this paper as they were published in languages other than English. A second limitation of this review was the decision by the authors to exclude robotic interventions for uses relating to cognitive decline/successful brain aging. Indeed, recent reviews have discussed the use of robotics for cognitive healthcare in the elderly [3]; however, the primary aim of this paper was to review evidence for robotics in addressing physical mobility to reduce disability and loss of independence in the home. Further, although outside the scope of this review and thus also excluded was the emergence of nanotechnology. It is plausible to suggest that progress in nanotechnology research (also known as nanorobotics) [53] could potentially reduce hazards in the home. Robotics will improve, in a number of different directions, to the point of assisting older people to live independently and safely in their homes, and enjoy excellent quality of life in their communities.

The recently released (April 2012) Living Longer. Living Better Report from the Australian Federal Government [54] in response to the Productivity Commission's Report on Care of Older Australians [55] recommends the major expansion of home care supportive services, although these are largely conceptualized as intensive case management services. However, the aged housing and care industry in Australia is moving ahead with the rapid take up of new technologies to assist older people to live more independently at home and in supported accommodation in association with the rollout of a new broadband network nationally [55].

Robotics are perhaps one of the newest technology areas to have entered the home care market, being previously largely developed for application in heavy industry and acute health. Looking forward, however, the potential for robotic application in the home is wide open. Some of the major barriers relate to cost of development, the incorporation of artificial intelligence in new design applications, and the encouragement of greater interdisciplinary convergence between the many research fields now involved in the development of new robotic technologies. At this point in time in Australia, progress on home grown robotic applications is limited, given the substantial infrastructure required in the start-up phase [56].

In light of the research reviewed, a number of key recommendations can be provided as follows:

4.1. Applying Research into Home Environments. The evidence from the current systematic review has clearly demonstrated that robotics research needs to be conducted in the home environment. To date, only four studies have attempted to conduct research within the home environment [28, 32, 40, 51]. These studies have demonstrated positive outcomes, providing a good rationale to take robotics into environments outside of laboratories or hospital clinics.

4.2. Diversifying Robotics. The majority of robotic technology studies found in the current review were directed at movement rehabilitation. However, for the elderly population, healthy living includes prompting and reminding for effective monitoring. Development of robotic technologies should include technologies that can provide gentle reminders for medications, continually scan the environment to ensure no falls have taken place, and have a protocol in place to advise relevant authorities if an incident has occurred. Similarly, robotics has the potential to allow for social connectedness by providing company for elderly people living alone, or to serve as interfaces for connecting with family and friends using existing technologies (e.g., Skype).

4.3. Reducing Costs. The final recommendation would be to investigate ways of reducing the costs of technologies. As shown in this paper, robotic technologies are still in development and trial phases. It would be anticipated that with commercial development and mass production, these costs would reduce significantly. However, at the present time costs appear to be a barrier towards broad adoption of robots in the home environment.

In conclusion, this systematic review has shown that robotic technologies have the potential to assist older people and people with disabilities to remain mobile and to live safe and healthy lives at home. Further research and training of the heath and disability workforces is needed to the adoption of robotics as an effective, routine, and practical option within the home environment. The evidence demonstrates that robots already exist to assist with movements, obstacle-avoidance, and functional rehabilitation, but require further development to realise their full potential for safety monitoring, falls, and social connectedness. Future robot design needs to consider development from a different perspective, considering not only assisted mobility, but also interfacing artificial intelligence for interaction with older individuals, to monitor their health, provide medication prompts, encourage exercise, and provide them with confidence to maintain independent living.

Conflict of Interests

The authors declare that they have no conflict of interests.

Acknowledgments

This work was supported by a Grant from the Institute for a Broadband-Enabled Society (IBES). The authors would like to thank Ms. Erin Hickingbotham for her assistance in preliminary data collection.

References

[1] United Nations, *World Population Prospects: The 2006 Revision*, United Nations, New York, NY, USA, 2007.

[2] Chronic Diseases, Australian Institute of Health and Welfare, http://www.aihw.gov.au/chronic-diseases/.

[3] M. E. Morris, E. Ozanne, K. Miller, N. Santamaria, A. J. Pearce, C. Said et al., *Smart Technologies for Older People: A Systematic Literature Review of Smart Technologies That Promote Health and Wellbeing of Older People Living at Home*, Institute for a Broadband-Enabled Socity, Melbourne, Australia, 2012.

[4] M. A. Groves and V. F. Wilson, "To move or not to move? Factors influencing the housing choice of elderly persons," *Journal of Housing for the Elderly*, vol. 10, pp. 33–47, 1992.

[5] A. Shumway-Cook, A. M. Ciol, J. Hoffman, J. B. Dudgeon, K. Yorkston, and L. Chan, "Falls in the medicare population: incidence, associated factors, and on health care," *Physical Therapy*, vol. 89, no. 4, pp. 324–332, 2009.

[6] J. W. Rowe and R. L. Kahn, "Successful aging," *The Gerontologist*, vol. 37, no. 4, pp. 433–440, 1997.

[7] C. Kuzma, "The human touch," *Science and Spirit*, vol. 4, pp. 15–17, 2006.

[8] L. Carelli, A. Gaggioli, G. Pioggia, F. de Rossi, and G. Riva, "Affective robot for elderly assistance," *Studies in Health Technology and Informatics*, vol. 144, pp. 44–49, 2009.

[9] S. Thiel, D. Häbe, and M. Block, "Co-operative robot teams in a hospital environment," in *Proceedings of the IEEE International Conference on Intelligent Computing and Intelligent Systems (ICIS'09)*, pp. 843–847, Shanghai, China, November 2009.

[10] E. Broadbent, I. H. Kuo, Y. I. Lee et al., "Attitudes and reactions to a healthcare robot," *Telemedicine Journal and E-Health*, vol. 16, no. 5, pp. 608–613, 2010.

[11] C. Ray, F. Mondada, and R. Siegwart, "What do people expect from robots?" in *Proceedings of the IEEE/RSJ International Conference on Intelligent Robots and Systems (IROS'08)*, pp. 3816–3821, Nice, France, September 2008.

[12] M. Kassler, "Robotics for health care: a review of the literature," *Robotica*, vol. 11, no. 6, pp. 495–516, 1993.

[13] A. J. Rentschler, R. A. Cooper, B. Blasch, and M. L. Boninger, "Intelligent walkers for the elderly: performance and safety testing of VA-PAMAID robotic walker," *Journal of Rehabilitation Research and Development*, vol. 40, no. 5, pp. 423–431, 2003.

[14] J. Broekens, M. Herrink, and H. Rosendal, "Assistive social robots in elderly care: a review," *Gerontechnology*, vol. 8, no. 2, pp. 94–103, 2009.

[15] Merriam-Webster Dictionary (Online), 2011, http://www.merriam-webster.com/netdict.htm.

[16] NHMRC, NHMRC levels of evidence and grades for recommendations for developers of guidelines, 2009, https://www.nhmrc.gov.au/_files_nhmrc/file/guidelines/developers/nhmrc_levels_grades_evidence_120423.pdf.

[17] M. L. Aisen, H. I. Krebs, N. Hogan, F. McDowell, and B. T. Volpe, "The effect of robot-assisted therapy and rehabilitative training on motor recovery following stroke," *Archives of Neurology*, vol. 54, no. 4, pp. 443–446, 1997.

[18] J. S. Morvan, J. P. Guichard, and V. Torossian, "Technical aids for the physically handicapped: a psychological study of the master robot," *International Journal of Rehabilitation Research*, vol. 20, no. 2, pp. 193–197, 1997.

[19] H. I. Krebs, N. Hogan, M. L. Aisen, and B. T. Volpe, "Robot-aided neurorehabilitation," *IEEE Transactions on Rehabilitation Engineering*, vol. 6, no. 1, pp. 75–87, 1998.

[20] J. A. Cozens, "Robotic assistance of an active upper limb exercise in neurologically impaired patients," *IEEE Transactions on Rehabilitation Engineering*, vol. 7, no. 2, pp. 254–256, 1999.

[21] B. T. Volpe, H. I. Krebs, N. Hogan, L. Edelsteinn, C. M. Diels, and M. L. Aisen, "Robot training enhanced motor outcome in patients with stroke maintained over 3 years," *Neurology*, vol. 53, no. 8, pp. 1874–1876, 1999.

[22] D. J. Reinkensmeyer, J. P. A. Dewald, and W. Z. Rymer, "Guidance-based quantification of arm impairment following brain injury: a pilot study," *IEEE Transactions on Rehabilitation Engineering*, vol. 7, no. 1, pp. 1–11, 1999.

[23] C. G. Burgar, P. S. Lum, P. C. Shor, and H. F. M. van der Loos, "Development of robots for rehabilitation therapy: the Palo Alto VA/Stanford experience," *Journal of Rehabilitation Research and Development*, vol. 37, no. 6, pp. 663–673, 2000.

[24] B. T. Volpe, H. I. Krebs, N. Hogan, L. Edelstein, C. Diels, and M. Aisen, "A novel approach to stroke rehabilitation: robot-aided sensorimotor stimulation," *Neurology*, vol. 54, no. 10, pp. 1938–1944, 2000.

[25] S. Jezernik, R. Schärer, G. Colombo, and M. Morari, "Adaptive robotic rehabilitation of locomotion: a clinical study in spinally injured individuals," *Spinal Cord*, vol. 41, no. 12, pp. 657–666, 2003.

[26] R. Loureiro, F. Amirabdollahian, M. Topping, B. Driessen, and W. Harwin, "Upper limb robot mediated stroke therapy—GENTLE/s approach," *Autonomous Robots*, vol. 15, no. 1, pp. 35–51, 2003.

[27] P. Winchester, R. McColl, R. Querry et al., "Changes in supraspinal activation patterns following robotic locomotor therapy in motor-incomplete spinal cord injury," *Neurorehabilitation and Neural Repair*, vol. 19, no. 4, pp. 313–324, 2005.

[28] M. Spenko, H. Yu, and S. Dubowsky, "Robotic personal aids for mobility and monitoring for the elderly," *IEEE Transactions on Neural Systems and Rehabilitation Engineering*, vol. 14, no. 3, pp. 344–351, 2006.

[29] J. F. Israel, D. D. Campbell, J. H. Kahn, and T. G. Hornby, "Metabolic costs and muscle activity patterns during robotic- and therapist-assisted treadmill walking in individuals with incomplete spinal cord injury," *Physical Therapy*, vol. 86, no. 11, pp. 1466–1478, 2006.

[30] J. Mehrholz, C. Werner, J. Kugler, and M. Pohl, "Electromechanical-assisted training for walking after stroke," *Cochrane Database of Systematic Reviews*, no. 4, Article ID CD006185, 2007.

[31] E. Rocon, J. M. Belda-Lois, A. F. Ruiz, M. Manto, J. C. Moreno, and J. L. Pons, "Design and validation of a rehabilitation robotic exoskeleton for tremor assessment and suppression,"

IEEE Transactions on Neural Systems and Rehabilitation Engineering, vol. 15, no. 1, pp. 367–378, 2007.

[32] S. Saeki, Y. Matsushima, and K. Hachisuka, "Cortical activation during robotic therapy for a severely affected arm in a chronic stroke patient: a case report," *Journal of UOEH*, vol. 30, no. 2, pp. 159–165, 2008.

[33] J. Hidler, L. F. Hamm, A. Lichy, and S. L. Groah, "Automating activity-based interventions: the role of robotics," *Journal of Rehabilitation Research and Development*, vol. 45, no. 2, pp. 337–344, 2008.

[34] T. W. J. Janssen and D. D. Pringle, "Effects of modified electrical stimulation-induced leg cycle ergometer training for individuals with spinal cord injury," *Journal of Rehabilitation Research and Development*, vol. 45, no. 6, pp. 819–830, 2008.

[35] H. I. Krebs, S. Mernoff, S. E. Fasoli, R. Hughes, J. Stein, and N. Hogan, "A comparison of functional and impairment-based robotic training in severe to moderate chronic stroke: a pilot study," *NeuroRehabilitation*, vol. 23, no. 1, pp. 81–87, 2008.

[36] J. Patton, D. A. Brown, M. Peshkin et al., "KineAssist: design and development of a robotic overground gait and balance therapy device," *Topics in Stroke Rehabilitation*, vol. 15, no. 2, pp. 131–139, 2008.

[37] R. G. Querry, F. Pacheco, T. Annaswamy, L. Goetz, P. K. Winchester, and K. E. Tansey, "Synchronous stimulation and monitoring of soleus H reflex during robotic body weight-supported ambulation in subjects with spinal cord injury," *Journal of Rehabilitation Research and Development*, vol. 45, no. 1, pp. 175–186, 2008.

[38] A. J. Rentschler, R. Simpson, R. A. Cooper, and M. L. Boninger, "Clinical evaluation of Guido robotic walker," *Journal of Rehabilitation Research and Development*, vol. 45, no. 9, pp. 1281–1294, 2008.

[39] F. Galluppi, C. Urdiales, I. Sanchez-Tato, F. Sandoval, and M. O. Belardinelli, "A study on a shared control navigation system: human/robot collaboration for assisting people in mobility," *Cognitive Processing*, vol. 10, supplement 2, pp. S215–S218, 2009.

[40] H. Shimada, T. Hirata, Y. Kimura et al., "Effects of a robotic walking exercise on walking performance in community-dwelling elderly adults," *Geriatrics & Gerontology International*, vol. 9, no. 4, pp. 372–381, 2009.

[41] N. A. Flinn, J. L. Smith, C. J. Tripp, and M. W. White, "Effects of robotic-aided rehabilitation on recovery of upper extremity function in chronic stroke: a single case study," *Occupational Therapy International*, vol. 16, no. 3-4, pp. 232–243, 2009.

[42] Q. Zeng, E. Burdet, and C. L. Teo, "Evaluation of a collaborative wheelchair system in cerebral palsy and traumatic brain injury users," *Neurorehabilitation and Neural Repair*, vol. 23, no. 5, pp. 494–504, 2009.

[43] A. C. Lo, P. D. Guarino, L. G. Richards et al., "Robot-assisted therapy for long-term upper-limb impairment after stroke," *The New England Journal of Medicine*, vol. 362, no. 19, pp. 1772–1783, 2010.

[44] A. Frizera Neto, J. A. Gallego, E. Rocon, J. L. Pons, and R. Ceres, "Extraction of user's navigation commands from upper body force interaction in walker assisted gait," *BioMedical Engineering Online*, vol. 9, article 37, 2010.

[45] V. Sharma, R. Simpson, E. Lopresti, and M. Schmeler, "Evaluation of semiautonomous navigation assistance system for power wheelchairs with blindfolded nondisabled individuals," *Journal of Rehabilitation Research and Development*, vol. 47, no. 9, pp. 877–890, 2010.

[46] J. R. Wolpaw, "Brain-computer interface research comes of age: traditional assumptions meet emerging realities," *Journal of Motor Behavior*, vol. 42, no. 6, pp. 351–353, 2010.

[47] J. A. Galvez, A. Budovitch, S. J. Harkema, and D. J. Reinkensmeyer, "Trainer variability during step training after spinal cord injury: implications for robotic gait-training device design," *Journal of Rehabilitation Research and Development*, vol. 48, no. 2, pp. 147–160, 2011.

[48] M. Turiel, S. Sitia, S. Cicala et al., "Robotic treadmill training improves cardiovascular function in spinal cord injury patients," *International Journal of Cardiology*, vol. 149, no. 3, pp. 323–329, 2011.

[49] I. Schwartz, A. Sajina, M. Neeb, I. Fisher, M. Katz-Luerer, and Z. Meiner, "Locomotor training using a robotic device in patients with subacute spinal cord injury," *Spinal Cord*, vol. 49, pp. 1062–1067, 2011.

[50] S. S. Conroy, J. Whitall, L. Dipietro et al., "Effect of gravity on robot-assisted motor training after chronic stroke: a randomized trial," *Archives of Physical Medicine and Rehabilitation*, vol. 92, no. 11, pp. 1754–1761, 2011.

[51] T. Carlson and Y. Demiris, "Collaborative control for a robotic wheelchair: evaluation of performance, attention, and workload," *IEEE Transactions on Systems, Man, and Cybernetics B*, vol. 42, no. 3, Article ID Article number6135817, pp. 876–888, 2012.

[52] S. H. Downs and N. Black, "The feasibility of creating a checklist for the assessment of the methodological quality both of randomised and non-randomised studies of health care interventions," *Journal of Epidemiology and Community Health*, vol. 52, no. 6, pp. 377–384, 1998.

[53] R. Frietas Jr., "Comprehensive nanorobotic control of human morbidity and aging," in *The Future of Aging*, G. M. Fahey, M. D. West, L. S. Coles, and S. B. Harris, Eds., chapter 23, Spinger, Dordrecht, The Netherlands, 2010.

[54] Department of Health and Ageing, Living longer, living better, 2012, http://www.health.gov.au/internet/main/publishing.nsf/Content/ageing-hacc-living.htm.

[55] Department of Broadband, Communications and the Digital Economy, National digital economy strategy: leveraging the national broadband network to drive Australia's digital productivity, 2011, http://www.nbn.gov.au/files/2011/05/National_Digital_Economy_Strategy.pdf.

[56] Academy of Technological Sciences and Engineering, Smart technology for healthy longevity, 2010, http://www.atse.org.au/news/featured-articles/155-smart-tech-for-health-longevity/.

11

The Use of Multiple Correspondence Analysis to Explore Associations between Categories of Qualitative Variables in Healthy Ageing

Patrício Soares Costa,[1,2] Nadine Correia Santos,[1,2] Pedro Cunha,[1,2,3] Jorge Cotter,[1,2,3] and Nuno Sousa[1,2]

[1] *Life and Health Sciences Research Institute (ICVS), School of Health Sciences, University of Minho, 4710-057 Braga, Portugal*
[2] *ICVS/3B's, PT Government Associate Laboratory, Guimarães, 4710-057 Braga, Portugal*
[3] *Centro Hospital Alto Ave, EPE, 4810-055 Guimarães, Portugal*

Correspondence should be addressed to Nuno Sousa; njcsousa@ecsaude.uminho.pt

Academic Editor: F. Richard Ferraro

The main focus of this study was to illustrate the applicability of multiple correspondence analysis (MCA) in detecting and representing underlying structures in large datasets used to investigate cognitive ageing. Principal component analysis (PCA) was used to obtain main cognitive dimensions, and MCA was used to detect and explore relationships between cognitive, clinical, physical, and lifestyle variables. Two PCA dimensions were identified (general cognition/executive function and memory), and two MCA dimensions were retained. Poorer cognitive performance was associated with older age, less school years, unhealthier lifestyle indicators, and presence of pathology. The first MCA dimension indicated the clustering of general/executive function and lifestyle indicators and education, while the second association was between memory and clinical parameters and age. The clustering analysis with object scores method was used to identify groups sharing similar characteristics. The weaker cognitive clusters in terms of memory and executive function comprised individuals with characteristics contributing to a higher MCA dimensional mean score (age, less education, and presence of indicators of unhealthier lifestyle habits and/or clinical pathologies). MCA provided a powerful tool to explore complex ageing data, covering multiple and diverse variables, showing if a relationship exists and how variables are related, and offering statistical results that can be seen both analytically and visually.

1. Introduction

Analysis of research data requires unique considerations depending on the type of data collected and/or on the main purpose of the research. For instance, while in some cases data is collected in ordinal mode, often it is also obtained in categorized groups. Or, as opposed to the traditional hypothesis testing designed to verify *a priori* hypotheses about relations between variables, exploratory data analysis is used to identify systematic relations between variables, when there are incomplete *a priori* expectations as to the nature of those relations. Falling in the latter category, the method correspondence analysis (CA), a (multivariate) descriptive data analytic technique, allows simplifying complex data and provides a detailed description of the data, yielding a simple, yet exhaustive analysis (a review of the development of the correspondence analysis methodology can be found in [1]). Specifically, multiple CA (MCA) allows for the analysis of categorical or categorized variables encompassing more than two categorical variables (whereas "simple" correspondence analysis pertains to the more "simple" dataset, a two-way contingency table) [2–7].

Summarily, MCA is part of a family of descriptive methods (e.g., clustering, factor analysis, and principal component analysis (PCA)) that reveal patterning in complex datasets. However, specifically, MCA is used to represent and model datasets as "clouds" of points in a multidimensional Euclidean space; this means that it is distinctive in describing the patterns geometrically by locating each variable/unit of analysis as a point in a low-dimensional space. The results are interpreted on the basis of the relative positions of the points and their distribution along the dimensions; as categories become more similar in distribution, the closer (distance between points) they are represented in space [2–6]. Although it is mainly used as an exploratory technique, it can be a particularly powerful one as it "uncovers" groupings of variable categories in the dimensional spaces, providing key insights on relationships between categories (i.e., multivariate treatment of the data through simultaneous consideration of multiple categorical variables), without needing to meet assumptions requirements such as those required in other techniques widely used to analyze categorical data (e.g., Chi-square analysis, Fischer's exact test, *G*-statistics, and ratio test) [8]. The use of MCA is, thus, particularly relevant in studies where a large amount of qualitative data is collected, often in pair with quantitative data, and where qualitative variables can become suboptimized in the data analysis. This is often the case in epidemiological and system studies where variables in the datasets may be quantitative or qualitative, temporal or nontemporal, and/or objective or subjective. As such, CA has been beneficial in areas ranging from the health and medicine to social sciences, archeology, ecology, software development, and market research (see reviews [7, 9, 10]).

In this context, among population-based studies, cognitive ageing studies can be particularly difficult to address. Foremost, data collection itself must consider and account for the multiple factors (variables) that might explain cognitive trajectories throughout ageing. Biologically, this is crucial because cognitive ageing results from a complex and adaptive interaction of endogenous and exogenous variables, ranging from physicostructural, clinical, genetic, and biochemical factors to psychological, social inclusion/continued intellectual stimulation, lifestyle, and sociodemographic indicators or measures [11–17]. In fact, altogether, these are at the basis of the inter- and intraindividual cognitive variability observed throughout ageing [18]. Subsequently, the large and diverse nature of the data renders analysis strategies decisions difficult. For example, while cognition is traditionally assessed via a battery of neurocognitive/psychological tests often on a continuous scale, other aspects, such as sociodemographic clinical variables, are often categorical or obtained in the form of questionnaires. Furthermore, even quantitative variables are often transformed into categorical ones (e.g., height and weight parameters to yield a BMI class). In this context, exploratory insights that maximize the use of all the qualitative information in the identification of categorical groupings of factors and reveal their relationship are needed if not crucial. In fact, illustrating its still surprisingly limited use albeit direct and valuable applicability in ageing studies, Sourial et al. [19] used MCA, encompassing data on several binary variables, from three separate studies, to examine the relationships among seven frailty domains in the elderly. The proof-of-concept study not only indicated that frailty is a multidimensional concept but also that MCA permits to efficiently gather separate large sets of data and/or to investigate for consistency between datasets, providing considerable insights in population studies.

Upon this, commonly used analysis strategies may be either unfeasible or when used alone only reveal that a relationship exists but not which response categories are related. For example, pairwise strategies are rendered impossible when dealing with a large number of categorical variables, and multivariate approaches (e.g., PCA) require the use of continuous variables. Furthermore, multivariate analysis results (despite their analysis power) do not allow exploring the individual response categories of the categorical variables. On the other end, MCA can account for these problems and preserve the categorical nature of the variables [2–6, 9]; the analysis is conducted at the level of the response categories themselves and not at the variable level. Furthermore, an important feature of CA is the graphical display of row and column points in biplots, which can help in detecting structural relationships among the variable categories and objects providing a visual map whose structuring can be interpreted (this duality is not present in other multivariate approaches to graphical data representation). Finally, CA has highly flexible data requirements, where the only strict data requirement is a rectangular data matrix with nonnegative entries. In fact, in a way, CA may be considered as a special case of PCA of the rows and columns of a table, especially applicable to a cross-tabulation; however, CA and PCA are used under different circumstances. Principal components analysis is used for tables consisting of continuous measurement, whereas correspondence analysis is applied to contingency tables (cross-tabulations). In CA the primary goal is to transform a table of numerical information into a graphical display, in which each row and each column are depicted as a point. The usual procedure for analyzing a cross-tabulation is to determine the probability of global association between rows and columns. The significance of association is tested by the Pearson chi-square test, but this test provides no information as to which are the significant individual associations between row-column pairs of the data matrix (i.e., it does not divulge how the association is constructed, nor does the statistic allow for an investigation of similar or different categories). Conversely, CA shows how the variables are related, not just that a relationship exists [2–6].

Based on the MCA technique, herein, we aim to obtain a global picture of the salient relationships among cognitive, clinical, physical, and lifestyle variables to explore their dimensional relationship to healthy ageing. The present work is based on the cognitive and clinical and sociodemographic assessment of older community-dwelling individuals in the Minho cohort in Northern Portugal [11, 20]. The study participants were representative of the Portuguese population in terms of age, gender, and educational status; on measures of sociodemographic characteristics the country ranks close to the OECD (Organisation for Economic Cooperation and Development; http://www.oecd.org/) average [21].

2. Material and Methods

2.1. Ethics Statement. The study was conducted in accordance with the Declaration of Helsinki (59th Amendment) and was approved by national and local ethics committees.

The study goals and the neurocognitive, clinical, and lifestyle assessments were explained to potential participants. All volunteers provided a written informed consent. Further exclusion/inclusion selection criteria are described elsewhere [11, 12].

2.2. Sample Characteristics. Participants (n = 1051) were randomly selected from the Guimarães and Vizela local area health authority registries; however, the cohort was representative of the health registries (less than 2% difference) and of the general Portuguese population with respect to gender (females, n = 560 or 53.3%) and age (range: 50–97 years; M = 67.2, SD = 9.24; age categories: [50–60[, 25.4% (females, 52.8%); [60–70[, 31.2% (females, 53.7%); [70+[, 43.4% (females, 53.3%)). All participants were community-dwellers and the majority was in the medium socioeconomic stratum (61.6%, females 47.3%; Class III in the Graffar measure [22]) and retired (n = 763, females 51.8%). Literacy rate was 92.2% (able to read and write), and the median years of the schooling was 4; specifically, 34.7 (females 71.0%), 49.4 (females 47.4%), and 15.9% (females 32.9%) of the cohort attended school for [0–4[, 4, and [4+[years.

2.3. Neurocognitive Evaluation. Tests were selected to provide cognitive (general cognitive status and executive and memory functions) profiles, as previously reported [11, 12, 20]. The following measures were used: mini-mental state examination (MMSE) to assess global cognitive status [23]; digit span forward test (subtest of the Wechsler adult intelligence test WAIS III, 1997) to evaluate short-term verbal memory [24]; digit span backward test (subtest of the Wechsler adult intelligence test WAIS III, 1997) for verbal working memory [24]; the selective reminding test (SRT, parameters: consistent long-term retrieval (CLTR), long-term storage (LTS), delayed recall, and intrusions) to evaluate multiple trial verbal learning and memory [25]; Stroop color and word test (parameters: words, colors, and words/colors) to measure response inhibition/cognitive flexibility [26]; and the controlled oral word association test F-A-S (COWAT-FAS, parameters: admissible and nonadmissible) to assess verbal fluency [27]. A team of trained psychologists conducted the neurocognitive/psychological assessments.

2.4. Clinical, Physical, and Lifestyle Characteristics. General health aspects considered included clinical history of stroke (ischemic or hemorrhagic stroke or transient ischemic attack), cardiac pathology (this designation is here used to include coronary bypass, cardiac insufficiency, myocardial infarction, and/or coronary disease), diabetes (diabetes mellitus type I or II), dyslipidemia, and/or hypertension. Clinical measures are those self-reported by the participants in response to the standardized clinical interview. Physical measures included weight (Kg), height (m), and abdominal perimeter (cm). BMI (Kg/m^2) was categorized as underweight, normal, overweight, and obese (resp., BMI: [0–18.5], [18.6–24.9], [25.0–29.9], and [30.0+[) [28]. For statistical procedures, the underweight and normal categories were combined due to the small sample size for underweight (n = 5). Metabolic complication risk was categorized none, increased, and substantially increased (resp., abdominal perimeter: females, [0–80.0], [80.1–88.0], and [88.1+[; males, [0–94.0], [94.1–102.0], and [102.1+[) [28]. Lifestyle, alcohol consumption (none, 50 or less, and more than 50 gr/day), physical activity status (none, less than 3, and over 3 times per week), and smoking habits (nonsmoker, former smoker, and smoker) were considered. A team of experienced clinicians performed a standardized clinical interview, including physical and lifestyle measures.

2.5. Analysis Methodology. Data analysis followed previously reported strategies [11, 12, 20] and was structured as follows.

(1) Conversion of all neurocognitive test scores into z scores to express all variables in the same scale.

(2) Exclusion of participants that met the previously established MMSE criteria for cognitive impairment (i.e., with a total score <17 if individual with ≤4 years of formal school education and/or ≥72 years of age or total score <23 if individual with more than 4 years of formal school education and/or ≤71 years of age).

(3) Principal component analysis (PCA) for allocation of the neurocognitive multiple test parameters into single or composite cognitive dimensions.

(4) Allocation of participants into cognitive categories according to quartile score for each of the identified PCA dimensions (below Q1 "poor"; middle 50% "normal"; above Q3 "good").

(5) Discretization of quantitative variables.

(6) Multiple correspondence analysis (MCA) to explore the association between qualitative variables categories (cognitive, clinical, physical, and lifestyle).

(7) Cluster analysis with object scores of each dimension to group subjects.

(8) Crosstabulations with relevant variables in the MCA and cluster variable (proportion z-test).

The SPSS package v20 (IBM SPSS Statistics) was used to conduct all statistical analysis.

2.6. Principal Component Analysis (PCA). PCA was used to reduce neurocognitive information through a linear function. All neurocognitive measures were considered in the analysis (extraction method: principal component analysis; rotation method: Varimax with Kaiser Normalization), and all individuals that met the established MMSE threshold and had no missing values in any of the considered neurocognitive measures (n = 684) were considered to identify the cognitive dimensions that grouped the neurocognitive variables. The parameters GDS, COWAT-FAS nonadmissible and SRT intrusions, and digit span forward were sequentially excluded from the analysis due to low component loadings (<0.400). The remaining parameters formed composites: "GENEXEC" (general cognition and executive function, Cronbach's alpha 0.793) composed of the parameters MMSE, Stroop (parameters: words, colors, and words/colors), FAS (parameter:

admissible), and digits (parameter: backward); and "MEM" (memory function, Cronbach's alpha 0.890) composed of the SRT test variables (parameters: CLTR, LTS, and delayed recall). Next, we allowed and imputed values for the dimensions cases with only one missing value, yielding a total of $n = 859$ individuals with calculated scores in the identified cognitive dimensions (the sample was representative of the initial study population except regarding literacy rate, 99.4% able to read and write). Dimensions were calculated based on the weighted arithmetic mean of each cognitive test. The analysis followed and was in agreement with previously reported observations [11, 20].

2.7. Multiple Correspondence Analysis (MCA). The object of correspondence analysis (CA) is to analyze categorical/categorized data that are transformed into cross tables and to demonstrate the results in a graphical manner. In CA, both relations between row and column variables and relations between different levels of each variable can be obtained [2–7]. Some considerations regarding CA are warranted particularly regarding the influence of cells and responses [1]. For instance, some reports have (i) explored the impact on the analysis by including and excluding/deleting categories [29, 30]; (ii) examined methods for identifying columns (attributes) that highlight row (incidence) differences [31]; and (iii) compared the theoretical similarities between CA and log-linear models [32]. Here, for MCA, from the initial total sample, $n = 239$ participants were excluded due to missing values in at least one of the considered clinical, general lifestyle, and/or physical variables, yielding, altogether, a total of $n = 812$ individuals (from the $n = 859$ from the cognitive analysis step) with no missing values which were included in all the remaining analysis. Since the missing values were assumed to be missing completely at random (MCAR) [33] and the range of the sample size was still above 250 after the exclusion of the missing data, this was considered the adequate strategy to follow, since there would be no prejudice to the adequacy, validity, or power of the present study [34, 35]. The sample remained representative of the initial study population for the measures considered.

Two solutions were explored using variable principal (VPrincipal) normalization method. The first solution included the maximum number of possible MCA dimensions (calculated from the difference between the sum of variables categories and the number of variables (39 minus 15, to yield 24 MCA dimensions)). The calculated total inertia was 1.6 (the maximum number of MCA dimensions ($n = 24$) divided by the number of variables ($n = 15$)). This step allowed exploring the number of dimensions to be included in the analysis and to obtain the reference value for total inertia (meaning that the contribution of each factor should now be calculated using the total inertia score as the denominator). The main use of inertia is as an indicator of the number of axes to retain for further analysis. To define the number of dimensions to retain, the following criteria/considerations were employed: (i) scree test [36]; (ii) eigenvalue (inclusion of MCA dimensions with inertia above 0.2 [3]); (iii) Cronbach's alpha score [3]; and (iv) although no defined number of dimensions is firmly established, some authors recommend two-dimensional pictures of data (which facilitates and allows for data interpretation) [37]. Based on these criteria, a second solution was explored with two MCA dimensions: the first accounting for 11.9% (0.190/1.6) of the variance and the second for 8.3% (0.132/1.6), yielding a total variance of 20.2% (0.323/1.6). Discrimination measures and a joint plot of category points were obtained. Category quantification plots constitute an alternative method of displaying discrimination of variables that can identify category relationships. The coordinates of each category on each dimension are displayed in order to determine which categories are similar for each variable. In the discrimination measures plot, the length and steepness of the lines indicate the discrimination measures of each variable for the two considered dimensions (another element for dimensions interpretation allowing to assess the relation system of the indicators and indicating its importance for each dimension). Specifically, in the MCA graphical representation, the squared distance of the ith row profile from the origin is

$$d_I^2(i,O) = \sum_{m=1}^{M*} f_{im}^2 \tag{1}$$

and is the Euclidean distance of the ith row profile coordinate from the origin [1], where, in the M-dimensional correspondence plot, the larger the distance of the ith row profile from the origin, the larger the weighted discrepancy between the profile of category i to the average profile of the column categories. As such, the further a point is from the origin, the greater the deviation from the expected under complete independence (a point near the origin indicates that the frequencies in row i of the contingency table fit the independence hypothesis). That is, the distance from an object to the origin is the reflection of the variation from the "average" pattern (the most frequent category for each variable). Objects with many characteristics corresponding to the average pattern lie near the origin, whereas objects with unique characteristics are located far from the origin (in this sense, the object scores plot is particularly useful for detecting outliers and typical groups of objects or revealing special patterns). Furthermore, by using confidence circles, it can be further graphically represented whether the position of a particular category contributes to the hypothesis of independence for the contingency table [38]. If the origin lies outside of the confidence circle, then the category can be considered to contribute to the dependency, whereas if the origin lies within the circle, it does not make such a contribution. The same conclusion can be made for the Euclidean distance of the column profile coordinates to the origin.

2.8. Cluster Analysis with Object Scores. Cluster analysis with object scores was used to classify subjects into groups (clustering variables: object scores of the MCA dimensions). Clusters are derived from the two MCA dimensions object scores. These values are based on the quantification of all qualitative variables (or treated as such) that define the individual profile. Since these are composite scores, the multidimensionality of the input (object scores) is preserved when performing cluster analysis. The "method of reciprocal averaging," that marks the MCA approach of the Leiden University in IBM SPSS software, is used to transform objects and variables categories. This method relates the quantifications between the variable categories and the object scores. The quantification of a certain category is the average of all the respective objects, and each object score is proportional to the average of all categories that the object is associated with. The quantification of the p categories of the m variables is calculated based on the formula $Y = D^{-1}G'X$, where Y is the categories quantification matrix; D is frequency of the p category; G is the binary matrix; and X is the object score matrix. Cluster analysis defines homogeneous subjects profiles based on the MCA dimensions assuming that they have substantive coherence.

Four separate clustering solutions, comprised of 2–5 clusters, were tested. Three criteria were considered to choose the best cluster solution: (i) the solution explained ≥5% of the dependent variables compared to the previous applied solution; (ii) the variance was greater than that of the previous solution; and (iii) the individuals were evenly distributed among the clusters (for each cluster solution). ANOVAs were performed on each cluster solution, using the MCA dimensions as dependent variables and cluster membership as a factor variable (independent variable). General effect size η^2 was derived by dividing the sum of all between-groups sum of squares by the sum of the total sum of groups; for the 2-, 3-, 4-, and 5-cluster solutions, η^2 was 0.33, 0.60, 0.74, and 0.77, respectively. While an increase in cluster solutions corresponded to an increase in variance, the five-cluster solution only explained 3.6% more than the four-cluster solution, compared with the four-cluster solution explaining 13.7% more than the three cluster solution. In the four-cluster solution, group membership varied between 20.8% ($n = 169$) and 27.6% ($n = 224$). The 4-membership clustering solution was considered to provide the best cluster solution.

3. Results

3.1. Multiple Correspondence Analysis. Clinical, general lifestyle, physical, and cognitive characterization of the MCA study sample ($n = 812$) is presented in Table 1. From the MCA analysis, a two-dimension MCA solution was considered the most adequate. The first and second dimensions presented are, respectively, eigenvalue, 2.857 and 1.984; inertia, 0.190 and 0.132; and Cronbach's alpha, 0.696 (95% CI 0.665, 0.726) and 0.531 (95% CI 0.483, 0.577). Although the generally accepted lower limit for Cronbach's alpha is 0.70, a smaller value is acceptable in exploratory research [2] where a small alpha score can be due to a reduced number of questions, poor interrelatedness between items, or heterogeneous constructs. Here, we are dealing with heterogeneous constructs to capture a two-dimensional picture of the data, and the methodological procedure was conducted assuming for this limitation. Discrimination measures (Table 2 and Figure 1(a)) and a joint plot of category points were obtained (Figure 1(b)). There were no clear differentiating values allocated to each of the obtained dimensions (Table 2); all discrimination measures were

TABLE 1: Clinical, general lifestyle, physical, and cognitive characterization.

	Count	Column n (%)
Sociodemographic characteristics		
Gender		
Male	410	50.5%
Female	402	49.5%
Age		
[50–60[	239	29.4%
[60–70[	281	34.6%
[70–...[	292	36.0%
School years		
Less than 4 years	191	23.5%
4 years	465	57.3%
More than 4 years	156	19.2%
Clinical characteristics		
Stroke		
Yes	42	5.2%
No	770	94.8%
Cardiac pathology		
Yes	75	9.2%
No	737	90.8%
Diabetes		
Yes	153	18.8%
No	659	81.2%
Dyslipidemia		
Yes	449	55.3%
No	363	44.7%
Hypertension		
Yes	452	55.7%
No	360	44.3%
Lifestyle and physical characteristics		
Smoking habits		
Former smoker	200	24.6%
Smoker	63	7.8%
Nonsmoker	549	67.6%
Alcohol consumption		
50 or less gr/day	379	46.7%
More than 50 gr/day	200	24.6%
None	233	28.7%
Physical activity		
Less than 3 times per week	134	16.5%
Over 3 times per week	178	21.9%
None	500	61.6%
BMI		
Normal/underweight	188	23.2%
Overweight	389	47.9%
Obese	235	28.9%

Table 1: Continued.

	Count	Column n (%)
Metabolic risk		
Increased	199	24.5%
Substantially increased	483	59.5%
None	130	16.0%
Cognitive dimensions		
GENEXEC		
Poor	201	24.8%
Normal	409	50.4%
Good	202	24.9%
MEM		
Poor	176	21.7%
Normal	406	50.0%
Good	230	28.3%

Table 2: MCA dimensions discrimination measures.

	MCA dimension		Mean
	1	2	
Gender	0.419	0.350	0.384
Age	0.150	0.332	0.241
School years	0.409	0.063	0.236
Stroke	0.005	0.073	0.039
Cardiac	0.006	0.139	0.073
Diabetes	0.022	0.083	0.053
Dyslipidemia	0.029	0.011	0.020
Hypertension	0.110	0.061	0.086
Smoking habits	0.333	0.272	0.302
Alcohol consumption	0.169	0.136	0.152
Physical activity	0.052	0.048	0.050
BMI	0.216	0.017	0.117
Metabolic risk	0.462	0.053	0.258
Cognitive dimension GENEXEC	0.352	0.125	0.239
Cognitive dimension MEM	0.122	0.221	0.171
Active total	2.857	1.984	2.421
% of variance	19.045	13.229	16.137

below 0.5 with a maximum value of 0.462 (metabolic risk) for the first dimension and 0.350 (gender) for the second dimension. Gender also contributed to the eigenvalue of the first dimension (value 0.419). The most discriminant variables for dimension 1 hierarchically were metabolic risk, school years, general cognition/executive function, and BMI; regarding dimension 2, the most discriminant variables were age, cardiac pathology, and memory (Table 1 and Figures 1(a)–1(d)). The variables gender, smoking, and alcohol presented relevant and similar discrimination measures in both dimensions. From the results and their graphical visualization, dimension 1 was termed "General/Executive, Lifestyle, and Education" and the second dimension "Memory, Clinical, and Age."

In dimension 1, gender correlated (transformed variables) significantly with smoking ($r = 0.583$, $P < 0.001$), alcohol ($r = 0.459$, $P < 0.001$), and metabolic risk ($r = 0.514$, $P < 0.001$); age correlated with school years ($r = 0.334$, $P < 0.001$), GENEXEC ($r = 0.304$, $P < 0.001$), and MEM ($r = 0.316$, $P < 0.001$); school years with GENEXEC ($r = 0.452$, $P < 0.001$); BMI correlated with metabolic risk ($r = 0.529$, $P < 0.001$); and GENEXEC correlated with MEM ($r = 0.380$, $P < 0.001$). Similar correlations were found for dimension 2, except for BMI with metabolic risk where no correlation was found. Only correlations above 0.30 were considered to have meaningful practical significance.

3.2. Cluster Analysis. The clustering analysis with object scores method was used to identify groups sharing similar characteristics within each of the identified dimensions ("General/Executive, Lifestyle, and Education" and "Memory, Clinical, and Age"). Specifically, analysis revealed 4 distinct clusters (cluster 1 to 4, C1 to C4) for each dimension (Figure 2). For GENEXEC, the different clusters showed a progressive decrease in performance (C1 > C2 > C3 > C4, all significantly different from each other; z-test for proportions comparisons adjusted with Bonferroni method, $P < 0.05$), while for MEM, the clusters C1 and C2 were comparable and the clusters C3 and C4 as well (C1 = C2 > C3 = C4, no significant difference between C1and C2 and between C3 and C4, but significant difference between C1/C2 and C3/C4 was found, $P < 0.05$). The relevant variables in the MCA dimensions were next cross-tabulated with cluster variable. Regarding age categories, C1 and C2 were significantly different from C3 and C4, specifically the proportion of older participants "[70+[" was significantly higher in the latter two clusters (C4 = C3 > C2 = C1, $P < 0.05$). A similar pattern was present regarding school education; specifically, for the "less than 4 school years" category C4 > C3 > C2 = C1 ($P < 0.05$). For "metabolic risk significantly increased," all clusters significantly differed from each other (C4 > C2 > C3 > C1, $P < 0.05$), with a similar pattern noted for "BMI obese" (C4 > C2 = C3 > C1, $P < 0.05$). Finally, for presence of "cardiac pathology," C3 > C4, C2, and C1, with C4 > C2 and = C1 and C2 = C1. Although not a discriminant variable in MCA, interestingly for gender the proportion of females was significantly higher in C2 and C4 compared to C1 and C3 ($P < 0.05$).

4. Discussion

Correspondence analysis is a technique that represents graphically the row and column categories and allows for a comparison of their "correspondences" (associations) at a category level. The development of CA has not been exclusively confined to statisticians; its diversity of development and application range has allowed for its application in, for example, the fields of health, social sciences and archaeology [1]. As such, altogether, CA makes a very relevant method of data analysis when an exploratory or even more in-depth analysis of categorical data is required, making it a particularly useful technique as it (i) is versatile, in part because no underlying distributional assumptions are

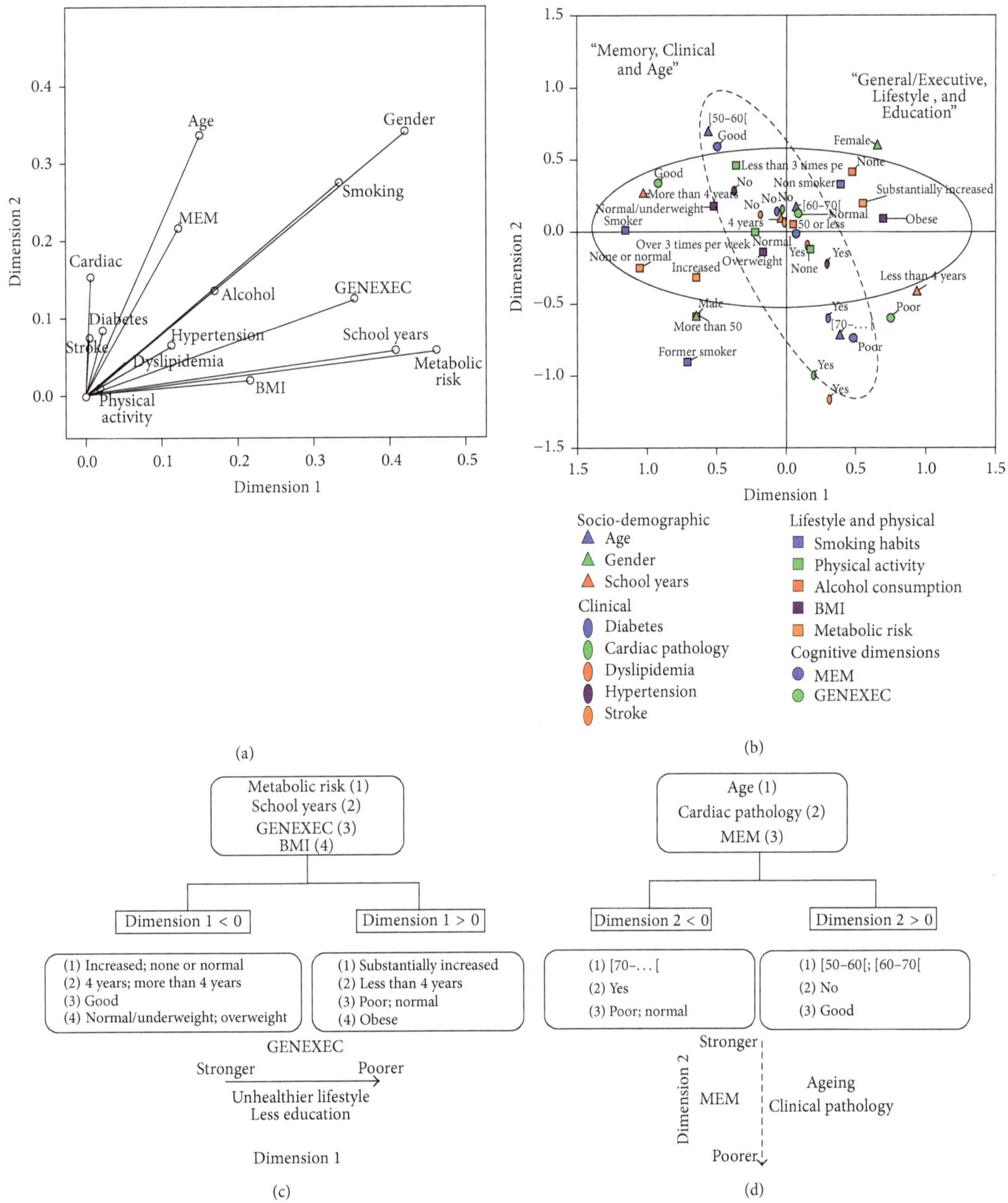

FIGURE 1: MCA dimensions. (a) MCA dimensions discrimination measures. (b) Joint category plot of the explored variable categories. (c) Positive and negative centroid coordinates for dimension 1. (d) Positive and negative centroid coordinates for dimension 2.

required, thus accommodating any type of categorical variable whether binary, ordinal, or nominal; (ii) gives a graphical output (often two-dimensional) for representing the associations between the variables in a low-dimensional space, thus providing key exploratory insights on the relationships between the collected data; and (iii) can be a complement or used in pair with other methods such as multidimensional scaling, biplots, and PCA (strategies followed in this report) [2–6].

Herein, we used a combined approach of PCA and MCA to a cross-sectional analysis in order to, upon identifying main cognitive dimensions, explore relationships between

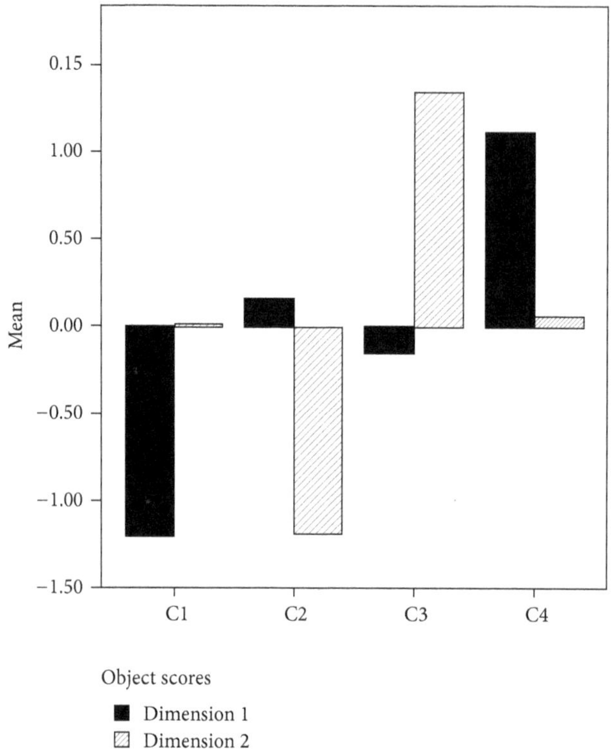

(a)

	Cluster				Total
	C1	C2	C3	C4	
	n (%)	*n* (%)	*n* (%)	*n* (%)	*n* (%)
Age categories: [70–. . .[	33 (15.4%)	15 (7.3%)	115 (68%)	129 (57.6%)	292 (36%)
School years: less than 4 years	4 (1.9%)	14 (6.8%)	45 (26.6%)	128 (57.1%)	191 (23.5%)
Metabolic risk: substantially increased	43 (20.1%)	165 (80.5%)	72 (42.6%)	203 (90.6%)	483 (59.5%)
BMI: obese	22 (10.3%)	68 (33.2%)	40 (23.7%)	105 (46.9%)	235 (28.9%)
Cardiac pathology: yes	10 (4.7%)	3 (1.5%)	41 (24.3%)	21 (9.4%)	75 (9.2%)
GENEXEC: good	118 (55.1%)	62 (30.2%)	17 (10.1%)	5 (2.2%)	202 (24.9%)
MEM: good	95 (44.4%)	95 (46.3%)	16 (9.5%)	24 (10.7%)	230 (28.3%)
Gender: female	7 (3.3%)	196 (95.6%)	1 (0.6%)	198 (88.4%)	402 (49.5%)

(b)

FIGURE 2: Cluster analysis with object scores. (a) Clusters (clusters 1 to 4, C1 to C4) identified for the MCA dimensions "General/Executive, Lifestyle, and Education" (dimension 1) and "Memory, Clinical, and Age" (dimension 2). (b) Crosstabulations with relevant variables in the MCA (and gender) and cluster variable.

cognitive, lifestyle, physical, and clinical variables among community-dwelling older individuals. The combination of the two methodologies is here favorable, with neither method used in detriment of the other but rather complementarily. First, PCA allowed grouping neurocognitive test variables (measures of cognition, each retaining a calculated weight in the final dimension) into cognitive dimensions, subsequently permitting the establishment of the "cognitive" score/class of each individual in regard to the entire cohort. Following previous findings [11, 20], two main cognitive dimensions were identified that represented general cognition and executive function (GENEXEC) and memory (MEM), each of which forming composites of multiple neurocognitive test variables. Thereafter, cognitive performance (categorized as "poor," "normal," and "good") could be explored in relation to the mixture of binary, categorical, discrete, or continuous variables (these suitably categorized) that comprised the sociodemographic, clinical, lifestyle, and physical aspects. Evidence of these relationships is necessary to elucidate whether particular characteristics belong to the construct of stronger versus poorer cognitive performance, with foreseeable value in our ageing society. In fact, albeit today's older adults being generally considered healthier and, likely consequently, more independent and active—with a significant positive implication in their continued contribution to society (particularly if with an accompanying proper allocation/restructuring of resources, policies, and interventions [39]), an increase in concurrent medical conditions can have detrimental consequences, causing excess (co)morbidity, disability, and decline in functional performance [40]. Furthermore, even if considering that gender, educational, and clinical aspects may remain "fixed" parameters (e.g., an individual either has or not a cardiac pathology), their association/combinatory effect with other more "modifiable" lifestyle parameters (e.g., physical activity) is of relevant interest.

From data analysis, and its graphical representation, two MCA dimensions—termed "General/Executive, Lifestyle, and Education" and "Memory, Clinical, and Age"—were identified. For the first, a more unhealthy lifestyle (as indicated by higher BMI and metabolic risk, among other measures) and lower education level were associated with poorer general cognition and executive function, while clinical aspects and ageing itself appeared to cluster with memory performance in a second dimension. Cluster analysis further added to the findings; with an increase in the overall dimension (object) score (meaning the contribution of age, pathologies, and indicators of more unhealthy lifestyle factors), the overall cognitive performance decreased. Particularly, when clusters were analyzed for the relevant measures, the weaker clusters in terms of cognition (C3 and C4), across memory and executive function domains, were those that comprised a combination of older participants, with lower school education, obese, with substantially increased metabolic risk, and with presence of cardiac pathology. Interestingly, while executive function appeared more particularly susceptible to indicators of an unhealthier lifestyle measures (which is particularly interesting in the case of C1 and C2 clusters, where, with no significant differences in age and school years, the GENEXEC performance is significantly different, together with indicators of lifestyle), memory seemed equally sensitive to these and to the presence of clinical pathology (especially, cardiovascular pathology). While pathologies such as diabetes, metabolic syndrome (and its individual components), and vascular-related pathologies have been associated with cognitive decline, deficits, and/or impairment, the maintenance of a "healthy" lifestyle and introduction of beneficial interventional measures have been associated with cognitive improvements, including the overall pathology and isolated disease components [41–46]. Specifically, risk factors for cerebrovascular and cardiovascular pathologies or disease are thought to reduce blood flow to the frontal and subcortical brain regions and therefore impact (negatively) cognitive function [47]. Additionally, the lifestyle indicators, BMI, and metabolic risk have been associated with memory performance [48, 49]. However, it is the interdependency/relation between the variables, possibly explaining unique trajectories of cognitive ageing, which actually enforces the need for encompassing exploratory studies and appropriate methodology. For instance, unhealthy behavior can act as a risk factor for chronic disease itself with impact on negative mood that, in turn, can trigger further unhealthy habits and consequently worsening of chronic conditions [50].

These observations are in line with a recently published longitudinal study indicating that the combined effect of multiple risk factors may be of greater concern than individual triggers on cognitive decline in older adults [51]. Specifically, it was shown that smoking had the most consistent longitudinal impact linked with lower cognitive performance on multiple cognitive outcomes (including memory and executive function). Here, interestingly, the variable smoking had relevant and similar discrimination measures in both dimensions, followed by alcohol. Regarding alcohol, published data relating its intake with cognition among older adults is mixed. On one hand, studies comparing drinkers and nondrinkers report lower cognitive functioning among nondrinkers and heavier drinkers compared to "average" (7–14 drinks per week) drinkers (e.g., [52]); however, even among longitudinal studies reporting statistically significant associations between better cognition and moderate alcohol consumption, the magnitudes of the associations can be small. Another limitation is that domain-specific measures of cognition are not often employed (as discussed, [53]). Still, recent work, which addresses these drawbacks, indicates that moderate alcohol intake through midlife and into later life confers the best cognitive outcomes in old age, as defined by word-finding ability. The relationships were independent of age, smoking status, hypertension, and gender. The authors also indicate that heavy drinkers had the lowest phonemic fluency scores, which is consistent with other tests of executive function and may precede declines in memory [53]. Finally, it was interesting that here gender itself was not a relevant measure in MCA and neither was it the variable that discriminated between clusters of performance (cluster analysis). In fact, the impact of gender on cognitive ageing is not clear in the literature. Studies that appear contradictory may simply just indicate that age classes may particularly matter when considering gender (e.g., regarding neuroendocrine aspects or menopause [54]), and/or that gender may have an indirect effect. For instance, if in the past females had a more secondary role in terms of participation in society and/or access to education, this might be manifested in poorer cognitive performance compared with the male peers, including the older years.

Following other studies across a breadth of epidemiological research that either also used MCA as the primary analysis tool or as a basis to building statistical models (e.g., [55–61]), here the strategy was meaningful, yielding results in agreement with the literature, revealing that MCA is a relevant methodological approach for a valuable first insight into medium-size datasets consisting of multiple domains (e.g., cognitive, clinical, and sociodemographic). Nonetheless, a few considerations are warranted. Although one of the advantages of the MCA technique is that qualitative information is transformed into quantitative information to be used in further analysis, when quantitative variables are transformed into qualitative ones some of its properties may be lost as well as the measurement precision. However, unlike most complex statistical methods, for the MCA procedure there are not any preconditions (such as multivariate normality and linearity). This technique allows the analysis of the relations between variables and between different categories/levels of each variable, offering at the same time, in comparison to other methods, statistical results that can be seen both analytically and visually. Furthermore, since it is based on the variable categories (distance), the directionality of the relationship is not applicable. Nonetheless, CA does remain an exploratory tool for the analysis of association(s) between categorical variables. Finally, here, the analysis is cross-sectional; however, CA can equally be used in longitudinal data. When there is one categorical variable measured at two-time points, a transition matrix can be constructed; in this case, the aim of a correspondence analysis of a transition matrix is to get an insight into the transitions from time 1 to time 2. Given that different questions about these transitions exist, these lead to different forms of CA (the same reasoning applies to CA of more than two time points). We refer to the Van der Heijden 2005 [62] article for more details on the applicability and considerations of CA in longitudinal studies.

The methodology should now be replicated across European cohorts to explore the findings in other study populations. Findings are expected to have direct implications in the clinic, identifying groups at risk for cognitive decline and decrease in functionality.

Authors' Contribution

Patrício Soares Costa and Nadine Correia Santos contributed equally in the authorship and should be listed as cofirst authors.

Acknowledgments

The authors are thankful to all study participants. The authors would like to acknowledge all colleagues who assisted with participants recruitment and evaluation. The authors are also thankful to Pedro Moreira for the careful reading of the paper. This work was funded by the European Commission (FP7): "SwitchBox" (Contract HEALTH-F2-2010-259772). NCS is supported by a SwitchBox postdoctoral fellowship (UMINHO/BPD/013/2011).

References

[1] E. J. Beh, "Simple correspondence analysis: a bibliographic review," *International Statistical Review*, vol. 72, no. 2, pp. 257–284, 2004.

[2] R. A. Johnson and D. W. Wichern, *Applied Multivariate Correspondence Analysis*, Prentice-Hall, Upper Saddle River, NJ, USA, 6th edition, 2007.

[3] J. F. Hair, R. L. Tatham, R. E. Anderson, and W. Black, *Multivariate Data Analysis*, Prentice-Hall, Upper Saddle River, NJ, USA, 5th edition, 1998.

[4] B. G. Tabachnick and L. S. Fidell, *Using Multivariate Statistics*, Allyn and Bacon, Boston, Mass, USA, 4th edition, 1996.

[5] S. E. Clausen, *Applied Correspondence Analysis: An Introduction*, Quantitative applications in the social science, Sage, Thousand Oaks, Calif, USA, 1998.

[6] M. Greenacre and T. Hastie, "The geometric interpretation of correspondence analysis," *Journal of the American Statistical Association*, vol. 82, no. 398, pp. 437–447, 1987.

[7] K. M. van Meter, M. A. Schiltz, P. Cibois, and L. Mounier, "Correspondence analysis: a history and French sociological perspective," in *Correspondence Analysis in the Social Sciences: Recent Developments and Applications*, M. Greenacre and J. Blasius, Eds., Academic Press, San Diego, Calif, USA, 1994.

[8] D. Aktürk, S. Gün, and T. Kumuk, "Multiple correspondence analysis technique used in analyzing the categorical data in social sciences," *Journal of Applied Sciences*, vol. 7, no. 4, pp. 585–588, 2007.

[9] N. Sourial, C. Wolfson, B. Zhu et al., "Correspondence analysis is a useful tool to uncover the relationships among categorical variables," *Journal of Clinical Epidemiology*, vol. 63, no. 6, pp. 638–646, 2010.

[10] P. Loslever, "Using multiple correspondence analysis with membership values when the system study yields miscellaneous datasets," *Cybernetics and Systems*, vol. 40, no. 7, pp. 633–652, 2009.

[11] N. C. Santos, P. S. Costa, P. Cunha et al., "Mood is a key determinant of cognitive performance in community-dwelling older adults: a cross-sectional analysis," *Age*, 2012.

[12] A. C. Paulo, A. Sampaio, N. C. Santos et al., "Patterns of cognitive performance in healthy ageing in northern portugal: a cross-sectional analysis," *PLoS One*, vol. 6, no. 9, Article ID e24553, 2011.

[13] K. Anstey and H. Christensen, "Education, activity, health, blood pressure and apolipoprotein E as predictors of cognitive change in old age: a review," *Gerontology*, vol. 46, no. 3, pp. 163–177, 2000.

[14] R. A. Parslow, V. J. Lewis, and R. Nay, "Successful aging: development and testing of a multidimensional model using data from a large sample of older Australians," *Journal of the American Geriatrics Society*, vol. 59, no. 11, pp. 2077–2083, 2011.

[15] T. Archer, A. Fredriksson, E. Schütz, and R. M. Kostrzewa, "Influence of physical exercise on neuroimmunological functioning and health: aging and stress," *Neurotoxicity Research*, vol. 20, no. 1, pp. 69–83, 2011.

[16] F. Marcellini, C. Giuli, R. Papa, C. Gagliardi, M. Malavolta, and E. Mocchegiani, "BMI, life-style and psychological conditions in a sample of elderly Italian men and women," *Journal of Nutrition, Health and Aging*, vol. 14, no. 7, pp. 515–522, 2010.

[17] P. A. Reuter-Lorenz and C. Lustig, "Brain aging: reorganizing discoveries about the aging mind," *Current Opinion in Neurobiology*, vol. 15, no. 2, pp. 245–251, 2005.

[18] T. A. Salthouse, "Selective review of cognitive aging," *Journal of the International Neuropsychological Society*, vol. 16, no. 5, pp. 754–760, 2010.

[19] N. Sourial, C. Wolfson, H. Bergman et al., "A correspondence analysis revealed frailty deficits aggregate and are multidimensional," *Journal of Clinical Epidemiology*, vol. 63, no. 6, pp. 647–654, 2010.

[20] P. S. Costa, N. C. Santos, P. Cunha, J. A. Palha, and N. Sousa, "The use of Bayesian latent class cluster models to classify patterns of cognitive performance in healthy ageing," *PLoS One*, 2013.

[21] OECD, "Country statistical profile—Portugal," 2011, http://dx.doi.org/10.1787/csp-prt-Table-2011-1-en.

[22] M. Graffar, "Une methode de classification sociale d'echantillon des populations," *Courrier*, vol. 6, pp. 455–459, 1956.

[23] M. F. Folstein, S. E. Folstein, and P. R. McHugh, "'Mini mental state'. a practical method for grading the cognitive state of patients for the clinician," *Journal of Psychiatric Research*, vol. 12, no. 3, pp. 189–198, 1975.

[24] D. Wechsler, *Wechsler Adult Intelligence Scale (WAIS-III)*, Harcourt Assessment, San Antonio, Tex, USA, 1997.

[25] H. Buschke, M. Sliwinski, G. Kuslansky, and R. B. Lipton, "Aging, encoding specificity, and memory change in the Double Memory Test," *Journal of the International Neuropsychological Society*, vol. 1, no. 5, pp. 483–493, 1995.

[26] E. Strauss, E. M. S. Sherman, and O. Spreen, *A Compendium of Neuropsychological Tests: Administration, Norms and Commentary*, Oxford University Press, New York, N, USA, 2006.

[27] M. Lezak, D. Howieson, and D. Loring, *Neuropsychological Assessment*, Oxford University Press, New York, NY, USA, 2004.

[28] World Health Organization, "Waist circumference and waist-hip ratio," Report of a WHO Expert Consultation, WHO Library Cataloguing-in-Publication Data, Geneva, Switzerland, 2008.

[29] H. Kim, "Measures of influence in correspondence analysis," *Journal of Statistical Computation and Simulation*, vol. 40, pp. 3201–4217, 1992.

[30] H. Kim, "Influence functions in multiple correspondence analysis," *Korean Journal of Applied Statistics*, vol. 7, no. 1, pp. 69–74, 1994.

[31] W. J. Krzanowski, "Attribute selection in correspondence analysis of incidence matrices," *Applied Statistics*, vol. 42, no. 3, pp. 529–541, 1993.

[32] J. C. Gower, "Discussion of "a combined approach to contingency table analysis using correspondence analysis and log-linear analysis"," *Applied Statistics*, vol. 38, no. 1, pp. 249–292, 1989.

[33] D. B. Rubin, "Inference and missing data," *Biometrika*, vol. 63, no. 3, pp. 581–592, 1976.

[34] P. Kline, *An Easy Guide to Factor Analysis*, Routledge, London, UK, 2002.

[35] R. J. A. Little and D. B. Rubin, *Statistical Analysis with Missing Data*, Wiley, Hoboken, NJ, USA, 2nd edition, 2002.

[36] R. B. Cattell, "The meaning and strategic use of factor analysis," in *Handbook of Multivariate Experimental Psychology*, R. B. Cattell, Ed., Rand McNally, Chicago, Ill, USA, 1996.

[37] A. Gifi, *Non-Linear Multivariate Analysis,*, John Willey & Sons, Chichester, UK, 1996.

[38] L. Lebart, A. Morineau, and K. M. Warwick, *Multivariate Descriptive Statistical Analysis*, Wiley, New York, NY, USA, 1984.

[39] J. Beddington, C. L. Cooper, J. Field et al., "The mental wealth of nations," *Nature*, vol. 455, no. 7216, pp. 1057–1060, 2008.

[40] L. Ferrucci, F. Giallauria, and J. M. Guralnik, "Epidemiology of Aging," *Radiologic Clinics of North America*, vol. 46, no. 4, pp. 643–652, 2008.

[41] N. Yamamoto, G. Yamanaka, E. Takasugi et al., "Lifestyle intervention reversed cognitive function in aged people with diabetes mellitus: two-year follow up," *Diabetes Research and Clinical Practice*, vol. 85, no. 3, pp. 343–346, 2009.

[42] K. G. M. M. Alberti and P. Zimmet, "The metabolic syndrome—a new worldwide definition," *The Lancet*, vol. 366, no. 9491, pp. 1059–1062, 2005.

[43] T. N. Akbaraly, M. Kivimaki, M. J. Shipley et al., "Metabolic syndrome over 10 years and cognitive functioning in late midlife: the Whitehall II study," *Diabetes Care*, vol. 33, no. 1, pp. 84–89, 2010.

[44] M. Kivipelto, E.-L. Helkala, T. Hänninen et al., "Midlife vascular risk factors and late-life mild cognitive impairment: a population-based study," *Neurology*, vol. 56, no. 12, pp. 1683–1689, 2001.

[45] I. Skoog, B. Lernfelt, S. Landahl et al., "15-year longitudinal study of blood pressure and dementia," *Lancet*, vol. 347, no. 9009, pp. 1141–1145, 1996.

[46] M. F. Elias, P. K. Elias, L. M. Sullivan, P. A. Wolf, and R. B. D'Agostino, "Obesity, diabetes and cognitive deficit: the Framingham Heart Study," *Neurobiology of Aging*, vol. 26, supplement 1, pp. S11–S16, 2005.

[47] W. Dai, O. L. Lopez, O. T. Carmichael, J. T. Becker, L. H. Kuller, and H. M. Gach, "Abnormal regional cerebral blood flow in cognitively normal elderly subjects with hypertension," *Stroke*, vol. 39, no. 2, pp. 349–354, 2008.

[48] G. A. Dore, M. F. Elias, M. A. Robbins, M. M. Budge, and P. K. Elias, "Relation between central adiposity and cognitive function in the Maine-Syracuse study: attenuation by physical activity," *Annals of Behavioral Medicine*, vol. 35, no. 3, pp. 341–350, 2008.

[49] J. Gunstad, A. Lhotsky, C. R. Wendell, L. Ferrucci, and A. B. Zonderman, "Longitudinal examination of obesity and cognitive function: results from the baltimore longitudinal study of aging," *Neuroepidemiology*, vol. 34, no. 4, pp. 222–229, 2010.

[50] C. H. van Gool, G. I. J. M. Kempen, B. W. J. H. Penninx, D. J. H. Deeg, A. T. F. Beekman, and J. T. M. van Eijk, "Relationship between changes in depressive symptoms and unhealthy lifestyles in late middle aged and older persons: results from the longitudinal aging study Amsterdam," *Age and Ageing*, vol. 32, no. 1, pp. 81–87, 2003.

[51] A. Dregan, R. Stewart, and M. C. Gulliford, "Cardiovascular risk factors and cognitive decline in adults aged 50 and over: a population-based cohort study," *Age Ageing*, vol. 42, no. 3, pp. 338–345, 2013.

[52] I. Lang, R. B. Wallace, F. A. Huppert, and D. Melzer, "Moderate alcohol consumption in older adults is associated with better cognition and well-being than abstinence," *Age and Ageing*, vol. 36, no. 3, pp. 256–261, 2007.

[53] A. L. Gross, G. W. Rebok, D. E. Ford et al., "Alcohol consumption and domain-specific cognitive function in older adults: Longitudinal data from the johns hopkins precursors study," *Journals of Gerontology B*, vol. 66, no. 1, pp. 39–47, 2011.

[54] G. A. Greendale, C. A. Derby, and P. M. Maki, "Perimenopause and cognition," *Obstetrics & Gynecology Clinics of North America*, vol. 38, no. 3, pp. 519–535, 2011.

[55] B. F. M. Bakker, "A new measure of social status for men and women: the social distance scale," *Netherlands Journal of Social Sciences*, vol. 29, no. 2, pp. 113–129, 1993.

[56] C. Guinot, J. Latreille, D. Malvy et al., "Use of multiple correspondence analysis and cluster analysis to study dietary behaviour: food consumption questionnaire in the SU.VI.MAX. cohort," *European Journal of Epidemiology*, vol. 17, no. 6, pp. 505–516, 2001.

[57] M. L. Burton, E. Greenberger, and C. Hayward, "Mapping the ethnic landscape: personal beliefs about own group's and other groups' traits," *Cross-Cultural Research*, vol. 39, no. 4, pp. 351–379, 2005.

[58] S. M. Cavalcante, L. R. Kerr, S. M. Brignol et al., "Sociodemographic factors and health in a population of children living in families infected with HIV in Fortaleza and Salvador, Brazil," *AIDS Care*, vol. 25, no. 5, pp. 550–558, 2012.

[59] D. B. Panagiotakos and C. Pitsavos, "Interpretation of epidemiological data using multiple correspondence analysis and log-linear models," *Journal of Data Science*, vol. 2, pp. 75–86, 2004.

[60] L. D. Howe, B. Galobardes, A. Matijasevich et al., "Measuring socio-economic position for epidemiological studies in low- and middle-income countries: a methods of measurement in epidemiology paper," *International Journal of Epidemiology*, vol. 41, no. 3, pp. 871–886, 2012.

[61] P. Traissac and Y. Martin-Prevel, "Alternatives to principal components analysis to derive asset-based indices to measure socio-economic position in low- and middle-income countries: the case for multiple correspondence analysis," *International Journal of Epidemiology*, vol. 41, no. 4, pp. 1207–1208, 2012.

[62] P. G. M. Van der Heijden, "Correspondence Analysis of Longitudinal Data," in *Encyclopedia of Biostatistics*, P. Armitage and T. Colton, Eds., John Wiley & Sons, Chichester, UK, 2005.

12

Cumulative Weight Exposure Is Associated with Different Weight Loss Strategies and Weight Loss Success in Adults Age 50 or Above

Martin Sénéchal,[1,2] Jana Slaght,[3] and Danielle R. Bouchard[3,4]

[1] *Children's Hospital Research Institute of Manitoba, Winnipeg, MB, Canada R3E 3P4*
[2] *Department of Pediatrics and Child Health, Faculty of Medicine, University of Manitoba, Winnipeg, MB, Canada R3E 3P4*
[3] *Faculty of Kinesiology and Recreation Management, University of Manitoba, Winnipeg, MB, Canada R3T 2N2*
[4] *Health, Leisure, and Human Performance Research Institute, Winnipeg, MB, Canada R3T 2N2*

Correspondence should be addressed to Martin Sénéchal; martin.senechal@me.com

Academic Editor: F. R. Ferraro

Objectives. To evaluate if cumulative weight exposure is associated with weight loss strategy choices and weight loss success. *Methods.* Data from the National Health and Nutrition Examination Survey were used; a total of 4,562 people age 50 years or older who reported trying to lose weight in the last year were studied. Cumulative weight exposure (CWE) score was defined as the sum of body mass index points above 25 kg/m^2 at the age of 25, 10 years ago, 1 year ago, and now. Weight loss strategies were self-reported and weight loss success was defined as reaching a 5% weight loss in the last year. *Results.* Chosen strategies for weight loss vary across tertiles of CWE. Participants in the highest CWE tertile were about 4 to 20 times more likely to lose at least 5% of body weight in the past year compared to those in the lowest CWE tertile ($P < 0.05$). *Discussion.* Strategies used to lose weight and weight loss success using different weight loss strategies vary considerably across cumulative weight exposure. Thus, cumulative weight exposure might be a variable worth considering when intervening with this population.

1. Introduction

The prevalence of obesity has increased in all age groups in the past decades [1–3]. There is a body of evidence showing that body weight usually increases in a linear fashion with age and peaks around 65 years [4]. As a result, the number of years spent carrying extra body weight will inevitably increase in the next generations as well as the prevalence of obesity in middle age adults and youth. Cumulative weight exposure (CWE) score which is defined as the sum of units of body mass index (BMI) over (positive) or under (negative) the upper limit of the optimal weight BMI category (25 kg/m^2) for each of the available time points is one way to quantify the accumulation of weight over years [5, 6]. Prospective data from our group and others showed that CWE is associated with an increased likelihood of developing type 2 diabetes [5, 6], premature mortality [7, 8], and mobility impairment [9]. In addition, a recent study has reported that CWE was strongly associated with the increased likelihood of developing atherosclerosis in older adults [10]. These results suggest that CWE significantly impacts health in older adults and consequently it is imperative to study the implications of CWE for clinical settings.

The benefits of weight loss have been debated in older adults [11, 12]. However, a large randomized controlled trial of 585 older adults clearly demonstrated that the advantages of voluntary weight loss, using diet as a strategy, surpass the potential harms after 12 years of follow-up [13]. Regardless of that debate, more than 55% of adults over the age of 50 are trying to lose weight [14]. Although many strategies of weight loss are used, the first-line approach remains lifestyle modification including diet and exercise [15–17]. However, only 20% of obese individuals are currently able to maintain an initial 10% body weight loss for a period of two to five years using diet and exercise as the primary intervention [18]. Additionally, a recent study revealed that some weight loss strategies were more effective than others to reach a weight loss greater than 5% or 10% among obese adults [19].

It is likely that the CWE will increase in future generations of older adults and, so far, no one has verified if CWE is associated with weight loss strategy choices or if it is related to weight loss success. As a result, the first aim of this study was to evaluate whether weight loss strategy choices varied across different tertiles of CWE in older adults. The second objective was to investigate if CWE was associated with weight loss success (≥5% of total body weight between the self-reported weight 1 year ago and current body weight) stratified by weight loss strategies.

2. Methods

2.1. Study Population. The study sample consisted of 4,562 men and women aged 50 years and above who self-reported voluntarily trying to lose weight in the previous year in the U.S. National Health and Nutrition Examination Survey (NHANES: cycle 1999–2010). This cross-sectional study was completed in the noninstitutionalized population. Detailed survey operation manuals and consent forms are available on the NHANES website [20]. Briefly, the NHANES survey consisted of a home interview and a thorough health examination performed in a mobile exam center. During the home interview, participants were asked questions about their health status, disease history, and lifestyle behaviours. All participants provided written and informed consent. The protocol was approved by the National Center for Health Statistics.

Initially, 15,812 individuals were eligible based on age, but 3,877 were excluded because they were missing one or more time points for either body weight or height, precluding us from measuring CWE. In addition, those having a BMI below 18.5 kg/m^2 ($N = 273$) at the tested cycle or the previous year were excluded from the dataset. Out of the remaining 11,616 individuals, only the 4562 individuals (39.3%) who reported trying to lose weight in the previous year were kept for the final analysis. Using Chi-square tests, no significant differences ($P > 0.05$) were observed for age (66.3 ± 10.1 versus 63.9 ± 9.2), sex (52% versus 54% women), ethnicity (non-Hispanic white 57.5% versus 58.5%; non-Hispanic black 18.8% versus 18.0%; Hispanic 20.8% versus 20.6%), income ≥ $55,000 (22.5% versus 23.0%), or education level (36.1% versus 34.6%) between participants included in the current study compared to the participants not included in this study.

2.2. Measurement of Cumulative Weight Exposure. Body mass was measured at the tested cycle but was self-reported for 1 and 10 years ago, as well as at 25 years of age. Height was self-reported at age 25 and measured at the tested cycle. BMI was calculated for each of the four time points. When calculating BMI at age 25, the self-reported height at age 25 was used. However, for calculating BMI 10 years ago, the mean between the self-reported height at age 25 and the measured height was used.

The CWE score was calculated as the sum of units of BMI over (positive) or under (negative) the upper limit of the optimal weight BMI category (25 kg/m^2) for each of the available time points. For example, someone with a BMI of 26 kg/m^2 at age 25, 23 kg/m^2 10 years ago, 32 kg/m^2 last year, and 31 kg/m^2 at the measured cycle was given a CWE of 12 (1-2 + 7 + 6). CWE was recently used by our group in a previous prospective study by considering the number of years between objective measures of body weight and height [6]. However, in the case of this study, it seemed imprudent to weigh each measure differently because the data on body weight and height were self-reported up to 60 years ago, and the exact years or the exact dates of measurement were not recorded.

2.3. Strategies for Weight Loss. All individuals who reported trying to lose weight the year prior to the measured cycle (in a previous question) were asked to give details about the strategies used. The question was how did you try to lose weight? This question was asked using an interviewer-administered computer-assisted personal interviewing system and completed at home. The participants have read all the options. In each option, the participants answered "yes" or "no" whether he or she tried to lose weight in the past year. A list of 14 to 20 options was given depending on the cycle. For cycles 1999 to 2004, 14 options were listed: eating less food, consuming less calories, eating less fat, doing exercise, skipping meals, eating diet food, eating a liquid diet, joining a weight loss program, using prescribed medication, using nonprescribed medication, vomiting, drinking more water, using a special diet (e.g., Atkins), or "others." The participants could list as many "other" strategies as they wished. For cycles 2005 to 2010, six more options were available: eating fewer carbohydrates, smoking, consuming more fruits and vegetables, changing bad habits, eating less sugar, or seeking help from professionals. For analysis, individuals were given a value of 1 when answering positively to a strategy and a value of 0 when answering negatively to a strategy. Strategies reported by less than 5% of the sample were combined and labelled as "others." The strategies include using prescribed medication, using nonprescribed medication, vomiting, smoking, and using a special diet. As a result, 14 individual strategies are described in Results in addition to the "other" variables.

2.4. Weight Loss Success. Weight loss success was measured as losing a minimum of 5% of total body weight between the self-reported weight 1 year ago and the current weight as proposed elsewhere [21]. In this study the amount of weight loss was calculated as the difference between self-reported weight one year ago and measured weight at the evaluation.

2.5. Confounding Variables. Covariates included in the analyses were age (continuous variable), sex, race/ethnicity (non-Hispanic white, non-Hispanic black, Hispanic, and other), smoking status (currently smoking or not), education level (<high school, high school, and college or more), family income (<$20 000, $20 001–$54 999, and >$55 000), and marital status (single or partner).

2.6. Statistical Analysis. Data management and statistical analyses were performed using SAS version 9.3 (SAS Institute,

TABLE 1: Characteristics of the 4562 study participants.

	Low CWE ≤6.56	Mid CWE 6.57–20.86	High CWE ≥20.87	P value
General characteristics				
Age (years)	64.2 ± 9.6	64.6 ± 9.2	62.9 ± 8.6	<0.01
Men (%)	550 (36.2)	820 (53.9)	730 (48.0)	<0.01
BMI (kg/m^2)	26.3 ± 2.5	30.8 ± 2.6	37.8 ± 5.7	<0.01
Obesity status				
Obese at age 25	3 (0.2)	19 (1.2)	279 (18.3)	<0.01
Obese 10 years ago	11 (0.7)	339 (22.3)	1239 (87.5)	<0.01
Obese 1 year ago	96 (6.3)	1009 (66.3)	1496 (98.4)	<0.01
Currently obese	94 (6.2)	907 (59.6)	1466 (96.4)	<0.01
Successful weight loss	502 (33.0)	684 (45.0)	842 (55.4)	<0.01
Race/ethnicity				0.01
Non-Hispanic white	1006 (66.2)	852 (56.0)	767 (50.4)	
Non-Hispanic black	174 (11.4)	281 (18.5)	404 (26.6)	
Hispanic	272 (17.9)	357 (23.5)	319 (20.9)	
Other	68 (4.5)	31 (2.0)	31 (2.0)	
Education level				0.61
Less than high school	636 (41.8)	624 (41.0)	616 (40.5)	
High school	339 (22.3)	318 (20.9)	349 (20.9)	
College or above	533 (35.1)	565 (37.1)	547 (36.1)	
Smoking level				
Currently smoking	323 (21.3)	327 (21.1)	316 (20.8)	0.99
Household annual income				0.01
≤$20,000	314 (20.7)	336 (22.1)	386 (25.4)	
$20,000–54,999	573 (37.7)	556 (36.6)	597 (39.3)	
≥55,000	374 (24.6)	354 (23.3)	397 (19.5)	
Marital status				0.02
Married/partner	805 (53.0)	858 (56.4)	784 (51.5)	

Data are presented as mean (SD) for continuous variables and n (%) for categorical variables.
CWE = cumulative weight exposure.

Carry, NC) and SPSS version 18. Because of the complex survey design used in NHANES, traditional methods of statistical analysis based on the assumption of a simple random sample are not applicable. Briefly, NHANES provides additional variables to be included in regression models to adjust for sample weights and complex survey design (strata, probability sampling units). In each regression model performed in the current study, three extra variables were added to the model. For weight, as indicated on the NHANES website, we used the smallest subpopulation that includes all the variables in the analysis (i.e., 2-year MEC exam weight [22]). For variance, the variables named variance pseudo-PSU and pseudostratum were added as indicated to the NHANES guidelines for variance [23]. More details are provided on their website [24]. Chi-square, one-way ANOVA, and general linear models were used to compare characteristics of our sample as well as the chosen weight loss strategies across tertiles of CWE. Linear regression models were used to test the association between the continuous CWE and each of the reported weight loss strategies. These models were adjusted for age, sex, race/ethnicity, smoking status, family income, marital status, education level, dataset weight, dataset variance, and BMI. Thereafter, logistic regression models were performed to investigate the likelihood of using different strategies of weight loss across tertiles of CWE. In addition, we performed logistic regression models to investigate if the CWE was an independent predictor of weight loss success. All the logistic regression models were adjusted for age, sex, race/ethnicity, smoking status, family income, marital status, education level, dataset weight, dataset variance, and either obesity status or BMI. Significance was set at $P < 0.05$.

3. Results

Table 1 describes general characteristics of the sample stratified by tertiles of CWE. There was a significant difference among tertiles of CWE for age, sex, obesity status, race/ethnicity, annual income, and marital status (all $P < 0.05$), while no difference was observed among groups education level and current smokers.

Table 2 shows that eating less food (68.7%) and doing more exercise (46.2%) were the most reported weight

TABLE 2: Reported strategies to lose weight in the past year.

Strategies	Prevalence	Low CWE	Mid CWE	High CWE	*P* value
Less food	3132 (68.7)	1041 (68.5)	1013 (66.6)	1078 (70.9)	0.04
Less calories	1651 (36.2)	551 (36.2)	531 (34.5)	569 (37.4)	0.36
Less fat	1978 (43.4)	334 (9.0)	616 (15.5)	1028 (25.9)	0.19
Less sugar	264 (5.8)	80 (5.3)	86 (5.7)	98 (6.4)	0.36
Less carbohydrates	732 (16.0)	217 (14.3)	242 (15.9)	273 (17.9)	0.02**
Skip meals	663 (14.5)	177 (11.6)	213 (14.7)	263 (17.3)	0.19
Diet food products	404 (8.9)	116 (7.6)	133 (8.7)	155 (10.2)	0.19
Drink more water	1247 (27.3)	361 (23.8)	414 (27.2)	472 (31.0)	0.04**
Liquid diet	229 (5.0)	87 (5.7)	74 (4.9)	68 (4.5)	0.27
More fruits and vegetables	336 (7.4)	87 (5.7)	105 (6.9)	144 (9.5)	<0.01**
Modify bad habits	219 (4.8)	59 (3.9)	70 (4.6)	90 (5.9)	0.03
Join a weight loss program	260 (5.7)	80 (5.3)	75 (2.9)	105 (6.9)	0.04
More exercise	2106 (46.2)	756 (49.7)	715 (47.0)	635 (41.7)	<0.01**
Consult health professional	265 (5.8)	60 (3.9)	89 (5.9)	116 (7.6)	0.04
Others*	287 (6.3)	87 (5.7)	93 (6.1)	107 (7.0)	0.31

Data are presented as *n* (%); Chi-square tests were used across tertiles of CWE.
P value is unadjusted.
*Others included using prescribed medication, using of nonprescribed medication, vomiting, smoking, and using a special diet.
**Remained significant once adjusted for confounders.
CWE = cumulative weight exposure.

loss strategies in older adults. Significant differences were observed across tertiles of CWE for 8 out of the 15 possible self-reported strategies. However, only four strategies across CWE tertiles were significant after adjustments for confounders: exercising more ($P = 0.01$), drinking more water ($P = 0.04$), consuming more fruits and vegetables ($P = 0.04$), and eating fewer carbohydrates ($P = 0.02$).

Linear regression models were used to test the association between the continuous CWE and each of the reported weight loss strategies. The results showed that the same four strategies (i.e., exercising more, drinking more water, consuming more fruits and vegetables, and eating fewer carbohydrates) were associated with the CWE expressed as a continuous variable ($P < 0.05$) once adjusted for all confounders, including BMI.

Figures 1(a), 1(b), 1(c), and 1(d) describe the likelihood of exercising more, drinking more water, eating fewer carbohydrates, or eating more fruits and vegetables as strategies to lose weight across CWE tertiles. Older adults in the highest tertile of CWE were 42% less likely to use exercise as a strategy to lose weight OR (95% CI) 0.58 (0.67–0.77). On the other hand, older individuals in the highest tertile of CWE were 1.48 (1.26–1.75) times more likely to drink more water, 1.69 (1.29–2.24) times more likely to eat more fruits and vegetables, and 1.33 (1.09–1.62) times more likely to reduce carbohydrates consumption, as strategies to lose weight compared with the low tertile of CWE ($P = 0.01$).

Table 3 represents the odds of achieving at least 5% body weight loss during the past year (≥5% of total body weight between the self-reported weight 1 year ago and the current body weight). When adjusted for obesity status, age, sex, race/ethnicity, smoking, household annual income, and marital status older adults in the highest CWE were 13.74 (95% CI: 7.23–26.14; $P < 0.01$) times more likely to do so if they increased exercise level as strategy compared with their counterparts in the lowest CWE group. The odds increased

TABLE 3: Odds of losing at least 5% of body weight in the past year.

	Low CWE	Mid CWE	High CWE
Doing more exercise			
Model with obesity status	1.00	3.27 (2.10–5.09)	13.74 (7.23–26.14)
Model with BMI	1.00	3.69 (2.30–5.94)	19.66 (9.60–40.23)
Drinking more water			
Model with obesity status	1.00	1.92 (1.06–3.48)	5.00 (2.29–10.94)
Model with BMI	1.00	1.41 (0.80–2.49)	3.84 (1.71–8.64)
Eating less carbohydrates			
Model with obesity status	1.00	3.62 (1.76–7.44)	8.82 (3.20–24.26)
Model with BMI	1.00	2.53 (1.26–5.09)	4.61 (1.70–12.52)
Eating more fruits and vegetables			
Model with obesity status	1.00	2.10 (0.57–7.69)	3.02 (0.62–14.68)
Model with BMI	1.00	1.48 (0.45–4.92)	2.22 (0.48–10.29)

Odds ratio (95% confidence interval).
All models were adjusted for age, sex, race/ethnicity, smoking status, family income, marital status, education level, dataset weight, dataset variance, and either obesity status or BMI.
CWE = cumulative weight exposure.

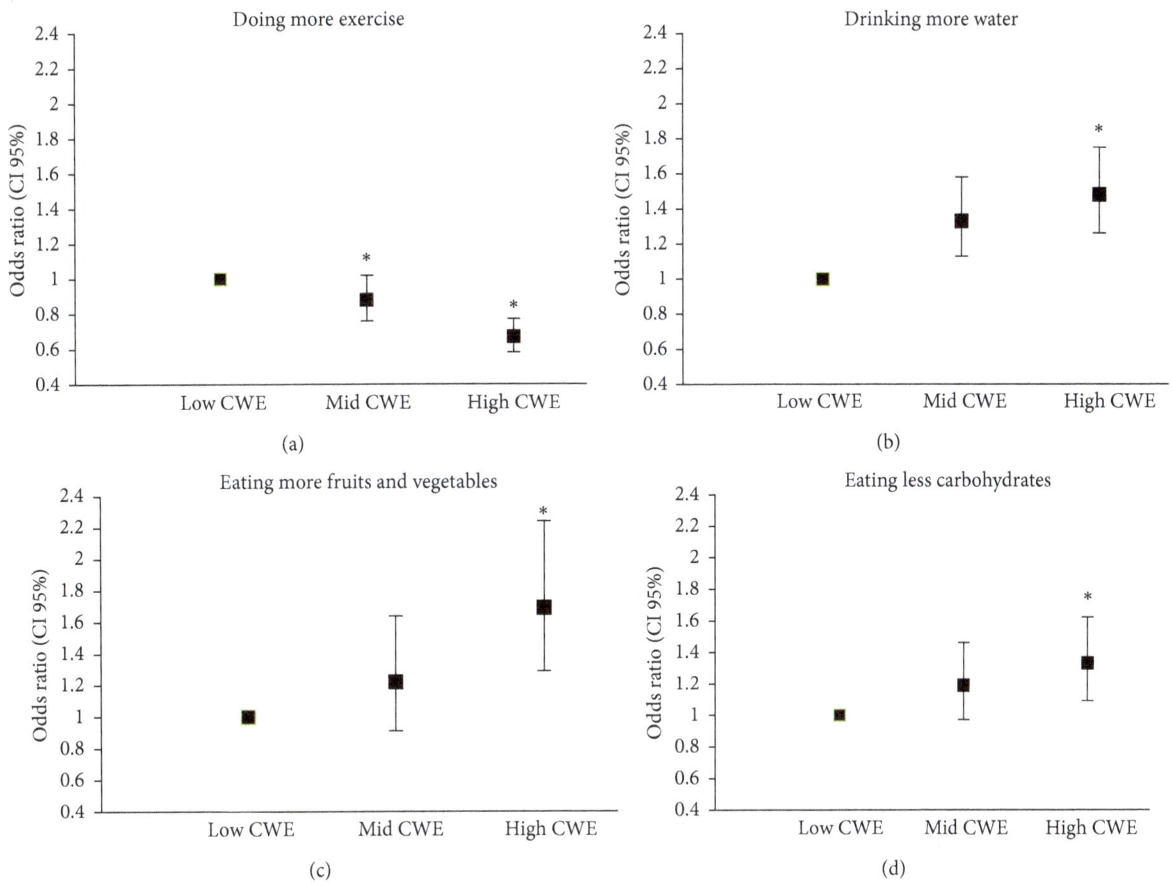

FIGURE 1: Strategies used to lose weight across CWE groups. *Significantly different from the low CWE group.

to 19.66 (95% CI: 9.60–40.23; $P < 0.01$) when using BMI instead of the obesity status in the model. Older adults in the highest CWE are 5.00 (2.29–8.99) times more likely to reach at least 5% weight loss if they increased water consumption and 8.82 (3.20–24.26) times more likely if they decreased carbohydrates, but not more likely to increase consumption of fruits and vegetables. The same significance level was observed when using BMI instead of obesity status in models. The respective numbers were 3.84 (1.71–8.64), 4.61 (1.70–12.52), and 2.22 (0.48–10.29).

4. Discussion

This study revealed novel insights into the management of obesity among adults age 50 or above. The first novel finding of the current study is that CWE is associated with the choice of weight loss strategies among adults age 50 years old and above. More specifically, people with the highest CWE are more likely to choose diet strategies such as drinking more water, eating fewer carbohydrates, and eating more fruits and vegetables and less likely to choose exercise as a strategy to achieve weight loss. The second novel finding is that CWE is associated with weight loss success in the past year when using these three specific strategies to lose weight. Collectively, these findings suggest that adults 50 years old or above who have accumulated extra body weight over the years might choose different weight loss strategies, and their weight loss success might differ based on the level of CWE.

As previously mentioned, reducing caloric intake and increasing exercise levels are the cornerstones for successful weight loss [15–17]. Based on the literature, the most popular weight loss strategy is to take fewer calories and eating smaller portions (less food) [14, 16, 19]. In the current study, when considering confounders, eating less food was not a weight loss strategy associated with CWE. This suggests that eating less food might be a strategy that adults are doing in general; however, our results support that older adults having accumulated extra body weight over the years are not more or less likely to decrease food portions in order to achieve weight loss. On the other hand, our results show that CWE was associated with two specific diet strategies to lose weight (i.e., drinking more water and reducing carbohydrates) even once adjusted for current obesity status or current BMI. This could be explained by the fact that older adults who have accumulated more excessive weight have already tried the most popular diet strategies (e.g., reducing fat, reducing calories, and increasing fruits and vegetables consumption) and are now looking for a new way to induce weight loss. To support this hypothesis, a study done with 20,000 people reported that BMI was positively associated with the number of attempts to lose weight in older adults [25]. In our study BMI was associated with the CWE ($r = 0.78$, $P < 0.01$)

increasing the challenge to distinguish if a greater CWE was associated with weight loss strategies to reach 5% of weight loss in the past year independent of BMI. We tried to address this issue by using obesity status (Yes/No BMI $\geq 30\,kg/m^2$). When logistic regression models to predict if doing more exercise, drinking more water, and eating fewer carbohydrates were associated with weight loss equal or above 5% in the past year, the high CWE group was more likely to have used these weight loss strategies compared with the low CWE group regardless of being adjusted for obesity status or BMI.

Previous studies have reported that between 50 and 60% of people are using exercise as a weight loss strategy [15, 16, 19], while in adults age 50 or above, the prevalence is 56.3% [15]. In our study, we observed a lower proportion (46%) of older adults in the same range of age using exercise as a strategy to lose weight. This difference could be explained in part by the fact that studies from the literature analysed data collected between 1998 and 2006, while our study took the data from 1999 to 2010. Consequently, it is possible that using exercise as a strategy to lose weight has declined as a result of the reduction of exercise levels in the whole population in the past few years [26], or as a result of the popularity of new weight loss strategies [27]. Even though our results confirm that exercise is a popular strategy chosen to lose weight among adults in that age range, it also extends the current knowledge by showing that if someone has accumulated weight throughout their lifespan, he or she is less likely to choose this strategy to lose weight. CWE has been associated with chronic conditions [7, 8] and mobility impairments [9] in the past. This could help explain why we observed that people in the highest CWE category reported that they were less inclined to choose to exercise in order to achieve weight loss.

In terms of weight loss success, our results show that adults age 50 years old or above who choose at least one of these strategies: exercise more, eat less carbohydrates, and drink more water, have four to twenty times greater odds of losing a minimum of 5% body weight in the past year if they have accumulated high excessive weight over the years. These findings are in line with strategies associated with losing a minimum 5% body weight reported by Nicklas et al. [19] who reported using a sample of adults that was associated with exercising more and using prescription weight loss medications. This latter difference might be explained by the fact that prescribed weight loss medications for older adults is still not widespread because of the possible risk of medication interactions, poor adherence to drug prescription [28], and the fact that weight loss drugs are usually not covered by health insurance which can cause a financial burden. In addition, our study includes data since 1999, when medications prescribed for weight loss were scarce, especially for older adults.

It has been demonstrated in the past that diet compliance is more important than the strategy to reach caloric reduction and weight loss [29]. However, our study suggests that some weight loss strategies might be more effective in a subsample of the population. For example, our study suggests that choosing to increase water consumption as a strategy to lose weight is three times more effective for individuals that have accumulated more weight over the years, compared with those who have accumulated less weight over the years, in achieving a minimum of 5% weight loss. Similar findings were observed for increasing exercise level and decreasing carbohydrates. Consequently, CWE might help to determine which adults would be more likely to respond positively to a given weight loss attempt using specific strategies.

Our current study revealed interesting results; however, some limitations need to be mentioned. The exposure variable is mostly based on self-reported measures of body weight and height. It is possible that body weight was underestimated and height overestimated as commonly reported [30, 31], especially that some individuals self-reported their body weight up to 60 years ago. One limitation of this study is that the CWE score was not weighed based on the number of years that one would have accumulated BMI below or above $25\,kg/m^2$. We decided not to do this because of the weak association between objective and self-reported weight and height measurements, especially when the self-reported measures go up over the decades [31–34]. Because of the strong association between the CWE and BMI, it is impossible to test both variables in the same model and determine what variable is more associated with the studied outcomes. The interaction between different self-reported weight loss strategies was not evaluated in the current study. It is possible that participants used combinations of different strategies to attempt weight loss, and perhaps changing one strategy such as increasing water consumption solely might not be associated with weight loss. Three cycles provided 19 options of weight loss strategies plus a section called "others," while three cycles (1999–2004) provided only 13 strategies plus a section called "others." Even if the participants could have reported any other strategies in "others" from 1999 to 2004, less than 1% of the sample reported anything in that category. This is not surprising considering that some literature reports that the use of open questions versus choosing from a list of answers leads to different answers [35]. Thus, it is possible that the strategies reported in efforts to lose weight in the past year could have been different if the possible answers had been the same in all the cycles. The cross-sectional design of this study limits our observation to association conclusions instead of causal effect. This study included evaluation done between 1999 and 2010, so it is possible that reported weight loss strategies were influenced by different temporal trends. Also, even if a person reported using a specific strategy to lose weight in the past year, we have no method to measure if the strategy was used and to what extent. Finally, we were not able to quantify the exact time between measures.

5. Conclusion

CWE score is associated with the use of different weight loss strategies among adults age 50 years old or above. In addition, CWE is a determinant of weight loss success when using specific weight loss strategies among that population. Clinical trials are now needed to identify if CWE is associated with weight loss success when weight loss strategies are controlled and weight loss is objectively measured.

Acknowledgments

The authors acknowledge the Canadian Institute of Health Research (CIHR) and the Integrated and Mentored Pulmonary and Cardiovascular Training (IMPACT) that support the salary and the training of Dr. Martin Sénéchal. Jana Slaght received a scholarship from Research Manitoba.

References

[1] I. Janssen, M. Shields, C. L. Craig, and M. S. Tremblay, "Prevalence and secular changes in abdominal obesity in Canadian adolescents and adults, 1981 to 2007–2009," *Obesity Reviews*, vol. 12, no. 6, pp. 397–405, 2011.

[2] World Health Organization, *Obesity: Prevention and Management of the Global Epidemic*, World Health Organization, Geneva, Switzerland, 2003.

[3] K. M. Flegal, M. D. Carroll, C. L. Ogden, and C. L. Johnson, "Prevalence and trends in obesity among US adults, 1999-2000," *The Journal of the American Medical Association*, vol. 288, no. 14, pp. 1723–1727, 2002.

[4] M. S. Tjepkema, *Adult Obesity in Canada: Measured Height and Weight*, 2005, http://statcan.gc.ca/pub/82-620-m/2005001/article/adults-adultes/8060-eng.htm.

[5] A. Abdullah, J. Stoelwinder, S. Shortreed et al., "The duration of obesity and the risk of type 2 diabetes," *Public Health Nutrition*, vol. 12, no. 1, pp. 119–126, 2010.

[6] D. R. Bouchard, B. Porneala, I. Janssen et al., "Risk of type 2 diabetes and cumulative excess weight exposure in the Framingham Offspring Study," *Journal of Diabetes and Its Complications*, vol. 27, no. 3, pp. 214–218, 2013.

[7] A. Abdullah, R. Wolfe, J. U. Stoelwinder et al., "The number of years lived with obesity and the risk of all-cause and cause-specific mortality," *International Journal of Epidemiology*, vol. 40, no. 4, pp. 985–996, 2011.

[8] I. Janssen and E. Bacon, "Effect of current and midlife obesity status on mortality risk in the elderly," *Obesity*, vol. 16, no. 11, pp. 2504–2509, 2008.

[9] S. Stenholm, T. Rantanen, E. Alanen, A. Reunanen, P. Sainio, and S. Koskinen, "Obesity history as a predictor of walking limitation at old age," *Obesity*, vol. 15, no. 4, pp. 929–938, 2007.

[10] J. P. Reis, C. M. Loria, C. E. Lewis et al., "Association between duration of overall and abdominal obesity beginning in young adulthood and coronary artery calcification in middle age," *Journal of the American Medical Association*, vol. 310, no. 3, pp. 280–288, 2013.

[11] S. L. Miller and R. R. Wolfe, "The danger of weight loss in the elderly," *The Journal of Nutrition, Health and Aging*, vol. 12, no. 7, pp. 487–491, 2008.

[12] M. Zamboni, G. Mazzali, E. Zoico et al., "Health consequences of obesity in the elderly: a review of four unresolved questions," *International Journal of Obesity*, vol. 29, no. 9, pp. 1011–1029, 2005.

[13] M. K. Shea, B. J. Nicklas, D. K. Houston et al., "The effect of intentional weight loss on all-cause mortality in older adults: results of a randomized controlled weight-loss trial," *American Journal of Clinical Nutrition*, vol. 94, no. 3, pp. 839–846, 2011.

[14] E. C. Weiss, D. A. Galuska, L. K. Khan, and M. K. Serdula, "Weight-control practices among U.S. Adults, 2001-2002," *American Journal of Preventive Medicine*, vol. 31, no. 1, pp. 18–24, 2006.

[15] C. L. Bish, H. M. Blanck, M. K. Serdula, M. Marcus, H. W. Kohl III, and L. K. Khan, "Diet and physical activity behaviors among Americans trying to lose weight: 2000 behavioral risk factor surveillance system," *Obesity Research*, vol. 13, no. 3, pp. 596–607, 2005.

[16] J. Kruger, D. A. Galuska, M. K. Serdula, and D. A. Jones, "Attempting to lose weight: specific practices among U.S. Adults," *American Journal of Preventive Medicine*, vol. 26, no. 5, pp. 402–406, 2004.

[17] V. S. Malik and F. B. Hu, "Popular weight-loss diets: from evidence to practice," *Nature Clinical Practice Cardiovascular Medicine*, vol. 4, no. 1, pp. 34–41, 2007.

[18] R. R. Wing and J. O. Hill, "Successful weight loss maintenance," *Annual Review of Nutrition*, vol. 21, pp. 323–341, 2001.

[19] J. M. Nicklas, K. W. Huskey, R. B. Davis, and C. C. Wee, "Successful weight loss among obese U.S. adults," *American Journal of Preventive Medicine*, vol. 42, no. 5, pp. 481–485, 2012.

[20] Centers for Disease Control and Prevention, *National Health and Nutrition Examination Survey (NHANES)*, Centers for Disease Control and Prevention, 2015.

[21] S. Ramage, A. Farmer, K. A. Eccles, and L. McCargar, "Healthy strategies for successful weight loss and weight maintenance: a systematic review," *Applied Physiology, Nutrition and Metabolism*, vol. 39, no. 1, pp. 1–20, 2014.

[22] Centers for Disease Control and Prevention and National Health and Nutrition Examination Survey (NHANES), *How to Select the Correct Weights for NHANES Analysis*, 2010, http://www.cdc.gov/nchs/tutorials/NHANES/SurveyDesign/Weighting/Task1.htm.

[23] Centers for Disease Control and Prevention. National Health and Nutrition Examination Survey (NHANES), *Variance Estimation*, 2010, http://www.cdc.gov/nchs/tutorials/nhanes/surveydesign/VarianceEstimation/intro_i.htm.

[24] Centers for Disease Control and Prevention, *National Health and Nutrition Examination Survey (NHANES). Sample Design and Analysis Guidelines*, Centers for Disease Control and Prevention, 2002, http://archive.nlm.nih.gov/proj/dxpnet/nhanes/docs/doc/nhanes3/lab/LAB_sample_design_and_analysis_guidelines.txt.

[25] A. Hiartaker, P. Laake, and E. Lund, "Body mass index and weight change attempts among adult women: the Norwegian women and cancer study," *European Journal of Public Health*, vol. 11, no. 2, pp. 141–146, 2001.

[26] R. C. Colley, D. Garriguet, I. Janssen, C. L. Craig, J. Clarke, and M. S. Tremblay, "Physical activity of Canadian adults: accelerometer results from the 2007 to 2009 Canadian Health Measures Survey," *Health Reports*, vol. 22, no. 1, pp. 7–14, 2011.

[27] R. F. Kushner, "Weight loss strategies for treatment of obesity," *Progress in Cardiovascular Diseases*, vol. 56, no. 4, pp. 465–472, 2014.

[28] B. J. Turner, "Improving on a coin toss to predict patient adherence to medications," *Annals of Internal Medicine*, vol. 134, no. 10, pp. 1004–1006, 2001.

[29] M. L. Dansinger, J. A. Gleason, J. L. Griffith, H. P. Selker, and E. J. Schaefer, "Comparison of the Atkins, Ornish, Weight Watchers, and Zone diets for weight loss and heart disease risk reduction: a randomized trial," *The Journal of the American Medical Association*, vol. 293, no. 1, pp. 43–53, 2005.

[30] J. L. Engstrom, S. A. Paterson, A. Doherty, M. Trabulsi, and K. L. Speer, "Accuracy of self-reported height and weight in women: an integrative review of the literature," *Journal of Midwifery and Women's Health*, vol. 48, no. 5, pp. 338–345, 2003.

[31] G. S. Perry, T. E. Byers, A. H. Mokdad, M. K. Serdula, and D. F. Williamson, "The validity of self-reports of past body weights by U.S. adults," *Epidemiology*, vol. 6, no. 1, pp. 61–66, 1995.

[32] S. C. Gorber, M. Tremblay, D. Moher, and B. Gorber, "A comparison of direct vs. self-report measures for assessing height, weight and body mass index: a systematic review," *Obesity Reviews*, vol. 8, no. 4, pp. 307–326, 2007.

[33] J. Stevens, J. E. Keil, L. R. Waid, and P. C. Gazes, "Accuracy of current, 4-year, and 28-year self-reported body weight in an elderly population," *American Journal of Epidemiology*, vol. 132, no. 6, pp. 1156–1163, 1990.

[34] E. V. Villanueva, "The validity of self-reported weight in US adults: a population based cross-sectional study," *BMC Public Health*, vol. 1, no. 1, article 11, 2001.

[35] N. Schwartz, "How questions shape the answers," *The American Psychological Association*, vol. 54, no. 2, pp. 93–105, 1999.

13

Homeless Aging Veterans in Transition: A Life-Span Perspective

Carla J. Thompson[1,2] **and Nancy L. Bridier**[1]

[1] *University of West Florida, Pensacola, FL 32514, USA*
[2] *Research and Advanced Studies, University of West Florida, 11000 University Parkway, Building 78, Office 121, Pensacola, FL 32514, USA*

Correspondence should be addressed to Carla J. Thompson; cthompsonl@uwf.edu

Academic Editor: Astrid E. Fletcher

The need for counseling and career/educational services for homeless veterans has captured political and economic venues for more than 25 years. Veterans are three times more likely to become homeless than the general population if veterans live in poverty or are minority veterans. This mixed methods study emphasized a life-span perspective approach for exploring factors influencing normative aging and life-quality of 39 homeless veterans in Alabama and Florida. Seven descriptive quantitative and qualitative research questions framed the investigation. Study participants completed a quantitative survey reflecting their preferences and needs with a subset of the sample ($N = 12$) also participating in individual qualitative interview sessions. Thirty-two service providers and stakeholders completed quantitative surveys. Empirical and qualitative data with appropriate triangulation procedures provided interpretive information relative to a life-span development perspective. Study findings provide evidence of the need for future research efforts to address strategies that focus on the health and economic challenges of veterans before they are threatened with the possibility of homelessness. Implications of the study findings provide important information associated with the premise that human development occurs throughout life with specific characteristics influencing the individual's passage. Implications for aging/homelessness research are grounded in late-life transitioning and human development intervention considerations.

1. Introduction

The special population of homeless veterans has become an alarming concern within America's aging population challenges. According to the National Coalition for Homeless Veterans [1], while only 7% of the US population is comprised of veterans, approximately 13% of the adult homeless populations are veterans. Recent national survey efforts conducted by the Veterans' Administration and related government agencies report that 8.6% of homeless veterans are over the age of 62 with aging female homeless veteran populations increasing each year [2]. Veterans are three times more likely to become homeless than the general population if they live in poverty or are minority veterans in poverty. "Low income veterans are twice as likely to become homeless than the general population of low-income adults" [1, paragraph 2]. Almost half of homeless veterans in the United States are over the age of 51 and are comprised primarily of veterans representing the Baby Boomers and are veterans of the Vietnam War years [3]. This mixed methods study emphasized a life-span development perspective modeled by [4] for addressing the issue of aging homeless veterans. The study explored expressed needs and commentaries of 39 homeless veterans within two states in the southeast region of the United States (Alabama and Florida). Seven research questions provided the focus areas of exploration. Quantitative survey data retrieved from a sample of 39 homeless veterans, qualitative individual interview data from a subset of $N = 12$ of the homeless veteran participants, and additional quantitative survey data from $N = 32$ service providers and stakeholders were retrieved to represent multiple perspectives for conducting triangulation of data procedures and interpretation. Specific materials and methods, including the background and theoretical framing of the investigation, study results, implications, and conclusions comprise the discussion.

2. Materials and Methods

Key preliminary tasks for determining the materials and methods used in the study included an overview examination of the background and the literature considerations pertinent to the investigation and the theoretical underpinnings for the study. These preliminary efforts provided the impetus for the research questions and hypotheses as well as the rationale for the selection of specific materials and methods for the study.

2.1. Background and Statement of the Problem. The need for services for homeless veterans has captured political and economic venues for more than 25 years. Aging homeless veterans who are not identified as in need of services for substance abuse are not eligible for existing Veterans' Administration services that include safe housing or shelter services [5]. Often aging homeless veterans who are not classified with service-related medical or health issues are also not provided access to resources and needed services offered by the Veterans' Administration. According to the Department of Veterans Affairs [5], eligibility for the Housing and Urban Development-Veterans Affairs Supportive Housing (HUD-VASH) program requires recipients to participate in VA provided case management and clinical services. The term, homeless veteran, is often depicted as chronically homeless by The McKinney-Vento Homeless Assistance Act as amended by S. 896, The Homeless Emergency Assistance and Rapid Transition to Housing (HEARTH) Act of 2009 [5]. Chronically homeless refers to a homeless individual who meets three criteria:

> *(i) homeless and lives or resides in a place not meant for human habitation, a safe haven, or in an emergency shelter; (ii) has been homeless and living or residing in a place not meant for human habitation, a safe haven, or in an emergency shelter continuously for at least 1 year or on at least 4 separate occasions in the last 3 years; and (iii) has an adult head of household (or a minor head of household if no adult is present in the household) with a diagnosable substance use disorder, serious mental illness, posttraumatic stress disorder, cognitive impairments resulting from a brain injury, or chronic physical illness or disability, including the cooccurrence of 2 or more of those conditions [5, page 4].*

Recent efforts by the President Obama administration to prevent and end veteran homelessness by 2015 are in progress and are focused on the goal of "finding every veteran safe housing and access to needed services" [6, paragraph 6]. In addition, the VA has worked jointly with local communities since 1993 on the Community Homelessness Assessment, Local Education, and Networking Groups (CHALLENG) for Veterans project [7]. The primary mandate of the previous CHALENG studies has been to "bring together VA and community service providers to foster coordinated services for homeless veterans" [7, page 23]. However, there has been little effort by the government to explore characteristics of homeless aging veterans and their respective needs (and changing needs) for services associated with specific individual development needs, such as education, mental health assistance, and employment. Since 96 percent of homeless veterans are alone (individuals) as compared with 63 percent of the overall homeless population, the need for examining specific individual characteristics of homeless veterans is a necessary prerequisite for determining appropriate services for this special population [8]. Although combat may be one of the most stressful experiences a veteran faces, many veterans face homelessness for a period longer than their war zone service [9]. The Interagency Council on Homelessness [9] reports that the average length of homelessness for a veteran is six years compared with four years for a nonveteran. The number of years a veteran remains homeless is important because the longer a person stays on the streets, the greater the possibility of developing health problems including physical health illnesses, mental disorders, and substance abuse issues [10]. Although previous studies indicate combat exposure and posttraumatic stress disorder (PTSD) were not found to be significant predictors of veterans becoming homeless, the impact of PTSD and the associated literature is evolving and changing as new research findings are discovered [11].

The state of Florida is ranked third in the nation in 2011 for the largest number of aging homeless veterans (with California ranked as the greatest number of homeless veterans), yet the numbers of services and special needs provided for Florida aging homeless veterans is lower than many states that serve far fewer number of homeless aging veterans [1]. The Veterans' Administration (VA) provides "beds" and other related homeless services only for those homeless veterans who are identified as substance abusers or have medical problems. The literature review efforts of previous research studies aimed at homeless veterans within the Gulf Coast region and preliminary overview examinations of existing programs currently servicing homeless veterans within the Northwest Florida region produced very limited information, especially regarding specific target groups of aging homeless veterans and aging homeless female veterans. Currently, services for homeless veterans in the northwest Florida region are limited to services for VA eligible veterans and first response facilities. Since the Florida panhandle region hosts multiple military establishments and since large numbers of military retired persons live in the region, the numbers of homeless veterans within the region parallel this pattern. In addition, the need for determining specific empirical information regarding how aging affects the needs of homeless veterans, especially homeless veterans within northwest Florida is evidenced in the lack of statistical information currently available for this region. The current study focused on northwest Florida and the surrounding region (including Alabama) for accessing participants and agencies not serviced by the Veterans' Administration. Homeless veterans and associated stakeholders from this region comprised the participants for the study. The significance of the study for the northwest Florida region and for the field of research associated with aging homeless veterans is evidenced in the staggering numbers of aging homeless veterans in Florida (especially women veterans) and the lack of programs for assessment and service specifically located within the Florida panhandle region [7].

The current study addressed the need to focus on the individual. The study investigated factors contributing to the expressed needs of homeless aging veterans (who are potentially transitioning from homeless to nonhomeless status) relative to specific individual characteristics from a life-span perspective. The individual's reactions and interactions with the environment relative to the various gains and losses experienced by the individual in life are specific to the types of characteristics and descriptive information indicative of a life-span perspective. This premise has underpinnings within the context of the life-span perspective of human development theory.

2.2. Theoretical Framework. The theoretical framework for the study focuses on the individual and is grounded within the context of the life-span perspective of human development theory posited by Baltes [4, 12, 13]. The life-span perspective of human development premise describes development as lifelong, sociocultural, multidimensional, multidirectional, plastic, contextual, and influenced by biology and culture involving a process consisting of growth, maintenance, and regulation of loss [4, 12, 14]. Sociocultural influences are inherent within the setting or environment in which the individual lives. Multidirectional influences include the positive and negative events experienced by the individual within the course of human development. Multidimensionality is the perspective that there are multiple pathways in an individual's development [15, 16]. Plasticity is the ability of the individual to adapt to life changes. Contextual influences include the types of changes in resources that occur in response to the individual's needs for resources throughout a changing life-span. Life-span development involves biological considerations, cultural considerations, and individual factors working together. The life-span perspective emphasizes development across the course of a lifetime, and all stages of the lifetime span contribute to development. The life-span theoretical framework, as displayed in Figure 1, established the foundation for the research questions, hypotheses, instrumentation, methodology, and triangulation of data alignment used in the study.

2.3. Specific Purpose and Objectives of the Study. The specific purpose of this mixed methods study was to explore the individual characteristics and needs of aging homeless veterans in transition within Alabama and northwest Florida relative to a life-span perspective. The study included four focused objectives: (1) to examine homeless veterans' perspectives utilizing a quantitative survey research approach and a qualitative interview inquiry research approach framed within the life-span development theory perspective of Baltes [4, 12]; (2) to conduct an intense focused interviewing effort of a subgroup of 12 aging homeless veterans within Alabama and northwest Florida, to determine specific characteristics and needs of this special population with an emphasis on individual considerations; (3) to conduct a quantitative survey research effort to obtain specific demographic and needs assessment information relative to the special population of aging homeless veterans and their respective service providers using the Veterans' Administration CHALLENG 2010 survey; and (4) to triangulate survey and interview data for the purpose of examining study results and emerging thematic findings relative to the constructs of life-span development theory.

2.4. Research Questions and Hypotheses. The theoretical framework assisted in guiding the development of the study within the context of examining the various constructs related to the individual's perspective of life-span development regarding specific gains, losses, and other influences as presented in Figure 1. Seven research questions (five quantitative research questions and two qualitative research questions) were generated from the theoretical framework development efforts.

Research Question 1. Is there a relationship between homeless veterans' levels of depression and the number of months they served in a war zone?

Research Hypothesis 1. There is a relationship between homeless veterans' levels of depression and the number of months they served in a war zone.

Research Question 2. Is there a relationship between whether or not a veteran served in a war zone and the homelessness status of the veteran?

Research Hypothesis 2. There is a relationship between service or no service in a war zone and whether or not the veteran becomes homeless.

Research Question 3. Is there a difference in the median rankings of perceptions of homeless veterans and service providers concerning VA accessibility?

Research Hypothesis 3. There is a difference between homeless veterans and service providers in their median rankings perceptions concerning VA accessibility.

Research Question 4. Is there a difference between the average perceptions of service providers in northwest Florida and service providers in Birmingham, Alabama, regarding their perceptions of VA community partnership integration?

Research Hypothesis 4. There is a difference between the average perceptions of service providers in northwest Florida and service providers in Birmingham, Alabama, regarding their perceptions of VA community partnership integration.

Research Question 5. How do the expressed needs of veterans in the current study differ from the expressed needs of veterans in the 2010 CHALENG studies?

Research Hypothesis 5. There is a difference in the rank ordering of the expressed needs of current study homeless veteran participants (from the Birmingham, Alabama, and northwest Florida regions) as compared with the CHALENG 2010 study participants.

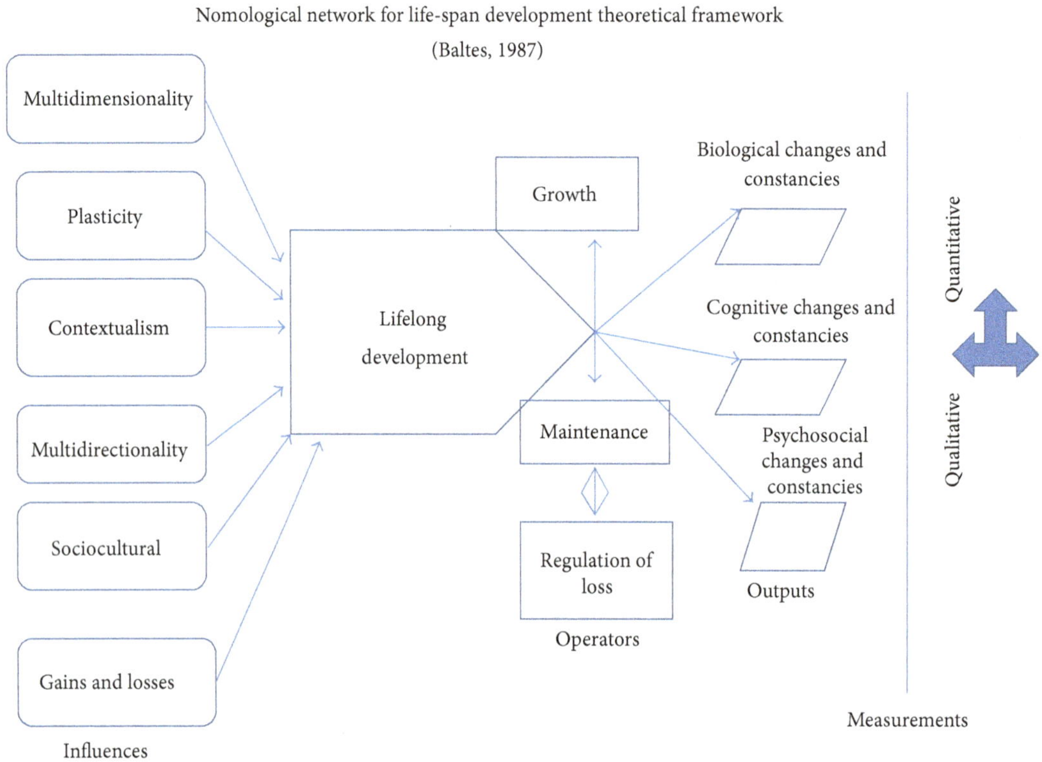

FIGURE 1: Nomological network for life-span development theoretical framework [4].

Research Question 6. What are the major contributing factors to veteran homelessness, focused on life and/or military experiences that have impacted homeless veterans' development considerations leading to their current living situations?

Research Question 7. What are the immediate needs of homeless veterans?

2.5. Methodology. The study utilized an exploratory mixed methods investigation focused on the characteristics and needs of the aging homeless military veteran population. The study involved two sequential procedural phases. The objective of the first phase was to determine the specific characteristics, perceptions, and needs of the homeless veteran participants. Phase one employed a survey instrument used to obtain demographic, perceptions, and needs information relative to aging homeless veterans who are currently not receiving housing services within the Birmingham, Alabama, and Northwest Florida regions. In addition, quantitative surveys were completed by service providers of homeless veterans. The second phase of the study consisted of qualitative interviews with a voluntary sample of aging, homeless veterans. Both quantitative and qualitative data were included in the data analysis procedures for the study.

2.6. Study Participants. Study participants included 39 homeless veterans and 20 service providers from the Birmingham, Alabama, and Pensacola, Florida, areas. Homeless veterans were recruited to participate from the resident population of nonprofit organizations servicing homeless veterans within the two locations. A subset of 12 homeless veterans (of the 39 homeless veterans who participated in the quantitative survey) agreed to participate in the one hour qualitative interview session within a private room with an interviewer. The 20 service providers who agreed to participate in the study were comprised of employees of shelters, ministers, counselors, attorneys, and anyone who had consistent service experiences with homeless veterans.

2.7. Instrumentation. Both quantitative and qualitative instruments were obtained prior to the research effort. The quantitative survey instrument aligned with the national CHALENG 2010 study [7]. The qualitative instrument consisted of a structured interview protocol developed for the study. Instruments used in both phases of the research effort are described individually.

2.7.1. Quantitative Instrumentation. The quantitative phase that employed the use of the Community Veteran Assessment instrument focused on the participant's demographic characteristics, length of time of homelessness status, length of military service/branch, psychological considerations, reported illnesses or mental health considerations, and expressed needs and services. The Community Veteran Assessment instrument was used in the Community Homelessness Assessment, Local Education, and Networking Groups

(CHALLENG) for Veterans project [7] and utilizes a five-point Likert scale. Service providers completed an analogous instrument, also using the same five-point Likert scale to assess providers' characteristics, perceptions of VA accessibility and coordination, perceived value of the strategies most commonly used for collaboration between the provider and the VA, and the provider's perception of the needs of veterans. Reliability for the quantitative instrument used in the study was obtained by computing a Cronbach Alpha measure of internal consistency for each of the subscales inherent in the instrument. The resulting internal consistency alpha values for each of the Community Veteran Assessment subscales include Veterans' Needs Subscale (.98), Provider Strategies Subscale (.85), VA-Community Partnership Subscale (.86), and Veterans' Depression Levels Subscale (.46).

2.7.2. Qualitative Instrumentation. A semistructured interview using ten open-ended questions conceptually based in Baltes [4, 12, 13] life-span perspective was used to elicit information from a subset of 12 homeless veterans (from the total 39 participants) who agreed to participate in the study. The qualitative interview focused on questions regarding homeless veterans' expressed life experiences, military history, mental and physical health concerns, needs, and future goals. The interview questions are located in the appendix.

2.8. Procedures. The mixed-methods research effort aligned with Baltes' [4] life-span development theory with procedures indicative of both quantitative and qualitative research procedures. Veterans were provided with informed consent forms, with an explanation of the purpose of the study and the information they would be asked to provide, and they were informed of the option not to participate. Confidentiality of provided information was explained, and participants were asked to complete a brief demographic form, followed by a request to complete the Community Veteran Assessment. After completing the quantitative survey, participants were asked if they were interested in completing an interview with one of the researchers. Homeless veterans who volunteered to participate ($N = 12$) were interviewed in a separate area for privacy. Participants were provided information regarding available counseling services if needed while participating in the interview. Participants were also advised that they may discontinue participation at any time during the interview. Using the qualitative interview questionnaire, personal interviews of approximately 45–60 minutes each were conducted with the homeless veterans and service providers. Interview transcriptions were completed, representing more than 20 hours of personal interview discussions.

2.9. Sample Description. The sample for the study was comprised of 39 homeless veterans between the ages of 33 and 67 years. Seventeen homeless veterans from the Birmingham, Alabama, area and 22 homeless veterans from the Pensacola, Florida, area volunteered to complete surveys. The distribution of participants included approximately 64% Caucasian, 28% African-American, 5% Hispanic, and 3% Native American. Males outnumbered the females 5 : 1 with 33 males and six females. A complete demographic breakdown is presented in Table 1.

Table 1: Descriptive information for gender and ethnicity of homeless veterans by location ($N = 39$).

	Birmingham, Alabama	Northwest Florida
Gender	$n = 17$	$n = 22$
Males ($n = 33$)	14	20
Female ($n = 6$)	3	2
Ethnicity		
Hispanic ($n = 2$)	1	1
African-American ($n = 11$)	4	7
Native-American ($n = 1$)	1	0
Caucasian ($n = 25$)	11	14

2.10. Data Analysis. Data retrieved from the quantitative and qualitative instruments were analyzed relative to each of the seven research questions posited in the study. Each of the research questions is discussed relative to specific analysis of data procedures and study findings.

3. Results and Discussion

Study findings are reported relative to each of the research hypotheses/questions and analysis of data discussions.

3.1. Research Hypothesis 1. There is a relationship between homeless veterans' levels of depression and the number of months they served in a war zone.

Research hypothesis one was analyzed using the Pearson correlation procedure to determine if there was a relationship between the veterans' levels of depression and the number of months served in a war zone. The results indicated no statistically significant relationship with $r(12) = .070$, $P > .05$. Therefore, study findings did not support a relationship between homeless veterans' depression levels and the length of time they served in a war zone.

3.2. Research Hypothesis 2. There is a relationship between service or no service in a war zone and whether or not the veteran becomes homeless.

Data from research question two were analyzed using the nonparametric Chi Square analysis of data procedure to determine whether veterans' becoming homeless was related to whether or not they served in a war zone. Expected cell frequencies were examined to see whether there were any expected frequencies less than 5; the smallest expected frequency was 3.0. Therefore a Fisher exact test was performed, and these results indicated that there was no statistically significant relationship between whether or not veterans served in a war zone and their potential for becoming homeless: $\chi^2(1) = .650$, $P = .689$. These results are also influenced by the small number of veteran participants in the study as demonstrated by the small cell frequencies resulting from the Chi Square Analysis findings.

3.3. Research Hypothesis 3. There is a difference between homeless veterans and service providers in their median rankings of their perceptions concerning VA accessibility.

Research question three was analyzed using the Mann-Whitney U test to determine the difference between homeless veterans and service providers in their median rankings of perceptions concerning VA accessibility. The results of the Mann-Whitney test indicated that there was a statistically significant difference between the homeless veterans (Mdn = 3.0) and service providers (Mdn = 4.0), $U = 258.50$, $Z = -2.06$, $P = .04$, and $r = .27$. The median rank for providers was significantly higher than the median rank for homeless veterans, indicating that the VA accessibility was perceived to be positively accessible to service providers, while homeless veterans' perceptions of the VA reflected significantly less positive levels of accessibility.

3.4. Research Hypothesis 4. There is a difference between the average perceptions of service providers in Northwest Florida and service providers in Birmingham, Alabama, regarding their perceptions of VA community partnership integration.

Research question four was analyzed using the Independent t-test procedure to determine mean differences in VA-Community partnership integration between the service providers from Birmingham, Alabama, and northwest Florida. The assumption of homogeneity of variance was assessed by the Levene test, $F = 3.93$, $P = .064$; this indicated no significant violation of the equal variance assumption; therefore, the pooled variances version of the t-test was used. The t-test for partnership integration indicated a significant difference in the means between Birmingham, Alabama, and Northwest Florida service providers with $t(17) = -2.64$, $P < .05$, with Birmingham, Alabama, service providers M = 7.13, SD = 7.1 and northwest Florida service providers M = 8.73, SD = 8.7, on a scale of 0–10 (computed by the combined perceptions of VA accessibility and VA ability to coordinate services). The effect size, as indexed by η^2, was .05; this is a medium effect. The 95% CI for the difference between sample means, M_1-M_2, had a lower bound of −2.88 and an upper bound of −0.32. This outcome suggests a stronger partnership between the VA and community service providers in the northwest Florida region as compared with community service providers' partnerships with the VA within the Birmingham, Alabama, area.

3.5. Research Hypothesis 5. There is a difference in the rank ordering of the expressed needs of current study homeless veteran participants (from the Birmingham, Alabama, and northwest Florida regions) as compared with the national CHALENG 2010 study participants (from the Birmingham, Alabama, and northwest Florida regions).

Research question five was analyzed by comparing homeless veteran participant expressed needs from each location (Birmingham, Alabama, and northwest Florida) to the corresponding locations in the CHALENG 2010 study. The Mann-Whitney U procedure was used to determine the difference in rank ordering of expressed needs of homeless veterans between current study participants and 2010 CHALENG study participants. There were no statistically significant differences in rank ordering of expressed needs of the current study homeless veterans from the Birmingham, Alabama, group when compared with the rank orderings of the CHALENG 2010 Birmingham, Alabama, group: $U = 35.0$, $Z = 1.14$, ($P > .05$). Similarly, a comparison of the current study homeless veterans participants' rank orderings of expressed needs from the northwest Florida group relative to the CHALENG 2010 northwest Florida group yielded no statistically significant differences in rank ordering, $U = 50.0$, $Z = .00$, ($P > .05$). A descriptive listing comparison of the top ten needs for each group is located in Table 2.

3.6. Research Question 6. What are the major contributing factors to veteran homelessness conditions within Birmingham, Alabama, and northwest Florida?

The qualitative analysis of data for research question 6 is integrated within the context and interpretation of research question 7.

3.7. Research Question 7. What are the immediate needs of homeless veterans who are located within the Birmingham, Alabama, and northwest Florida regions?

Analysis of data procedures for research questions 6 and 7 involved the retrieval of qualitative data from the $N = 12$ homeless veterans (a subset of the 39 homeless veteran study participants) who agreed to participate in the private interview sessions conducted by the researchers. Data gathered from interviews, recorded, transcribed, and then coded using thematic assessment, a data-driven research approach based on developing themes that answer a research question [17], were analyzed to respond to research questions six and seven. The analysis of data procedures included an integrated analysis and triangulation of data for generating inquiry-based explanatory results aligned with the constructs of a life-span development perspective. Interview data retrieved from the 12 study participants provided emergent themes with interpretive alignment to Baltes's life-span development model [4, 12, 13]. The emergent themes include lifelong or intermittent depression, drug use, and joining the service to escape current home life. The alignment between the theoretical model tenets of the life-span development perspective and the transitional perspectives of homeless veterans is reflected in selected participants' quotes in the following interpretive alignment discussions. Pseudonyms were used to protect the identity of the interviewees.

3.7.1. Thematic Findings: Development Is Life-Long. The life-long tenet of the life-span development perspective posits that development does not peak or decline at a certain age and some elements of development occur across the life-span rather than in the first few years of life [4]. Life course does not decline with age; processes not present at birth emerge during the life-span in the form of problems, challenges, or adjustments to life. This life-long tenet was illustrated

Table 2: Top ten highest unmet needs identified by homeless veterans in 2010 and 2012.

	Birmingham, Alabama		Northwest Florida	
	2010 CHALENG project ($n = 59$)	2012 Current study ($n = 17$)	2010 CHALENG project ($n = 120$)	2012 Current study ($n = 22$)
1	Welfare payments	Dental care	Child care	Guardianship (financial)
2	Women's health care	Welfare payments	Legal assistance for child support issues	Long term/permanent housing
3	Guardianship (financial)	VA disability/pension	Family reconciliation assistance	Help with finding employment
4	VA disability-pension	Guardianship (financial)	Legal assistance to help restore driver's license	Child care
5	Family reconciliation assistance	Help managing money	Welfare payments	Help managing money
6	Legal assistance for outstanding warrants/fines	Credit counseling	Legal assistance for outstanding warrants/Fines	Family reconciliation assistance
7	Dental care	Job training	Dental care	Welfare payments
8	Legal assistance for child support issues	Legal assistance for outstanding warrants/fines	Reentry services for incarcerated veterans	Dental care
9	Help with finding employment	Family reconciliation assistance	SSI/SSD process	SSI/SSD process
10	Child care	Legal assistance for child support issues	Guardianship (financial)	Job training

in the interview data as many homeless veterans explained their reasons for joining the military. The primary reason expressed by study participants for joining the military was to escape a dysfunctional or otherwise unhappy home life. Carl, a veteran who served between the Gulf and Iraq wars said: "I dropped out of high school and joined the Navy at age 17 to get away from an abusive father. Ray, who served 10 years in the Air Force reported, "I got my GED and joined the Army to get away from home." A female veteran who joined the Army at age 22 (Rita) stated, "I was shooting for retirement, but [after 15 years] had to come out for health reasons." Another veteran (Victor) whose life had been filled with problems of mental and physical illnesses and criminal charges stated, "I refuse to die until I reach happiness."

3.7.2. Thematic Findings: Development Is Sociocultural. According to the life-span development perspective [4], the setting and the time period of the individual's situation impacts his/her development. Sociocultural events can impact an individual's development in positive or negative ways, and for some individuals the inability to adapt may hinder the progress of development. Lifelong or intermittent depression was reported by all twelve of the homeless veterans who were interviewed. Depression may be a response to current life circumstances, environmental influences, or biological predispositions and may manifest immediately or as a delayed response [18]. Monty, a 31-year veteran of active Army and reservist service was recently shot in Afghanistan and forced to return home, but his grief has disrupted his ability to progress in every day civilian life: "I feel guilty leaving my buddies and I pray for them every night... I'm depressed more now than ever." Cassie, a veteran of Desert Storm reported, "In a war zone, you do not have time to be depressed. After you're home for while... it just hits you."

3.7.3. Thematic Findings: Development Is Contextual. The life-span development perspective model emphasizes the contextual tenet [4]. Changing of individual resources occurs in response to needs in three areas: (1) growth, (2) maintenance or recovery, or (3) dealing with loss. Contextual changes can be in response to death, substance abuse, or mental illness with individual resources typically related to talent, time, money, energy, or social support. Drug use was another prevalent theme among the homeless veterans interviewed. Harold, a veteran of Vietnam reported, "I struggled with alcohol and drugs following my discharge from the army and felt in limbo... thinking about *woulda, coulda, shoulda* led to my drug use and I eventually just hit the road." Rita reported she is recovering and "I haven't had a drink in over a month."

3.7.4. Thematic Findings: Development Is Multidimensional. The multidimensional tenet of the life-span development perspective [4] was exemplified in the interpretive interview data of study participants. Development cannot be described only in terms of increases or decreases in behavior but is comprised of multiple abilities and multiple pathways. Mitchell, an Army and Air Force veteran was a Licensed Practical Nurse (LPN) but lost his license because of a positive marijuana test. Although he cannot work as a nurse, he has used his social intelligence and life experiences to help other homeless veterans. "I do public speaking at different organizations to educate the community about homeless veterans. It is important for people to know that most people are just a couple of paychecks away from being homeless." (Mitchell).

3.7.5. Thematic Findings: Development Is Multidirectional. The multidirectional tenet of the life-span development perspective model [4] was demonstrated within participants' responses to interview questions. The development process consists of gains and losses, not necessarily in equal strength, and the balances between the two may change over time. Luke, a former Marine, reported "there is camaraderie between homeless veterans, regardless of branch of service and we talk about our issues—anger and anxiety—in a conversational environment, not in formal groups." He also stated that the support of his friends assists him in his recovery from drug abuse and depression and "I'm intelligent and I want to go back to college—I want a job I can be proud of and deserve."

3.7.6. Thematic Findings: Development Is Plastic. The plasticity tenet of the life-span development perspective model [4] was revealed in the qualitative data analyses. Plasticity is the within-person variability potential to adapt to life's changes in order to maintain a positive outlook. After a life of military service, the deaths of family members, depression, substance abuse, and homelessness, Harold focuses on the positive aspects of his current life, "I'm currently doing better than I have in 15 years… I am grateful for the military, God, and country." Mark acknowledged, "I'm the only one that can change my life." Mario also reported a desire to "feel better both physically and psychologically."

3.7.7. Thematic Findings: Development Is Influenced by Biology and Culture. The biology and culture tenet of Baltes's [4] model was exemplified in the interpretive alignment to the theory. Biological potential weakens with age as an individual's goals and/or cultural support may increase. Victor, who suffers from numerous physical ailments and is currently under VA medical care reported, "I worked as a welder and landscaper but can no longer do such physically demanding jobs, I need vocational training so I can get a job." Russell, a homeless veteran with a degree in Business Administration, was not coping as well as some of his peers and reported "I lost my job when the company I worked for closed. I just had surgery and the VA doctor is giving me antidepressants for depression, I cannot find a job and I cannot work construction or do any heavy lifting." Russell's weakened physical state and the cultural change in his employment status as a result of the declining economy have influenced his development leading to a loss of functioning.

4. Conclusions and Implications

Capturing empirical and inquiry-based results that substantiate the life-span perspective relative to homeless aging veterans was supported by the study. Interview data, survey data, and triangulation analysis of data with interpretation provided evidence of major influences depicting the tenets and characteristics of Baltes [4] theory of life-span development perspective. Homelessness, war, deployment, mental health issues, experiences prior to entering the military, drug and alcohol use, childhood and adolescent experiences, dysfunctional relationships, and other multidimensional and multidirectional factors were evidenced in the empirical and qualitative data findings. Quantitative and qualitative study findings align with the seven tenets of Baltes' theory of life-span development perspective and highlight several of the constructs (plasticity, context, maintenance, and regulation of loss) as key contributors to explanatory factors influencing the life-span development of homeless aging veterans.

The scholarly significance of the study is highlighted within three contexts: (1) the role of the current study within the context of sensitive populations for conducting research; (2) the practical need for the current study within the context of prevention efforts aimed at homelessness; and (3) the connection of the theory of life-span development with the population focus of aging homeless veterans as the framework for conducting research within the context of adding a robust perspective for adding to the body of research aimed at poverty, homelessness, and aging veterans.

Rosenheck et al. [19] support specific lessons for researchers aimed at special populations of homeless Americans; that is, (a) the diversity needs of these special populations must be "identified, respected, and addressed" (page 1); (b) the uniqueness of the specific subgroup needs (aging homeless veterans) must be "sensitively addressed" (page 1); (c) systematic assessments must be included in the effort with specific subgroup populations; (d) the basic needs for the subgroup must include "tangible needs for material resources" (page 1); and (e) the need to increase the "overall pool of resources" for special population subgroups (page 1). The current study amplifies the types of considerations scholars and researchers must address for the special population and subgroups within aging homeless veterans and highlights the diversity, uniqueness, assessment, and needs for resources of aging homeless veterans as a research population addressed with respect and sensitivity.

The practical major need for prevention efforts to end veteran homelessness moves beyond the scholarly significance for the study; that is, the need for research must address strategies that focus on the health and economic challenges of veterans before they are threatened with the possibility of homelessness. The Department of Veterans Affairs initiated the Veterans Homelessness Prevention Demonstration (VHPD) Program in five cities in the spring of 2011 and has targeted those veterans who have completed assignments in the Middleeast [20]. Thus, although prevention and immediate intervention are the current focus of the VA for veterans returning from service to prevent or intervene prior to homelessness occurrences, the need for programs to serve aging homeless veterans currently representing almost half of the veterans who are homeless and who will not be included in the targeted Veterans Homeless Prevention Demonstration Program is the focus of this research effort and aligns with the significance of the need for this timely study.

Connecting the application of research associated with homeless aging veterans to life-span development theory provides a strong venue for scholars interested in examining the constructs of the life-span development perspective. Aligning empirical and qualitative data with appropriate triangulation interpretive information to the seven tenets of Baltes life-span development perspective [4, 12, 13] provides researchers and scholars sound information for adding to the body of literature on poverty, aging, and homelessness.

President Obama's mandate to end veteran homelessness by 2015 is a strong declaration to the veterans who have served in the military and the providers who service them. In 2008 there were 154,000 homeless veterans and that number has been reduced to 59,000 in 2012 (Department of Veterans Affairs; National Coalition for Homeless Veterans). Although tremendous reduction in the number of homeless veterans has occurred since 2008, there remains much room for progress to reaching the 2015 goal. Findings of this study helped to frame the focus of research on homeless veteran experiences, specific characteristics, and needs, and how these factors influence life-span development. Understanding the contributing factors and how this unique population differs from nonveterans who are homeless is necessary to accomplishing this goal. In addition, service providers and the VA working cooperatively to establish programs aimed at assisting homeless veterans who may not have a physical, mental, or substance abuse diagnosis are recommended as an emerging need for future programs aimed at ending homelessness for veterans. Aging homeless veterans and female homeless veterans are two populations that have not been specifically addressed in the literature yet with the Vietnam generation nearing their mid-60s and increasing numbers of women serving in the military, these populations are among the most vulnerable to homelessness. Litz [21] suggested "the wars of Afghanistan and Iraq are the most sustained combat operations since the Vietnam war" (page 1). As these conflicts come to an end, a new generation of veterans will return home to a weakened economy to face joblessness and medical and mental health problems as well as possible homelessness.

Considering homeless veterans from a life-span development perspective may help service providers understand how sociocultural, contextual, and biological factors impact a veteran's development and adaptation to the changes from a structured military environment to life as a civilian. Each veteran can also contribute to helping fellow veterans as "occupational experts" with multidimensional knowledge. The issue of homeless veterans is not just a matter of finding homes for those who currently lack housing, but also establishing proactive programs aimed at preventing homelessness for those most at risk.

Appendix

Qualitative Interview Questions

(1) Tell me about your life story (any issues prior to service).

(2) What was your reason for joining the military?

(3) What can you tell me about the type of homecoming reception you received following your military discharge?

(4) What type of support system do you currently have?

(5) What is the biggest contributing factor to your current living situation?

(6) What are your immediate needs?

(7) What are your feelings regarding your military service and current circumstances?

(8) How have things changed for you since you became involved with Three Hots and a Cot?

(9) What do you want others to know about you and other veterans?

(10) What is most important to you?

Acknowledgment

This research was supported in part by a grant from University of West Florida Center on Aging.

References

[1] National Coalition for Homeless Veterans, "Facts and Media: Statistics," NCHV, Washington, DC, USA, 2012, http://nchv.org/index.php/news/media/background_and_statistics/#faq.

[2] L. Perl, "Veterans and homelessness," Library of Congress, Washington, DC, USA, 2013, http://www.fas.org/sgp/crs/misc/RL34024.pdf.

[3] J. Khadduri and D. Culhane, *2010 Annual Homeless Assessment Report to Congress*, Diane Publishing, Darby, Pa, USA, 2011.

[4] P. B. Baltes, "Theoretical propositions of life-span developmental psychology: on the dynamics between growth and decline," *Developmental Psychology*, vol. 23, no. 5, pp. 611–626, 1987.

[5] U.S. Department of Veterans' Affairs, "Homeless Veterans: HUD-VASH eligibility criteria," Department of Veterans Affairs: Washington, DC, USA, 2013, http://www.va.gov/homeless/hud-vash_eligibility.asp.

[6] U.S. Air Force, "Official issue first report on homeless veterans," 2011, http://www.af.mil/news/story.asp?id=123242565.

[7] J. Kuhn and J. Nakashima, "The seventeenth annual progress report: Community Homelessness Assessment, Local Education and Networking Group (CHALENG) for Veterans fiscal year 2010," 2011, http://www.va.gov/homeless/chaleng.asp.

[8] U.S. Department of Housing and Urban Development, "A supplemental report to the 2009 annual homeless assessment report to congress," Office of Community Planning and Development, US Department of Housing and Urban Development and the US Department of Veteran Affairs: Washington, DC, USA, 2011, https://www.onecpd.info/resources/documents/2009AHARVeteransReport.pdf.

[9] U.S. Interagency Council on Homelessness, "National survey of homeless veterans in 100,000 homes campaign communities," United States Interagency Council on Homelessness, Washington, DC, USA, 2011, http://100khomes.org/sites/default/files/images/NationalSurveyofHomelessVeterans.pdf.

[10] National Coalition for the Homeless, "Why are people homeless?" National Coalition for the Homeless: Washington,

DC, USA, 2009, http://www.nationalhomeless.org/factsheets/why.html.

[11] A. Fontana and R. Rosenheck, "The role of war-zone trauma and PTSD in the etiology of antisocial behavior," *Journal of Nervous and Mental Disease*, vol. 193, no. 3, pp. 203–209, 2005.

[12] P. Baltes, "Extending longevity: dignity gain—or dignity drain?" *MaxPlanck Research*, vol. 3, pp. 14–19, 2003.

[13] P. Baltes, *Life-Span Development and the Brain*, Cambridge University Press, Cambridge, UK, 2006.

[14] P. Baltes, U. Lindenberger, and U. Staudinger, "Life span theory in developmental psychology," in *Handbook of Child Psychology: Theoretical Models of Human Development*, W. Damon and R. Lerner, Eds., pp. 569–595, John Wiley & Sons, 2006.

[15] R. Dixon and R. Lerner, "History and systems in development psychology," in *Developmental Psychology: An Advanced Textbook*, M. H. Bornstein and M. E. Lamb, Eds., pp. 3–45, Lawrence Erlbaum Associates, Mahwah, NJ, USA, 1999.

[16] P. Baltes and M. Baltes, "Plasticity and variability in psychological aging: methodology and theoretical issues," in *Determining the Effects of Aging on the Central Nervous System*, G. Guski, Ed., pp. 41–66, Schering, Berlin, Germany, 1980.

[17] V. Braun and V. Clarke, "Using thematic analysis in psychology," *Qualitative Research in Psychology*, vol. 3, no. 2, pp. 77–101, 2006.

[18] N. Niv, K. Mueser, L. F. Smith, S. Glynn, S. Maruska, and N. Frousakis, "What is depression?" Department of Veterans Affairs Desert Pacific MIRECC, Long Beach, Calif, USA, 2011, http://www.mirecc.va.gov/visn22/depression_education.pdf.

[19] R. Rosenheck, E. Bassuk, and A. Salomon, "Special populations of homeless Americans," in *Proceedings of the National Symposium on Homelessness: Practical Lessons*, US Department of Housing and Urban Development, the US Department of Health and Human Services, Washington, DC, USA, 1999.

[20] U.S. Department of Veterans Affairs, "Veterans Homelessness Prevention Demonstration Program (VHPD)," Department of Veterans Affairs, Washington, DC, USA, 2011, http://www.va.gov/HOMELESS/NationalCenter_VHPD.asp.

[21] B. Litz, "A brief primer on the mental health impact of the wars in Afghanistan and Iraq," 2006, http://www.ptsd.ne.gov/pdfs/impact-of-the-wars-in-afghanistan-iraq.pdf.

14

Variations in Community Prevalence and Determinants of Recreational and Utilitarian Walking in Older Age

Elizabeth Procter-Gray,[1] Suzanne G. Leveille,[2] Marian T. Hannan,[3] Jie Cheng,[1] Kevin Kane,[1] and Wenjun Li[1]

[1]*Health Statistics and Geography Lab, Division of Preventive and Behavioral Medicine, University of Massachusetts Medical School, 55 Lake Avenue North, Worcester, MA 01655, USA*
[2]*College of Nursing and Health Sciences, University of Massachusetts Boston, 100 Morrissey Boulevard, Boston, MA 02125-3393, USA*
[3]*Institute for Aging Research, Hebrew SeniorLife/Harvard Medical School and Beth Israel Deaconess Medical Center, 1200 Centre Street, Boston, MA 02131-1097, USA*

Correspondence should be addressed to Wenjun Li; wenjun.li@umassmed.edu

Academic Editor: Elke Bromberg

Background. Regular walking is critical to maintaining health in older age. We examined influences of individual and community factors on walking habits in older adults. *Methods.* We analyzed walking habits among participants of a prospective cohort study of 745 community-dwelling men and women, mainly aged 70 years or older. We estimated community variations in utilitarian and recreational walking, and examined whether the variations were attributable to community differences in individual and environmental factors. *Results.* Prevalence of recreational walking was relatively uniform while prevalence of utilitarian walking varied across the 16 communities in the study area. Both types of walking were associated with individual health and physical abilities. However, utilitarian walking was also strongly associated with several measures of neighborhood socioeconomic status and access to amenities while recreational walking was not. *Conclusions.* Utilitarian walking is strongly influenced by neighborhood environment, but intrinsic factors may be more important for recreational walking. Communities with the highest overall walking prevalence were those with the most utilitarian walkers. Public health promotion of regular walking should take this into account.

1. Introduction

The benefits of regular physical activity for older adults, including reduced risk of chronic diseases and disabilities, are well known [1–6]. The Centers for Disease Control and Prevention (CDC) currently recommends 150 minutes per week of moderate-intensity (e.g., brisk walking) or 75 minutes of vigorous-intensity aerobic activity per week for adults aged 65 and older [7]. However, the most recent CDC data indicate that only 15.9% of American older adults met these guidelines in 2011 [7] and are far from reaching physical activity goals set by Healthy People 2020 [8].

Walking is the most common type of moderate-intensity physical activity among older adults [9–11]. It is inexpensive and achievable by people of a wide range of physical abilities. Walking may be done for two primary purposes: (1) for intentional exercise and recreation or (2) simply as a means of getting from place to place for utilitarian purposes (e.g., to accomplish errands or get to work). The biomechanics, optimal walking speed, and energy expenditure of these two types of walking may differ, as load or gradient differs [12–14]. Several previous studies have investigated how recreational walking and utilitarian walking are influenced by the walking environment [15–17]. Li et al. found that utilitarian walkers had significantly higher risks of falling and being injured in falls than recreational walkers [18]. However, to our knowledge, no study has looked at the wider range of determinants specifically to see how they might differ between the two types of walking, such as walkers' physical abilities, socioeconomic factors, environmental features, and neighborhood characteristics.

We examined the recreational and utilitarian walking habits of older adults living in 16 neighborhoods in the greater Boston, Massachusetts area. We investigated the extent and determinants of community-level variations in walking frequencies, and possible implications to public health practices.

2. Materials and Methods

2.1. Study Design and Participants. The MOBILIZE Boston Study has been described in detail elsewhere [18–20]. Briefly, it is a prospective cohort study to investigate risk factors and mechanisms of falls among community-dwelling persons, mainly aged 70 years and older. The cohort included 765 participants living in the Boston, MA area, who are able to read and speak in English and walk 20 feet without the assistance of another person, intending to stay in the Boston area for at least two years, and who are without moderate to severe cognitive impairment (score ≥18 on the Mini-Mental State Exam (MMSE)) [21]. Participants were recruited from September 2005 to December 2007, using door-to-door recruitment in randomly sampled households within 5 miles of the study clinic at Hebrew SeniorLife in Boston with at least one member aged 70 years or older as recorded in city and town lists [19]. Domestic companions aged 64 and older living with study participants (aged ≥ 70 years) were eligible to enroll in the study. This analysis excluded 20 participants who did not have data on walking habits or on covariates used in the analyses, for a final sample size of 745 participants. Written informed consent was obtained from study participants. The Institutional Review Board of Hebrew Senior Life approved this study.

2.2. Data Collection. The two-part baseline assessment included a home interview, followed within 4 weeks by a study clinic visit. During the baseline home interview, trained interviewers administered questionnaires to assess self-rated general health, cognitive function [21], physical function [22], health behaviors [23], fall history in the 12 months prior to baseline, medication use, comorbid conditions [24, 25], and sociodemographic characteristics.

During the home visit, participants were given a questionnaire to complete and bring to their clinic visit. The form was reviewed by research assistants for completion. On the questionnaire, participants were asked about their walking habits. The frequency of outdoor walking was assessed with the question, "Over the past seven days, how often did you take a walk outside your home or yard for any reason (never, seldom (1-2 days), sometimes (3-4 days), or often (5–7 days))?" Utilitarian walking was determined by the query, "Do you walk to the store, post office, bank or other businesses in your neighborhood?" Recreational walking was queried as, "Besides walking to stores or businesses, do you walk for exercise in your neighborhood?" The frequencies of utilitarian and recreational walking were categorized as "Never, less than once per month, 1–3 times per month, 1-2 times per week, and 3 or more times per week." For the purpose of the current analysis, three operational outcomes of walking habits were defined, namely, "habitual" walking (walking outside the home for any purpose five or more days per week), recreational walking at least once per week, and utilitarian walking at least once per week.

During the clinical examination at baseline, participant body height and weight were assessed to calculate body mass index (BMI, kg/m^2). Balance was measured with the Berg Balance Test [26]. An inability to stand from a chair without using arms was taken as an indicator of poor lower extremity muscle strength. Lower extremity function was assessed by the Short Physical Performance Battery (SPPB) [27, 28]. Gait speed (m/sec) was assessed by the shortest time taken to complete 2 trials of a 4-meter walk at self-selected walking speed.

2.3. Characteristics of Communities. Participants lived in Boston and a number of neighboring towns. A participant's community was defined as the town, city, or subdivision of a large city of residence. The city of Boston includes 16 communities according to neighborhood planning districts defined by the Boston Redevelopment Authority. In order to ensure the compatibility of community sizes and adequate sample sizes for each geographic unit of analysis, we combined several adjacent communities with similar sociodemographic profiles into a single community unit. Larger cities with larger sample sizes were divided into smaller units based on established geographic concepts (frequently used neighborhood names). As shown in Figure 1, 16 communities were defined for the purpose of this analysis.

Each of the participants' home addresses was geocoded using ArcGIS Desktop 10 (ESRI 2011, Redlands, CA) and their census blocks were determined by linking the geographic coordinates to US Census block maps. Participants' census block groups and census tracts were identified accordingly. Community-level demographic and SES data were derived by aggregating census track level data from 5 year rolling averages of 2005–2009 American Community Surveys of US Census. Participants' community-level characteristics of interest included measures of income, educational attainment, housing characteristics, community stability, and racial composition.

Measures of geographic access to community resources were derived using Geographic Information System (GIS) based road network distances to community amenities. From the Massachusetts Geographic Information System (Mass-GIS), we obtained GIS data layers of libraries (2005), town halls (2013), public parks (2014), transportation infrastructure (2012), and land use and housing density data (2010). GIS layer of food stores was obtained from InfoUSA (2012) and GIS layer of post offices, from United States Post Office (2014). Using ArcGIS 10.1 (ESRI, Redlands, CA), we calculated the road network distance in miles from the participant's residence to the closest amenity of each type and residential density as number of households per acre of residential land.

2.4. Statistical Analysis. Participant characteristics found to be associated with at least one of the walking outcomes of interest in previous studies [18] were summarized with descriptive statistics. Their associations with the three walking outcomes were estimated using unadjusted logistic regressions.

Multivariable logistic regression models adjusted for the personal composite score were used to estimate associations of selected community socioeconomic factors and amenity distances with the three walking outcomes. These measures were treated as linear continuous variables except for percentage of vacant housing units and percentage minority. Because of their U-shaped associations with utilitarian walking, we constructed three categories of each of these variables. We modeled participants in the same community as a cluster for the socioeconomic measures, because they shared the same SES values, but each participant had his/her own unique amenity-distance scores. A seemingly-unrelated-estimation test [29, 30] was used to assess the equality of the associations (odds ratios) of these community characteristics and distance-to-amenities measures with recreational versus utilitarian walking.

Community level differences in prevalence of walking habits were assessed using logistic regression models, where each of the three walking habit variables was the dependent variable, and community indicators were predictors. Four models were estimated for each walking habit: (1) community differences without adjustment; (2) with adjustment for personal characteristics; (3) with adjustment for personal characteristics and distances to amenities; and (4) with adjustment for personal characteristics, amenity distances, and community-level SES factors. In order to preserve degrees of freedom but still adjust for these factors, we derived a single composite adjustment score for each walking outcome for each individual using the entire set of characteristics as predictors in logistic models [22, 31]. A person's composite score was calculated as the summation of all the products of each specific regression coefficient multiplied by his/her value of the corresponding predictor. The area under the ROC (Receiver Operator Characteristic) curves of each model was used as a measure of model fit. A comparison between those participants aged 64 to 79 years and those 80 years and older revealed very similar community-level trends, so all ages were combined in the analysis. All statistical analyses were carried out using Stata MP 12 (Stata Corp LP, College Station, TX).

3. Results

One in three participants reported walking at least five days per week outside the home; 42% walked recreationally at least once a week; and 28% walked for utilitarian purposes at least once a week. About 18.3% walked for both utilitarian and recreational purposes at least once a week. Mean self-selected walking speed for this population was 0.92 m/sec for women and 0.99 m/sec for men.

The associations of selected personal characteristics with the three walking outcomes under investigation were strong, especially so with habitual walking (Table 1). Associations with the specific behaviors of recreational and utilitarian walking were less robust but were similar to each other, especially for traits related to physical impairments such as slow walking speed (<0.68 m/sec), poor lower-body strength, and poor balance which may make walking difficult or more dangerous.

Despite the fact that fairly similar determinants at the personal level. Recreational and utilitarian walking showed very different patterns of association with community-related factors, the communities differed greatly in the average walking distances to the nearest bus stop, subway, hospital, shopping center, post office, park, food store, town hall, and library, and each of these distances was negatively associated with utilitarian walking ($p < 0.01$, Table 2). None was associated with recreational walking, however. The difference between utilitarian walking and recreational walking with respect to these destination distances was significant in every case. Walking at least five days per week was associated with shorter distances to the nearest subway stop, hospital, post office, and food store (Table 2).

As with amenity distances, community SES characteristics were more likely to be associated with utilitarian walking than with recreational walking. Utilitarian walking was significantly associated with a lower community median household income, a lower proportion of owner-occupied housing units, and intermediate percentages of vacant housing units (5–10%) and minority population (20–50%) (Table 2). With the exception of median income, each of the above factors associated with utilitarian walking was thereby also associated with the likelihood of walking five or more days per week, but none of the factors was significantly associated with recreational walking.

A comparison of the prevalence of habitual walking across the 16 Boston-area communities showed great variation, ranging from 16.7% in Hyde Park to 48.1% in Boston Downtown (Table 3). This variation appeared to result mainly from community differences in utilitarian rather than recreational walking (Figure 1). Both before and after adjustment for personal characteristics (Table 3, Models 1 and 2), there were significant differences among communities in utilitarian walking at least once per week ($p < 0.001$ overall) but not in recreational walking ($p > 0.85$).

Further adjustment for distance from home to amenities diminished the magnitudes of community associations with utilitarian walking somewhat, such that the community variable was no longer a significant predictor overall ($p = 0.10$, Table 3, Model 3), and the final adjustment for community SES greatly decreased the overall association ($p = 0.94$, Table 3, Model 4), indicating that access to amenities and socioeconomic factors had accounted for a great deal of the community variation in utilitarian walking. Even after all adjustments, however, the odds ratios for community differences from the referent community remained higher in magnitude for utilitarian walking (range: 1.90–6.96) than for recreational walking (range: 0.72–1.14). Measures of community associations with walking at least five days per week (habitual) were diminished by adjustment for distance to amenities and community SES in a way similar to that of utilitarian walking, showing the importance of utilitarian walking in producing the patterns of total walking observed but community differences remained significant overall ($p = 0.01$, Table 2, Model 4). The three communities with the highest percentages of elders who walked five or more days per week for any purpose (Brookline North, Jamaica Plain,

TABLE 1: Participants' characteristics by walking habits.

	Overall (n = 745)	Walking ≥5 days/week Yes (n = 251)	Walking ≥5 days/week No (n = 494)	Recreational walking ≥once/week Yes (n = 310)	Recreational walking ≥once/week No (n = 429)	Utilitarian walking ≥once/week Yes (n = 208)	Utilitarian walking ≥once/week No (n = 530)
	Mean (SD) or %						
Demographic							
Age (years)	78.1 (5.4)	77.2 (5.2)**	78.6 (5.5)	77.4 (5.2)**	78.6 (5.5)	76.9 (5.0)**	78.5 (5.5)
Male gender	36.0	43.3**	32.2	37.1	35.0	38.5	34.9
White race/ethnicity	77.9	80.5	76.5	81.3	77.4	78.4	77.7
Education							
High school graduate or less	34.1	28.7*	36.8	31.3	36.4	33.7	34.5
Some college or college graduate	34.5	34.7*	34.4	34.2	34.3	32.7	34.9
Graduate studies	31.4	36.7*	28.7	34.5	29.4	33.7	30.6
Lifestyle							
Body mass index (kg/m^2)							
<25	32.1	37.9**	29.2	35.2**	29.8	37.5*	30.0
25–29.9	41.7	44.2**	40.5	44.5**	40.1	43.3*	41.5
30+	26.2	17.9**	30.4	20.3**	30.1	19.2*	28.5
Use of alcohol							
Every day use	13.3	19.5**	10.1	12.9	13.5	16.8	12.1
1–6 days/week	25.4	29.1**	23.5	29.7	22.4	26.4	24.9
1–3 days/month	22.0	24.7**	20.7	20.7	23.1	20.7	22.6
Not at all	39.3	26.7**	45.8	36.8	41.0	36.1	40.4
Physical disability							
Balance (Berg score)							
<48	21.6	13.2**	25.9	13.9**	27.3	15.9**	23.6
48–50	25.1	23.1**	26.1	26.1**	24.0	19.2**	27.2
51+	53.3	63.8**	48.0	60.0**	48.7	64.9**	49.3
Unable to do chair-stand test without arms	7.5	4.4*	9.1	2.9**	10.7	2.4**	9.4
Gait speed (m/sec)							
<0.68	13.3	6.0**	17.0	8.7**	16.6	3.9**	16.8
0.68–1.33	80.1	82.5**	79.0	81.3**	79.3	87.0**	77.6
>1.33	6.6	11.6**	4.0	10.0**	4.2	9.1**	5.7
Activities of daily living							
No difficulty	77.9	84.1*	74.7	83.9**	73.7	85.6**	75.3
Little/some difficulty	14.9	11.2*	16.8	10.0**	18.2	11.1**	16.0
Much difficulty/inability	7.3	4.8*	8.5	6.1**	8.2	3.4**	8.7
Short physical performance battery <10	40.5	30.3**	45.8	32.3**	45.9	27.4**	45.1
Reduced activity due to illness past year	28.3	25.9	29.6	29.4	27.5	23.6	30.0
Other health-related							
Moderate/severe bodily pain	39.1	29.9**	43.7	34.5*	42.4	35.6	40.4
Number of comorbid conditions	2.9 (1.5)	2.7 (1.4)*	3.0 (1.5)*	2.8 (1.5)	2.9 (1.5)	2.6 (1.4)**	3.0 (1.5)
Fair/poor self-rated health	14.4	7.2**	18.0	11.6	15.6	10.6	15.5
Peripheral neuropathy	12.1	7.2**	14.6	9.4	14.0	7.7*	13.6
Foot pain	23.9	18.7*	26.5	22.3	25.2	23.1	24.2
Number of medications							
0–4	34.9	41.4**	31.6	38.1	32.9	45.2**	31.1
5–8	45.2	43.8**	46.0	43.6	46.9	39.9**	47.4
9+	19.9	14.7**	22.5	18.4	20.3	14.9**	21.5
Impaired cognition (MMSE 18–23)	11.7	7.2**	14.0	10.3	12.4	9.1	12.3
Falls efficacy score <90	13.6	7.6**	16.6	12.9	13.8	11.1	14.3

*$p < 0.05$ in unadjusted logistic regression of the walking behavior on the characteristic. In the case of multicategory characteristics, for example, education level, the statistic applies to the characteristic overall, not to particular categories.
**$p < 0.01$.

TABLE 2: Associations of three measures of walking with geographic access to amenities and community-level socioeconomic characteristics.

Characteristic	Community mean (SD) or percent	Community range (min., max)	Odds ratio (95% confidence interval)[1] Walk at least 5 days per week	Recreation walk at least once per week	Utilitarian walk at least once per week	SUEST test[2] p-value
Mean distances (km) from home block centroid to nearest amenities						
Bus stop	0.48 (0.31)	0.20, 1.40	0.74 (0.52–1.04)	1.04 (0.76–1.43)	0.25 (0.15–0.43)**	<0.001
Subway	2.03 (1.42)	0.47, 5.23	0.88 (0.79–0.97)**	0.93 (0.85–1.02)	0.69 (0.61–0.78)**	<0.001
Hospital	2.14 (1.41)	0.56, 4.80	0.84 (0.76–0.94)**	0.92 (0.84–1.02)	0.69 (0.60–0.78)**	<0.001
Shopping center or mall	4.36 (1.71)	1.16, 7.32	0.93 (0.85–1.02)	1.00 (0.92–1.08)	0.85 (0.77–0.94)**	0.002
Post office	1.89 (1.17)	0.73, 4.75	0.82 (0.73–0.92)**	0.92 (0.83–1.02)	0.64 (0.55–0.74)**	<0.001
Public park (≥1 acre)	0.57 (0.23)	0.28, 1.10	0.77 (0.53–1.13)	0.82 (0.58–1.16)	0.41 (0.26–0.64)**	0.02
Grocery/convenience store	0.78 (0.44)	0.22, 1.65	0.77 (0.61–0.99)*	1.08 (0.87–1.34)	0.26 (0.17–0.39)**	<0.001
Town hall	3.69 (1.44)	1.49, 7.09	0.93 (0.86–1.02)	0.97 (0.89–1.05)	0.85 (0.77–0.94)**	0.03
Public library	1.18 (0.54)	0.62, 2.49	0.95 (0.76–1.18)	1.02 (0.83–1.26)	0.65 (0.50–0.83)**	0.002
Community-level socioeconomic factors						
Median household income ($10,000)	7.9 (3.3)	2.9, 12.7	0.95 (0.90–1.01)	0.98 (0.94–1.03)	0.87 (0.77–0.99)*	<0.001
% below federal poverty level	9.3 (8.1)	1.5, 28.8	1.25 (0.99–1.57)	1.07 (0.88–1.30)	1.66 (1.00–2.77)	0.007
% of adults unemployed	19.0 (5.1)	11.8, 28.4	1.07 (0.71–1.61)	1.12 (0.81–1.53)	1.06 (0.43–2.62)	0.38
% college graduates	54.4 (24.2)	12.3, 82.0	1.01 (0.92–1.10)	1.00 (0.94–1.07)	1.01 (0.83–1.22)	0.88
% of housing units owner-occupied	56.3 (21.5)	23.7, 89.2	0.89 (0.82–0.97)**	0.96 (0.89–1.03)	0.73 (0.63–0.86)**	<0.001
% housing units vacant, referent <5%	6.5 (2.9)	3.1, 12.5	Ref.	Ref.	Ref.	
5–10%			1.59 (1.11–2.29)*	1.29 (0.92–1.82)	3.14 (1.42–6.97)**	<0.001
>10%			1.31 (0.83–2.07)	1.21 (0.79–1.84)	2.05 (0.75–5.61)	
% minority (non-White), referent <20%	34.9 (28.0)	9.6, 93.9	Ref.	Ref.	Ref.	
20–50%			1.63 (1.13–2.36)**	1.36 (0.96–1.93)	3.98 (1.85–8.54)**	<0.001
>50%			1.06 (0.69–1.63)	1.25 (0.84–1.85)	1.74 (0.73–4.13)	

*$p < 0.05$.
**$p < 0.01$.
[1]Odds ratio estimates adjusted for personal characteristics.
[2]Seemingly-unrelated estimation testing the hypothesis that the odds ratio in the recreational walking regression equals that in the utilitarian walking regression.

and Boston Downtown) also had the highest percentages of persons who walked at least once per week for utilitarian purposes, and they were the only communities with more utilitarian than recreational walkers.

Areas under the ROC curve, indicating the goodness-of-fit of models in Table 3, show that community alone (Model 1) was a stronger predictor of a person's utilitarian walking habit (area = 0.70) than of recreational walking habit (area = 0.56, $p < 0.001$). Adjustments for personal characteristics and distances improved each model significantly, but the fit of the recreational walking model never became as good as that for utilitarian walking ($p < 0.001$ for each model).

Table 3: Personal walking habits of participants by community.

	N	Prev. (%)	Model 1 unadjusted		Model 2 adjusted for personal characteristics[2]		Model 3 adjusted for personal and distance to amenities[3]		Model 4 adjusted for personal, distance, and community SES[4]	
			OR[1]	95% CI	OR	95% CI	OR	95% CI	OR	95% CI
(A) Walking ≥5 days/week										
Boston: Hyde Park	36	16.7	Ref.		Ref.		Ref.		Ref.	
Boston: Mattapan	24	25.0	1.67	0.47–5.96	2.02	0.54–7.62	2.82	0.74–10.79	2.36	0.62–8.93
Boston: West Roxbury	71	25.4	1.70	0.61–4.74	1.96	0.67–5.68	2.57	0.87–7.57	2.40	0.81–7.17
Newton-Central	27	25.9	1.75	0.51–5.98	1.92	0.52–7.06	2.45	0.66–9.06	1.88	0.50–6.99
Boston: North/South Dorchester	60	26.7	1.82	0.64–5.18	2.39	0.80–7.12	2.25	0.74–6.80	2.08	0.69–6.28
Brookline-South	51	31.4	2.29	0.79–6.58	1.70	0.57–5.10	1.41	0.46–4.26	1.03	0.33–3.26
Newton-West	73	31.5	2.30	0.84–6.29	1.87	0.66–5.29	3.29	1.15–9.45*	2.48	0.85–7.23
Dedham, Needham	40	32.5	2.41	0.80–7.22	1.95	0.62–6.08	2.90	0.92–9.16	1.63	0.52–5.16
Milton	47	34.0	2.58	0.89–7.48	2.68	0.89–8.11	3.50	1.14–10.76*	2.72	0.89–8.31
Boston: Roslindale	37	35.1	2.71	0.90–8.19	3.33	1.04–10.66*	3.55	1.09–11.56*	3.41	1.05–11.10*
Boston: Roxbury	59	35.6	2.76	0.99–7.71	3.31	1.13–9.69*	2.82	0.96–8.31	2.23	0.74–6.72
Boston: Allston/Brighton	38	36.8	2.92	0.97–8.73	2.75	0.88–8.56	1.74	0.55–5.49	1.44	0.43–4.78
Newton-East	47	38.3	3.10	1.08–8.92*	2.27	0.76–6.82	2.82	0.93–8.54	1.82	0.60–5.57
Brookline-North	51	47.1	4.44	1.58–12.51**	3.89	1.32–11.50*	2.29	0.76–6.85	1.64	0.49–5.44
Boston: Jamaica Plain	57	47.4	4.50	1.62–12.47**	4.95	1.70–14.43**	3.37	1.15–9.89*	2.66	0.86–8.25
Boston: Downtown	27	48.1	4.64	1.46–14.76**	6.86	2.01–23.38**	3.24	0.95–11.09	2.22	0.55–8.99
	745									
Overall p value for community differences				$p = 0.10$		$p = 0.07$		$p = 0.56$		$p = 1.0$
Area under ROC curve				0.60		0.73		0.74		0.75
p value for change in area under ROC compared to previous model				NA		$p < 0.001$		$p = 0.004$		$p = 0.64$
(B) Walking for recreation ≥1 time/week										
Boston: Hyde Park	36	41.7	1.46	0.64–3.35	1.52	0.65–3.58	1.10	0.46–2.63	0.95	0.39–2.27
Boston: Mattapan	24	41.7	1.46	0.56–3.78	1.70	0.62–4.66	1.36	0.49–3.76	1.14	0.41–3.16
Boston: West Roxbury	70	32.9	Ref.		Ref.		Ref.		Ref.	
Newton-Central	26	38.5	1.28	0.50–3.25	1.14	0.43–3.00	1.04	0.39–2.74	0.79	0.30–2.11
Boston: North/South Dorchester	58	41.4	1.44	0.70–2.97	1.67	0.79–3.54	1.16	0.55–2.48	0.97	0.46–2.08
Brookline-South	50	46.0	1.74	0.82–3.67	1.44	0.66–3.12	0.88	0.40–1.95	0.86	0.39–1.92
Newton-West	73	38.4	1.27	0.64–2.53	1.20	0.59–2.45	1.14	0.55–2.33	1.06	0.52–2.18
Dedham, Needham	40	40.0	1.36	0.61–3.05	1.41	0.60–3.27	1.23	0.53–2.87	1.02	0.44–2.40
Milton	47	34.0	1.05	0.48–2.31	1.01	0.45–2.26	0.78	0.34–1.77	0.72	0.32–1.65
Boston: Roslindale	37	43.2	1.56	0.69–3.53	1.68	0.72–3.92	1.25	0.53–2.94	1.04	0.44–2.46
Boston: Roxbury	59	39.0	1.31	0.63–2.69	1.30	0.62–2.75	0.97	0.46–2.07	0.86	0.40–1.84
Boston: Allston/Brighton	38	47.4	1.84	0.82–4.13	1.59	0.68–3.69	0.96	0.41–2.28	0.99	0.42–2.33
Newton-East	47	53.2	2.32	1.09–4.96*	1.72	0.79–3.77	1.33	0.59–2.96	1.00	0.44–2.27
Brookline-North	51	49.0	1.96	0.94–4.13	1.87	0.86–4.05	1.09	0.49–2.42	0.96	0.43–2.14

TABLE 3: Continued.

	N	Prev. (%)	Model 1 unadjusted		Model 2 adjusted for personal characteristics[2]		Model 3 adjusted for personal and distance to amenities[3]		Model 4 adjusted for personal, distance, and community SES[4]	
			OR[1]	95% CI	OR	95% CI	OR	95% CI	OR	95% CI
Boston: Jamaica Plain	56	44.6	1.65	0.80–3.40	1.63	0.77–3.46	0.99	0.46–2.14	0.93	0.43–2.01
Boston: Downtown	27	48.1	1.90	0.77–4.69	1.83	0.71–4.72	1.01	0.39–2.66	0.92	0.35–2.43
	739									
Overall p value for community differences			$p = 0.86$		$p = 0.97$		$p = 1.0$		$p = 1.0$	
Area under ROC curve			0.56		0.66		0.68		0.68	
p value for change in area under ROC compared to previous model			NA		$p < 0.001$		$p = 0.007$		$p = 0.92$	

$^{*}p < 0.05$.
$^{**}p < 0.01$.
[1]Odds ratio estimates for the specified walking habit relative to a member of the referent community, obtained by logistic regression.
[2]Logistic regression model adjusted for a composite score predicted from the following personal characteristics: age, sex, self-rated health, bodily pain, alcohol consumption, education level, body mass index, short physical performance battery, falls efficacy, ADL (activities of daily life ability), race, foot pain, balance, number of comorbidities, gait speed, peripheral neuropathy, flights of stairs in the home, Mini-Mental State Examination Score, number of medications, illness causing reduced activity in past year, and strength to rise from a chair.
[3]Logistic regression model adjusted for a composite score predicted from the personal characteristics as listed in model 2 and for distances from the participant's block centroid to the following amenities: the nearest bus stop, subway station, hospital, shopping center, post office, public park, food store, town hall, and library.
[4]Logistic regression model adjusted for a composite score predicted from the personal and distances-to-amenities characteristics as listed in model 3 and for the following socioeconomic characteristics of the participant's community: median household income, percent below federal poverty level, percent of adults unemployed, percent of college graduates, percent of housing units owner-occupied, percent of housing units vacant, and percent of minority (non-White).

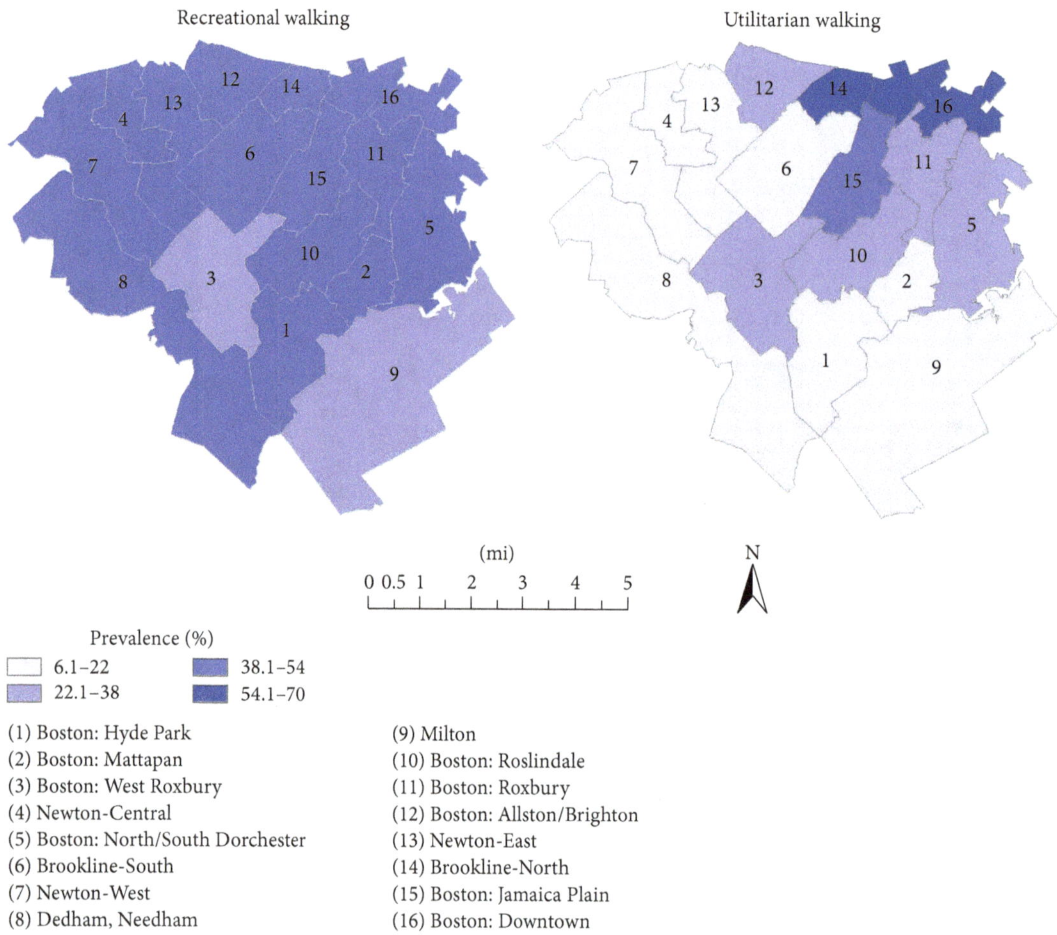

FIGURE 1: Community variations in prevalence of recreational and utilitarian walking.

4. Discussion

This study found variability among communities in the percentage of elders walking five or more times per week. Much of this variability could be attributed to differences in utilitarian rather than recreational walking habits. Prevalence of recreational walking at least once per week was low (40%) among elders in the area, regardless of socioeconomic and built environmental conditions. Prevalence of utilitarian walking was also generally low (28% overall) but varied significantly among communities, accounting for much of the difference in the percentage of elders walking regularly. The data imply, on one hand, the importance of utilitarian walking, and on the other hand, the limited contribution of recreational walking, to total physical activity.

While many personal characteristics, especially those concerning physical abilities and disabilities, were associated with recreational (and utilitarian) walking, we did not find any socioeconomic or environmental factors that were significant predictors of recreational walking. In contrast, utilitarian walking was strongly associated with many community characteristics including shorter walking distances from home to several amenities and neighborhood socioeconomic factors such as lower income and lower housing occupancy. This agrees with the findings for general adult populations [15, 32] and for older adults [16]. Van Holle and associates [16] made objective measures of the walkability of neighborhoods and found that neighborhood characteristics were associated with "walking for transport" or "walking for errands" but not with walking for recreation. It is worth noting that we found the same patterns of association and nonassociation of community characteristics with walking of the three types among those participants aged 80 and older as well as among those aged 64 to 79 years.

This analysis has several strengths. First, this study examined walking habits in a large cohort of community-dwelling elders aged 70 and above, with 37% aged 80 and older, a segment of the population that has been little studied with regard to walking. This older age of our cohort may account for the somewhat slower mean gait speed than that reported in the literature for healthy septuagenarians [33]. The MOBILIZE Boston participants were strategically recruited to represent a broad range of socioeconomic and residential conditions; the cohort resembled the underlying population well [19]. We obtained detailed measurement of a wide range of personal and socioeconomic characteristics and distances to amenities that might attract walkers in a well-characterized urban area. The distinction between walking for recreational versus utilitarian purposes afforded the opportunity to identify two different sets of determinants specific to the two types of walking, filling a knowledge gap in the elder population.

This study also has several limitations. It is limited to one urban area in the northeastern region of the country where the older adult population tended to be English-speaking, of white race and have higher income. Although the MOBILIZE Boston cohort matched the general older population according to sex, race, and ethnicity, the participants had somewhat higher education than the general community. Self-report of walking habits was subject to recall inaccuracies. Still, relative frequencies across communities should be fairly accurate, especially after adjustment for a wide range of demographic characteristics. Duration of walking activity was not collected except in very broad categories which did not allow for community-level or person-level comparisons. We also did not know whether or how often a load might have been carried by walkers. One might infer that this would be more common among utilitarian walkers (while shopping, etc.), possibly adding a physiological benefit of extra energy expenditure [13] but increasing risk of injury in a fall [34].

The unmeasured potential neighborhood self-selection and the cross-sectional design do not allow examination of longitudinal changes in walking habits which might elucidate causality. In addition, information on selection of walking routes was not collected. To address these issues, our current studies have been collecting detailed information on time and location of walking and selection of walking paths among older adults, using accelerometer and Global Positioning System devices.

Clearly, an older person's decision to walk regularly depends on a whole host of factors in addition to the built environment: necessary errands if they do not drive, access to public transportation, physical ability, time availability, feelings of fear, culture, and social influences being but a few [35]. However, the benefits of physical activity, in preventing obesity, arthritis, and their associated health problems and especially in warding off disability as people age [1–5], suggest that efforts to encourage walking to the extent possible by modifications of the environment may be worthwhile. Our findings point toward further investigation of communities like Brookline North, Jamaica Plain, and Downtown Boston to see which features distinguish them from other Boston communities in promoting physical activity by elders.

5. Conclusions

The primary finding of this study was that while the prevalence of recreational walking was relatively uniform across all communities, the prevalence of utilitarian walking varied widely and was more strongly associated with multiple factors at both the community and individual levels. In most communities examined in this study, the prevalence of regular walking behavior was low, which suggests a tremendous opportunity for health promotion. The challenge for public health is not only to find ways to promote utilitarian walking by elders using the knowledge gained to date but also to increase our understanding of factors that encourage recreational walking, so that both types of walking become more appealing, accessible, and safe.

List of Abbreviations

CDC: the Centers for Disease Control and Prevention, USA
MMSE: the Mini-Mental State Exam
BMI: Body mass index (BMI, kg/m^2)
SPPB: Short physical performance battery
SES: Socioeconomic status
GIS: Geographic information system
ROC: Receiver operator characteristic.

Conflict of Interests

The authors declare that they have no conflict of interests.

Authors' Contribution

Wenjun Li conceived of the study. Wenjun Li, Marian T. Hannan, and Suzanne G. Leveille obtained the funding. Elizabeth Procter-Gray and Wenjun Li carried out the analysis, interpreted the statistical results, and drafted the paper. Marian T. Hannan and Suzanne G. Leveille are investigators of the MOBILIZE Boston Study, who designed the study and collected the data. Kevin Kane and Jie Cheng derived demographic and GIS data and created the maps. All authors contributed to the paper writing and read and approved the final paper.

Acknowledgments

The study was funded by the National Institute on Aging (Grant nos. 5R01AG028738 and R01AG041525), which also funded the research that generated the data used in this study (Grant nos. 5R01AG026316, 5R37AG025037, and 5P01AG004390). Funding from Pfizer was used to code and classify medications. Neither the National Institutes of Health nor Pfizer played any role in the design or conduct of the study; the collection, management, analysis, or interpretation of the data; or the preparation, review, or approval of the paper.

References

[1] B. A. Stamford, "Exercise and the elderly," *Exercise and Sport Sciences Reviews*, vol. 16, pp. 341–379, 1988.

[2] C. Vallbona and S. B. Baker, "Physical fitness prospects in the elderly," *Archives of Physical Medicine and Rehabilitation*, vol. 65, no. 4, pp. 194–200, 1984.

[3] M. A. Fiatarone, E. C. Marks, N. D. Ryan, C. N. Meredith, L. A. Lipsitz, and W. J. Evans, "High-intensity strength training in nonagenarians. Effects on skeletal muscle," *Journal of the American Medical Association*, vol. 263, no. 22, pp. 3029–3034, 1990.

[4] S. H. Gueldner and J. Spradley, "Outdoor walking lowers fatigue," *Journal of Gerontological Nursing*, vol. 14, no. 10, pp. 6–12, 1988.

[5] I. Melzer, N. Benjuya, and J. Kaplanski, "Effects of regular walking on postural stability in the elderly," *Gerontology*, vol. 49, no. 4, pp. 240–245, 2003.

[6] M. Pahor, J. M. Guralnik, W. T. Ambrosius et al., "Effect of structured physical activity on prevention of major mobility disability in older adults: the LIFE study randomized clinical trial," *The Journal of the American Medical Association*, vol. 311, no. 23, pp. 2387–2396, 2014.

[7] U.S. Centers for Disease Control and Prevention, *How Much Physical Activity Do Older Adults Need?* CDC, 2015.

[8] Office of Disease Prevention and Health Promotion, *Healthy People 2020*, U.S. Department of Health and Human Services, Washington, DC, USA, 2010.

[9] D. R. Bassett Jr., "Scientific contributions of A. V. Hill: exercise physiology pioneer," *Journal of Applied Physiology*, vol. 93, no. 5, pp. 1567–1582, 2002.

[10] J. P. Hughes, M. A. McDowell, and D. J. Brody, "Leisure-time physical activity among US adults 60 or more years of age: results from NHANES 1999–2004," *Journal of Physical Activity & Health*, vol. 5, no. 3, pp. 347–358, 2008.

[11] C. H. Wong, S. F. Wong, W. S. Pang, M. Y. Azizah, and M. J. Dass, "Habitual walking and its correlation to better physical function: implications for prevention of physical disability in older persons," *Journals of Gerontology. Series A, Biological Sciences and Medical Sciences*, vol. 58, no. 6, pp. 555–560, 2003.

[12] G. J. Bastien, P. A. Willems, B. Schepens, and N. C. Heglund, "Effect of load and speed on the energetic cost of human walking," *European Journal of Applied Physiology*, vol. 94, no. 1-2, pp. 76–83, 2005.

[13] N. A. Gomeñuka, R. L. Bona, R. G. da Rosa, and L. A. Peyré-Tartaruga, "Adaptations to changing speed, load, and gradient in human walking: cost of transport, optimal speed, and pendulum," *Scandinavian Journal of Medicine & Science in Sports*, vol. 24, no. 3, pp. e165–e173, 2014.

[14] F. Saibene and A. E. Minetti, "Biomechanical and physiological aspects of legged locomotion in humans," *European Journal of Applied Physiology*, vol. 88, no. 4-5, pp. 297–316, 2003.

[15] B. E. Saelens, J. F. Sallis, J. B. Black, and D. Chen, "Neighborhood-based differences in physical activity: an environment scale evaluation," *The American Journal of Public Health*, vol. 93, no. 9, pp. 1552–1558, 2003.

[16] V. Van Holle, J. Van Cauwenberg, D. Van Dyck, B. Deforche, N. Van de Weghe, and I. De Bourdeaudhuij, "Relationship between neighborhood walkability and older adults' physical activity: results from the Belgian Environmental Physical Activity Study in Seniors (BEPAS Seniors)," *International Journal of Behavioral Nutrition and Physical Activity*, vol. 11, article 110, 2014.

[17] T. Sugiyama, S. Inoue, E. Cerin, T. Shimomitsu, and N. Owen, "Walkable area within which destinations matter: differences between Australian and Japanese cities," *Asia-Pacific Journal of Public Health*, vol. 27, no. 2, pp. NP2757–NP2763, 2015.

[18] W. Li, E. Procter-Gray, L. A. Lipsitz et al., "Utilitarian walking, neighborhood environment, and risk of outdoor falls among older adults," *American Journal of Public Health*, vol. 104, no. 9, pp. e30–e37, 2014.

[19] S. G. Leveille, D. P. Kiel, R. N. Jones et al., "The MOBILIZE Boston Study: design and methods of a prospective cohort study of novel risk factors for falls in an older population," *BMC Geriatrics*, vol. 8, article 16, 2008.

[20] E. J. Samelson, J. L. Kelsey, D. P. Kiel et al., "Issues in conducting epidemiologic research among elders: lessons from the MOBILIZE Boston Study," *American Journal of Epidemiology*, vol. 168, no. 12, pp. 1444–1451, 2008.

[21] M. F. Folstein, S. E. Folstein, and P. R. McHugh, "'Mini-mental state'. A practical method for grading the cognitive state of patients for the clinician," *Journal of Psychiatric Research*, vol. 12, no. 3, pp. 189–198, 1975.

[22] J. L. Kelsey, E. Procter-Gray, M. T. Hannan, and W. Li, "Heterogeneity of falls among older adults: implications for public health prevention," *American Journal of Public Health*, vol. 102, no. 11, pp. 2149–2156, 2012.

[23] R. S. Paffenbarger Jr., R. T. Hyde, C.-C. Hsieh, and A. L. Wing, "Physical-activity, other life-style patterns, cardiovascular-disease and longevity," *Acta Medica Scandinavica*, vol. 220, no. 711, pp. 85–91, 1986.

[24] G. A. Rose, "The diagnosis of ischaemic heart pain and intermittent claudication in field surveys," *Bulletin of the World Health Organization*, vol. 27, pp. 645–658, 1962.

[25] O. Sangha, G. Stucki, M. H. Liang, A. H. Fossel, and J. N. Katz, "The self-administered comorbidity questionnaire: a new method to assess comorbidity for clinical and health services research," *Arthritis Care & Research*, vol. 49, no. 2, pp. 156–163, 2003.

[26] Y. Zhang, L. Yao, W. Liu et al., "Bioinformatics analysis raises candidate genes in blood for early screening of Parkinson's disease," *Biomedical and Environmental Sciences*, vol. 27, no. 6, pp. 462–465, 2014.

[27] Centers for Disease Control and Prevention and National Center for Injury Prevention and Control, *Web-Based Injury Statistics Query and Reporting System (WISQARS)*, Centers for Disease Control and Prevention, National Center for Injury Prevention and Control, 2014.

[28] G. J. Bastien, B. Schepens, P. A. Willems, and N. C. Heglund, "Energetics of load carrying in Nepalese porters," *Science*, vol. 308, no. 5729, article 1755, 2005.

[29] C. C. Clogg, E. Petkova, and A. Haritou, "Statistical methods for comparing regression coefficients between models," *American Journal of Sociology*, vol. 100, no. 5, pp. 1261–1312, 1995.

[30] J. Weesie, "sg121: seemingly unrelated estimation and the cluster-adjusted sandwich estimator," *Stata Technical Bulletin*, vol. 52, pp. 34–47, 1999.

[31] R. L. Duckham, E. Procter-Gray, M. T. Hannan, S. G. Leveille, L. A. Lipsitz, and W. Li, "Sex differences in circumstances and consequences of outdoor and indoor falls in older adults in the MOBILIZE Boston cohort study," *BMC Geriatrics*, vol. 13, no. 1, article 133, 2013.

[32] N. Owen, E. Cerin, E. Leslie et al., "Neighborhood walkability and the walking behavior of Australian adults," *American Journal of Preventive Medicine*, vol. 33, no. 5, pp. 387–395, 2007.

[33] O. S. Mian, J. M. Thom, L. P. Ardigò, M. V. Narici, and A. E. Minetti, "Metabolic cost, mechanical work, and efficiency during walking in young and older men," *Acta Physiologica*, vol. 186, no. 2, pp. 127–139, 2006.

15

The Combined Effects of Tai Chi, Resistance Training, and Diet on Physical Function and Body Composition in Obese Older Women

S. A. Maris,[1] D. Quintanilla,[1] A. Taetzsch,[2] A. Picard,[3] J. Letendre,[1] L. Mahler,[3] I. Lofgren,[2] F. Xu,[1] and M. J. Delmonico[1]

[1]*Department of Kinesiology, University of Rhode Island, Kingston, RI 02881, USA*
[2]*Department of Nutrition and Food Sciences, University of Rhode Island, Kingston, RI 02881, USA*
[3]*Department of Communicative Disorders, University of Rhode Island, Kingston, RI 02881, USA*

Correspondence should be addressed to S. A. Maris; stephen.a.maris@gmail.com

Academic Editor: Wojtek Chodzko-Zajko

Obesity is a major health problem in the USA, especially in minority populations over the age of 60 years, and the aging process can cause adverse effects on physical function. Previous research has shown that Tai Chi, resistance training (RT), and diet result in overall health improvements. However, the combination of these specific interventions has yet to be translated to obese older women in an urban setting. The purpose of this study was to examine a combined intervention on the primary outcomes of physical function and body composition. Using a nonrandomized design, 26 obese women (65.2 ± 8.1 years) completed a 12-week intervention; participants were assigned to an intervention (EXD) group or a control (CON) group. The EXD group (n = 17) participated in Tai Chi, RT, and a dietary session. The CON group (n = 9) was asked to continue their normal lifestyle. Timed up and go (TUG) time was reduced by 0.64 ± 2.1 seconds (P = 0.04) in the EXD group while the CON group saw a borderline significant increase of 0.71 sec (P = 0.051). The combined intervention helped improve performance on TUG time, but there were no significant increases in other body composition or function measures.

1. Introduction

The prevalence of obesity, defined as a body mass index (BMI) greater than 30 kg/m^2, has doubled in the past 10 years in the general population and estimates indicate that 35% of adults over the age of 65 are obese in the USA [1]. Obese individuals are at a greater risk of developing health conditions including hypertension, cardiovascular disease, diabetes and some forms of cancer [2, 3]. Previous research [4] has shown that women have a higher prevalence of obesity compared to men, and the rates of obesity greatly differ across different racial groups. Over the age of 60 years, the prevalence rates of obesity for non-Hispanic White women, non-Hispanic Black women, Hispanic women, and non-Hispanic Asian women are 32.8%, 56.6%, 44.4%, and 11.4%, respectively [5].

In older women, obesity accelerates the decline of physical function that is associated with aging and has adverse effects on chronic disease risk [6]. The aging process has a negative effect on physical function and results in decreased muscular strength, and this decline in muscular strength associated with aging is known as sarcopenia [7, 8]. Sarcopenia is the age-related loss of muscle mass, and the decrease in muscular strength is considered to be a contributor to the decline in overall physical functioning in the older adult population [8]. Effective approaches targeting active lifestyles are needed as older adults have four times the physical limitations when compared to individuals less than 60 years of age [9].

Resistance training (RT) is a frequently used exercise modality in obese individuals and has been shown to improve muscle mass and strength, physical function, and body composition in older women [10–14]. However, RT is not considered an aerobic activity; in contrast, Tai Chi exercise is comparable to aerobic activities [15, 16]. Aerobic activities have greater influences on obesity reduction and promote greater weight loss when compared to anaerobic activities such as RT. Previous studies utilizing Tai Chi as an exercise intervention have demonstrated significant improvements in physical function and facilitate weight loss [17–21]. Resistance training and Tai Chi have also been found to have a very high adherence rate in older adults due to the low risk of injury associated when performed at a moderate intensity [12, 13, 20–22]. Along with increasing physical activity, older adults should improve their diet to augment the effects of exercise [2].

Combining an exercise program with a behavioral-based dietary intervention has been shown to significantly improve function and body composition [6, 23–25]. Previous dietary research has shown that the Dietary Approach to Stop Hypertension (DASH) diet improves total diet quality, blood pressure, and can facilitate weight loss [23, 26, 27]. The DASH diet has been shown to be an effective and reliable intervention tool in obese older adults [23, 25, 28]. Furthermore, the modified DASH diet (<35% fat versus <27% fat) combined with exercise results in significant decreases in fat mass and results in significant weight loss in older adults [15, 25].

There have been numerous studies that show combining exercise forms with a dietary intervention results in improved physical function, muscle strength, and body composition [6, 15, 24, 25, 29]. However, there is a lack of translational research on Tai Chi and RT in combination with dietary changes in an urban setting. In addition, a study combining these individually demonstrated interventions has not been evaluated in obese older women in an urban setting. We hypothesized that physical function, muscular strength, and body composition would significantly improve in the intervention (EXD) group as a result of a 12-week intervention compared to a control (CON) group. Thus, the purpose of this study was to examine the effects of Tai Chi, diet, and RT in obese older women on measures of physical and muscle function and body composition.

2. Methods

2.1. Study Design. This study used a nonrandomized intervention design to study changes in physical function and body composition in 26 obese older women. The intervention consisted of a 12-week design with a control group used as a comparison. The study took place at an urban senior center in Providence, Rhode Island. This study was approved by the Institutional Review Board at the University of Rhode Island, and a written informed consent was obtained from each participant prior to the start of the study.

2.2. Participants. Women living in the surrounding communities (within 1 mile of the senior center) were recruited for this study via flyers, press releases to local newspapers, and "word-of-mouth" at the local senior center. Eligibility criteria included (1) women ages of 50–80 years, (2) BMI of 30.0 to 50.0 kg/m^2, (3) being not involved in an exercise program in the past 6 months, and (4) postmenopausal women. The exclusionary criteria included (1) failure to provide informed consent, (2) significant or suspected cognitive impairment, (3) severe hearing loss, speech disorder, language barrier, or visual impairment, (4) progressive, degenerative neurologic disease, (5) terminal illness with life expectancy of <12 months as determined by physician, (6) severe pulmonary disease, uncontrolled diabetes, blood pressure, or anemia, (7) being not medically stable, (8) major surgery within 6 months, (9) significant cardiovascular disease, and (10) inability to safely engage in exercise. All of the inclusion and exclusion criteria were obtained via self-report, but height, weight, and BMI were measured during an orientation session. Verification of other exclusion criteria was accomplished by requesting medical clearance from each participant's primary care physician if the participant had one. However, medical clearance was not a requirement for the study as some participants were of lower income and did not have a primary care physician.

2.3. Outcome Measures. All testing procedures were performed at the senior center (intervention site) under standardized conditions to reduce variability in the results. Participants were given a familiarization trial before all physical performance testing procedures to ensure understanding of the test and to allow for practice.

2.3.1. Physical Function. The primary measure of physical function was the timed up and go (TUG) test. The TUG test has been shown to be a valid predictor of falls and mobility of the older adult population [30]. The TUG test requires that the participants rise from a chair and walk at normal gait speed around a cone eight feet away and then return and sit back down.

Another measure of function was the short physical performance battery (SPPB) that includes a standing balance test, 4-meter usual gait speed, and timed 5-chair stands. Each test was scored and analyzed individually with a score of 0–4, and a total score out of 12 was calculated. The SPPB is a portable and reliable measure that has been shown to be a strong predictor of mortality and overall function [31].

2.3.2. Flexibility. The chair-sit-and-reach test is a measure of flexibility used frequently in older adults [32]. This test required the participant to sit on the edge of a chair with one knee bent and the other knee extended straight in front, while reaching towards the toes. The score was the number of centimeters short of reaching the toes (negative number) or beyond the toes (positive number).

2.3.3. Muscle Function and Strength. Grip strength is a valid and reliable method and has been shown to be successful in measuring upper body strength in older adults [33]. Grip strength was measured using a hand-grip dynamometer (Jaymar Dynamometer, J.A. Preston, Corp., Jackson, MS) in the participants nondominant hand. The hand dynamometer is considered to be a very reliable tool and can be performed with little or no risk for the participants [34].

Knee extensor isometric strength was determined by using a handheld manual muscle dynamometer (Nicholas

Manual Muscle Tester—Lafayette Instrument Company, Lafayette, IN). This was measured as the peak amount of force that the examiner had to exert to break the isometric contraction held by the participant [35]. The device has been successful in determining strength in the older adult population and it is a portable, easy to use device [28]. The value recorded was leg extensor torque (kg-m) in order to account for variations in leg length.

2.3.4. Anthropometrics. Height and weight were measured with a stadiometer (Webb City, MO, USA) to calculate BMI and were following a 12-hour fast. Waist and hip measures were determined by utilizing a standard tape measure with an attached tensometer. Body composition was measured using a simple foot-to-foot bioelectrical impedance device (Tanita BF-556). This test has been shown to be a valid and reliable measure of body composition while having few associated risks [36].

2.3.5. Other Measures. The participants were asked to complete surveys about physical activity levels and dietary quality. The Yale Physical Activity Survey was used to estimate energy expenditure per week and time spent performing physical activity [37]. Dietary quality and patterns were assessed using the Dietary Screening Tool (DST). The DST was created to assess nutrition status and classify participants in relation to nutrition risk among older adults [38].

2.4. Group Assignment. Since this project was a translational study designed to benefit the participants, a nonrandomized design was chosen. After baseline testing was completed, participants were placed into either the EXD group or the CON group by the order in which they finished testing. Due to the limited space at the local senior center, there was a limit on how many participants could be placed in the EXD group. Those participants who wished to be involved in the study after the EXD group was full were asked to be in the CON group. The EXD group received all three aspects of the intervention, while the CON group was asked to maintain their normal lifestyle.

2.5. Intervention

2.5.1. DASH Dietary Education Intervention. A 45-minute behavior-based dietary education session was held once a week for the 12-week intervention period. The dietary sessions were instructed and led by a registered dietitian. A modified DASH-based diet was used as the diet plan and has been shown to have a high compliance rate with older adults [23, 26]. Dietary logs were used to evaluate participants' compliance throughout the 12 weeks and to provide feedback to the participants.

2.5.2. Tai Chi Exercise Intervention. Participants in the EXD group participated in Tai Chi exercise sessions 3 times per week for 12 weeks. The Tai Chi exercise was led by trained study staff who were trained in Tai Chi by an experienced principal investigator before the start of the intervention. The modified 24-movement Yang style form of Tai Chi was used since it has been shown to be an effective form of Tai Chi through previous research [15]. The Tai Chi sessions lasted approximately 45 minutes and included 10-minute warm up and 35 minutes of practice and exercise and were followed by a 5-minute cooldown period.

2.5.3. RT Exercise Intervention. The RT program was based on the American College of Sports Medicine RT Guidelines [3], and each session included approximately 45 minutes. The RT sessions were led by trained study staff who were trained by a principal investigator in the protocol prior to the beginning of the study. The program incorporated elastic tubing which may help avoid musculoskeletal injuries and can be used as a practical method of achieving strength gains in older adults [14]. Seven total upper and lower body exercises for major muscles were done with 1–3 sets of 10–15 repetitions for each exercise. The goal was for the exercise intensity to be moderate, with the final repetitions being at or near maximum voluntary effort. This intensity level has been shown to have positive effects on physical functioning in older adults [28].

2.6. Statistical Analysis. To assess our main hypothesis, the changes from baseline descriptive measures were analyzed to define differences between the groups. Independent samples t-tests for continuous data and a Fisher's exact test were used for categorical data. Next, the Shapiro Wilk test was used to determine if the data for changes in the outcome variables were normally distributed. If the data were normally distributed, a paired t-test was run to examine within-group changes from baseline. If the data were not normally distributed (TUG test and SPPB) a nonparametric equivalent was used, the signed rank test. A univariate analysis with outliers defined as data point 3 deviations higher or lower than the mean and Cook's distance [39] test (>1.0 for as a cut-point) were conducted with the data to determine outliers, but no outliers for changes in the main outcome variables were found. Analyses of covariance tests were utilized to examine the pre-/postchanges between the two groups, adjusted for baseline values. All data were expressed as means (±standard deviation).

3. Results

Figure 1 depicts the flow of participants that took place throughout the study. The total analytic sample consisted of 26 participants, with 17 in the EXD group, BMI = 38.8 (5.1) kg/m^2, and 9 in the CON group, BMI = 36.6 (3.4) kg/m^2. The mean attendance for all aspects of the intervention sessions was 67.5% in the EXD group.

Table 1 describes the baseline characteristics of the two groups. There were significant differences between groups in time spent performing physical activity [7965.5 (5696.5) kcal/week in the EXD group versus 3100.4 (3657.5) kcal/week in the CON group; $P = 0.038$] and average waist circumference [115.0 (8.9) cm in the EXD group versus 106.8 (9.8) cm in the CON group; $P = 0.042$].

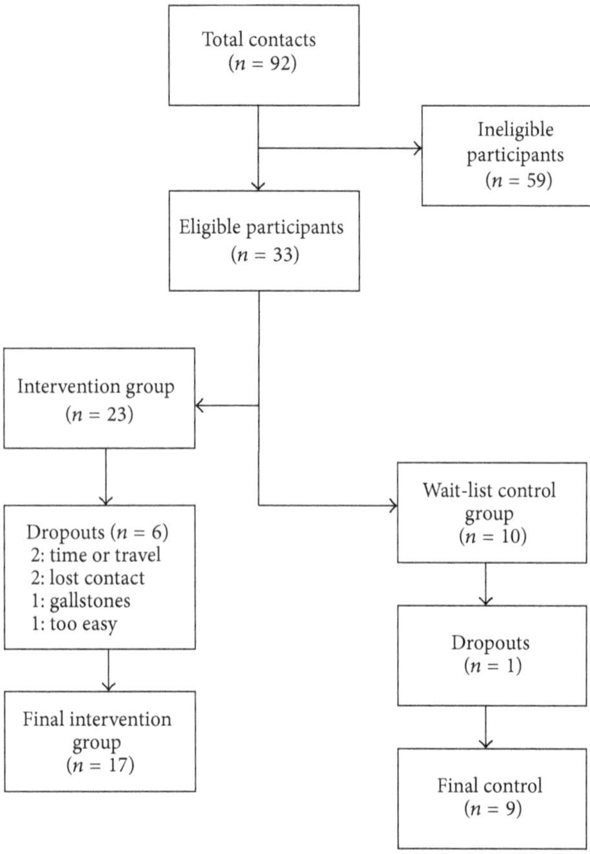

FIGURE 1: Flow chart of participants throughout the study. The total analytical sample consisted of 26 participants, with 17 in the EXD group and 9 in the control group.

TABLE 1: Baseline characteristics of the experimental group (EXD) and of the control group (CON).

Characteristic	EXD group (n = 17)	CON group (n = 9)	P value
Age (years)[1]	65.2 (8.1)	65.6 (8.6)	0.912
Education[2]			0.132
High school, GED, or less[*3]	10	5	
Associates/some college[*3]	6	1	
Bachelors or higher[*3]	1	3	
Weight (kg)[1]	97.9 (16.1)	94.5 (12.0)	0.578
Height (cm)[1]	158.3 (6.6)	159.8 (6.0)	0.593
BMI (kg/m^2)[1]	38.8 (5.1)	36.6 (3.4)	0.241
Waist circumference (cm)[1]	115.0 (8.9)	106.8 (9.8)	0.042
Hip circumference (cm)[1]	124.3 (11.1)	120.1 (6.2)	0.305
Waist to hip ratio[1]	0.93 (0.05)	0.89 (0.07)	0.167
Body fat (%)[1]	49.8 (3.3)	49.6 (2.9)	0.888
Race/ethnicity[1]			
Non-White[*1]	13 (76)	9 (100)	0.263
White[*1]	4 (24)	0 (0)	
Physical activity (kcal/week)[3,1]	7965.5 (5696.5)	3100.4 (3657.5)	0.038
Diet quality score[4,1]	72.6 (21.4)	76.4 (27.6)	0.716
At risk (<60)[*]	6 (40)	4 (44)	
Possible risk (60–75)[*]	8 (47)	4 (44)	
Not at risk (>75)[*]	2 (13)	1 (12)	

There were two baseline differences found in the physical activity kcal/week and in the waist circumference measures.
BMI: body mass index; %: percent.
All data are expressed as means with (standard deviations).
[1]Data analyzed using Student's t-test, [2]data analyzed using Fisher's exact test, [3]measured by Yale Physical Activity Survey, and [4]measured by Dietary Screening Tool.
[*]Data are expressed as "n" and (percentage).

Figure 2 depicts the changes that occurred in TUG time in both groups with the 12-week intervention. There were significant within-group changes in TUG time in the EXD and the CON groups, as the EXD group saw an improvement of −0.6 (2.1) sec (P = 0.04), and the CON group saw a decline of 0.7 (0.9) seconds with the 12-week period (P = 0.05).

Table 2 shows the changes that occurred from baseline to 12 weeks in both groups regarding function and muscle strength. There were no significant changes that occurred after baseline regarding between-group differences for muscle strength or SPPB scores. However, the EXD group had the tendency to improve flexibility by 2.3 (5.4) cm with the 12-week intervention (P = 0.07), while the CON group did not significantly change (P = 0.51).

Table 3 reports the changes that occurred in body composition between both groups. The EXD group had an unexpected increase in waist to hip ratio by 0.03 (0.01) (P = 0.04), but the CON group did not significantly change (P > 0.05). There were no other significant changes in measures of body composition.

4. Discussion

The major finding of the study was that significant improvements were observed in the TUG, a measure of mobility, after a 12-week Tai Chi, RT, and diet intervention in a mostly minority population. There was also a tendency for improved flexibility as assessed by a sit-and-reach test. To our knowledge, the current translational study is the first to test the combined interventions of Tai Chi, RT, and diet on physical function and body composition in obese older women living in an urban community setting.

The major finding of this current study has shown that TUG performance improved in the EXD group and declined in the CON group. The reduction in TUG time of 0.6 seconds in the EXD group was a 5.7% improvement from baseline in the EXD group, while an increase of 0.7 seconds was a worsening of 8.7% in the CON group. These findings in TUG improvement confirm the results of previous studies utilizing Tai Chi [18]. Tai Chi alone and Tai Chi combined with other interventions have been shown to result in positive improvements in function [15, 18, 22]. These changes in TUG time could be attributed to the tendency to improve flexibility, as well as improvements in balance that were seen in previous studies incorporating Tai Chi [23]. It is important to monitor

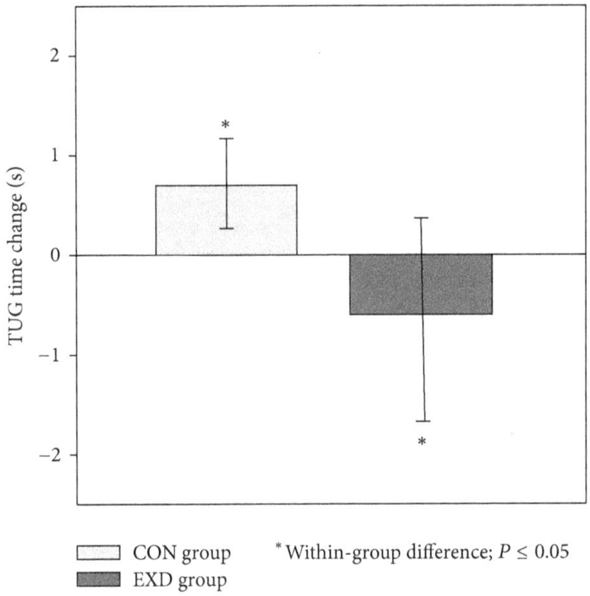

FIGURE 2: Changes in the EXD and CON groups in TUG time change with the 12-week intervention. The EXD group improved TUG time by of 0.6 (2.1) sec with the 12-week intervention (P = 0.04) and the CON group saw a decline of 0.7 (SD = 0.9) after the 12 weeks (P = 0.05). *Significant changes within groups ($P < 0.05$). TUG: timed up and go. All data were analyzed using analysis of covariance adjusted for baseline values. All data are expressed as least squared means (standard error).

TABLE 2: Baseline data and postintervention changes in physical and muscle function in the EXD and CON groups.

Variable	EXD group (n = 17)	CON group (n = 9)	P value between-group
SPPB score (0–12)			
Baseline	8.4 (2.5)	8.9 (2.9)	0.628
Postintervention	9.1 (2.9)	9.0 (2.6)	
Change	0.8 (2.4)	0.5 (1.9)	0.810
4 m gait speed time (s)			
Baseline	5.41 (1.47)	5.17 (1.20)	0.681
Postintervention	5.35 (1.67)	5.17 (1.26)	
Change	−0.06 (1.00)	−0.16 (0.37)	0.781
Five-chair stand (s)			
Baseline	10.75 (5.85)	14.24 (3.87)	0.122
Postintervention	11.08 (6.35)	14.63 (5.18)	
Change	0.33 (6.24)	−0.01 (2.98)	0.624
Flexibility score (cm)			
Baseline	9.6 (10.4)	3.8 (3.9)	0.124
Postintervention	6.4 (11.1)	2.0 (6.5)	
Change	−2.3 (5.4)	−1.7 (7.0)	0.930
Knee ext. torque (kg-m)			
Baseline	6.74 (2.2)	6.65 (1.10)	0.907
Postintervention	7.67 (5.68)	6.10 (2.21)	
Change	0.92 (5.51)	−0.54 (2.54)	0.477
Grip strength (kg)			
Baseline	19.38 (6.90)	18.93 (6.06)	0.871
Postintervention	20.12 (6.57)	19.13 (5.14)	
Change	0.72 (4.09)	0.95 (3.31)	0.969

The EXD group improved flexibility by 2.3 (5.4) cm with the 12-week intervention (P = 0.07); however, no significant changes occurred with the 12-week intervention.
Ext.: Extension.
All data were analyzed using analysis of covariance adjusted for baseline values.
All data are expressed as least squared means (standard error).

and improve physical function as it is a measure of functional independence in the elderly, and improving measures of function can assist with completion of everyday tasks [40]. By maintaining function and fitness capacity, older adults can continue to live independently and can better accomplish everyday activities [40]. Maintaining independence and a healthy lifestyle can reduce economic and personal burdens that are commonly associated with aging [40].

Unexpectedly, muscle strength did not significantly improve in the EXD group. The lack of change in muscle strength was an unexpected finding because previous studies observed improvements in muscle function and physical function in older women after combining resistance training and dietary modifications [12, 28]. This lack of change in strength in the current study could be attributed to the population cohort. It has been found that obese women have higher muscle strength measures when compared to lean women, which could have attributed to this lack of change [41].

Additionally the EXD group had a tendency to improve flexibility, as the participants in the EXD group improved in flexibility measures by 24% after baseline. This improvement was also demonstrated in previous studies combining Tai Chi and diet modification [15, 16]. The findings of the current study in flexibility are similar in comparison to the findings from a previous study by Katkowski et al. [15]. That 16-week study utilized Tai Chi combined with the DASH diet in obese older women, which resulted in significant within-group changes in flexibility (5.29 ± 2.16 cm; P = 0.022). A possible mechanism that explains these results is that Tai Chi involves the rotation of the head, trunk, and extremities while maintaining Tai Chi form, which can, therefore, improve flexibility in the arm, trunk, and hip [42].

Contrary to previous research, this study did not find significant changes in lean mass or body fat percentage between the two groups. Additionally, the current study found that anthropometric variables did not change in the EXD or CON group except for a slight, yet unexpected increase in waist to hip ratio in the EXD group. This finding is in contrast to the current literature, which has typically seen decreases in anthropometric measures after similar interventions [43, 44].

TABLE 3: Anthropometric changes with the 12-week intervention between the EXD and CON groups.

Variable	EXD ($n = 17$)	CON ($n = 9$)	Between-group: P value
Weight (kg)	0.08 ± 0.69	0.34 ± 0.95	0.829
BMI (kg/m^2)	1.10 ± 0.79	−0.34 ± 1.10	0.305
% Body fat	−0.30 ± 0.54	0.26 ± 0.74	0.549
Waist circumference (cm)	0.77 ± 1.56	3.19 ± 2.20	0.397
Waist to hip ratio	0.03 ± 0.01*	0.04 ± 0.01	0.542

The EXD group saw an increase in waist to hip ratio measures after the 12 weeks, and no other significant changes occurred in body composition.
*Significant changes within groups ($P < 0.05$). Ext: extension; %: percentage.
All data were analyzed using analysis of covariance adjusted for baseline values.
All data are expressed as least squared means (standard error).

This lack of change could have occurred because the primary goal of the dietary intervention was to improve dietary quality instead of weight loss, as well as the relatively short duration of the intervention.

This study adds to the current literature on the effects of combined exercise and dietary interventions. This is also the first study to combine RT, Tai Chi, and dietary changes in obese older minority women. The findings from the current study confirm those findings in previous studies in obese older women regarding the TUG test and flexibility measures [15, 29]. However, the studies done in obese older women [15, 29] did not incorporate minority women as a major part of their study population. The current study helps fill the gap in the current literature by including this minority population and by combining multiple intervention strategies into one program.

There are several strengths of this study. First, a primary strength was the inclusion of minority women (84% non-White women). Second, the current study also included a waitlist control group that was used as a comparison and to strengthen the study design. Third, this study utilized well-validated measures of physical function in older adults.

Despite the strengths listed above, there are some limitations to this study that need to be addressed. One limitation was that the final analytical sample was only 26 total participants. However, previous studies incorporating Tai Chi that found significant results in the TUG test (1.38 seconds: $P < 0.001$) over a 12-week period had as few as 14 women in the intervention group [18]. Second, the study groups were not randomized, which could have resulted in some bias with regard to the interpretation of the results. However, there were few baseline differences between the two groups and this was primarily a translational study with the main goal of improving health of the participants. Finally, whenever a combination of intervention strategies occurs, the results cannot be attributed to a single intervention strategy. However, previous studies [15, 25, 28] have shown that each of the interventions has been shown to improve obesity-related health and function outcomes.

In conclusion, the combination of Tai Chi, RT, and diet resulted in improved TUG times and improved measures of flexibility over 12 weeks in older obese women living in an urban setting, but not in measures of muscle strength or body composition. This translational research study was able to positively influence flexibility and function of the participants and the equipment used in the study was donated to the Senior Center for continuation of the program. This study resulted in improved mobility in obese older women, and the intervention program was performed at a low cost and can easily be adopted by a senior center. Future studies should examine this combined intervention strategy with a larger sample size in this population in order to confirm these findings and to better evaluate the combined effects on muscle strength.

Acknowledgments

This material and article is based upon work supported by the Cooperative State Research Service, U.S. Department of Agriculture under project number R100NE-1039-INT.

References

[1] T. H. Fakhouri, C. L. Ogden, M. D. Carroll, B. K. Kit, and K. M. Flegal, "Prevalence of obesity among older adults in the United States, 2007–2010," *NCHS Data Brief*, vol. 106, pp. 1–8, 2007.

[2] E. M. Mathus-Vliegen, A. Basdevant, N. Finer et al., "Prevalence, pathophysiology, health consequences and treatment options of obesity in the elderly: a guideline," *Obesity Facts*, vol. 5, no. 3, pp. 460–483, 2012.

[3] W. J. Chodzko-Zajko, D. N. Proctor, M. A. Fiatarone Singh et al., "Exercise and physical activity for older adults," *Medicine and Science in Sports and Exercise*, vol. 41, no. 7, pp. 1510–1530, 2009.

[4] C. L. Ogden, M. D. Carroll, B. K. Kit, and K. M. Flegal, *Prevalence of obesity among adults: United States, 2011–2012*, NCHS data brief, no 131, National Center for Health Statistics, Hyattsville, Md, USA, 2011.

[5] S. E. Fitzpatrick, S. Reddy, T. S. Lommel et al., "Physical activity and physical function improved following a community-based intervention in older adults in georgia senior centers," *Journal of Nutrition for the Elderly*, vol. 27, no. 1-2, pp. 135–154, 2008.

[6] S. D. Anton, T. M. Manini, V. A. Milsom et al., "Effects of a weight loss plus exercise program on physical function in overweight, older women: a randomized controlled trial," *Clinical Interventions in Aging*, vol. 6, no. 1, pp. 141–149, 2011.

[7] G. Onder, B. W. Penninx, P. Lapuerta et al., "Change in physical performance over time in older women: the women's health and aging study," *The Journals of Gerontology, Series A: Biological Sciences and Medical Sciences*, vol. 57, no. 5, pp. M289–M293, 2002.

[8] I. Rosenberg, "Epidemiologic and methodologic problems in determining nutritional status of older persons—Proceedings of a held in Albuquerque, New Mexico, October 19–21, 1988—Summary Comments," *The American Journal of Clinical Nutrition*, vol. 50, pp. 1231–1233, 1989.

[9] Z. Milanović, S. Pantelić, N. Trajković, G. Sporiš, R. Kostić, and N. James, "Age-related decrease in physical activity and functional fitness among elderly men and women," *Clinical Interventions in Aging*, vol. 8, pp. 549–556, 2013.

[10] L. Krist, F. Dimeo, and T. Keil, "Can progressive resistance training twice a week improve mobility, muscle strength, and quality of life in very elderly nursing-home residents with impaired mobility? A pilot study," *Clinical Interventions in Aging*, vol. 8, pp. 443–448, 2013.

[11] J. P. Botero, G. E. Shiguemoto, J. Prestes et al., "Effects of long-term periodized resistance training on body composition, leptin, resistin and muscle strength in elderly post-menopausal women," *The Journal of Sports Medicine and Physical Fitness*, vol. 53, no. 3, pp. 289–294, 2013.

[12] A. E. Mikesky, R. Topp, J. K. Wigglesworh, D. M. Harsha, and J. E. Edwards, "Efficacy of a home-based training program for older adults using elastic tubing," *European Journal of Applied Physiology and Occupational Physiology*, vol. 69, no. 4, pp. 316–320, 1994.

[13] U.-B. Flansbjer, J. Lexell, and C. Brogårdh, "Long-term benefits of progressive resistance training in chronic stroke: a 4-year follow-up," *Journal of Rehabilitation Medicine*, vol. 44, no. 3, pp. 218–221, 2012.

[14] M. E. Rogers, H. S. Sherwood, N. L. Rogers, and R. M. Bohlken, "Effects of dumbbell and elastic band training on physical function in older inner-city African-American women," *Women and Health*, vol. 36, no. 4, pp. 33–41, 2002.

[15] L. Katkowski, N. Beebe, S. Magnanti et al., "Effects of the addition of T'ai Chi to a dietary weight loss program on lipoprotein atherogenicity in obese older women," *The Journal of Alternative and Complementary Medicine*, vol. 19, no. 9, pp. 759–766, 2013.

[16] J. F. Audette, Y. S. Jin, R. Newcomer, L. Stein, G. Duncan, and W. R. Frontera, "Tai Chi versus brisk walking in elderly women," *Age and Ageing*, vol. 35, no. 4, pp. 388–393, 2006.

[17] P. A. Adler and B. L. Roberts, "The use of Tai Chi to improve health in older adults," *Orthopaedic Nursing*, vol. 25, no. 2, pp. 122–126, 2006.

[18] P. Intarakamhang and P. Chintanaprawasee, "Effects of Dao De Xin Xi exercise on balance and quality of life in Thai elderly women," *Global Journal of Health Science*, vol. 4, no. 1, pp. 237–244, 2012.

[19] R. E. Taylor-Piliae, K. A. Newell, R. Cherin, M. J. Lee, A. C. King, and W. L. Haskell, "Effects of Tai Chi and Western exercise on physical and cognitive functioning in healthy community-dwelling older adults," *Journal of Aging and Physical Activity*, vol. 18, no. 3, pp. 261–279, 2010.

[20] P. M. Wayne, D. P. Kiel, J. E. Buring et al., "Impact of Tai Chi exercise on multiple fracture-related risk factors in post-menopausal osteopenic women: a pilot pragmatic, randomized trial," *BMC Complementary and Alternative Medicine*, vol. 12, article 7, 2012.

[21] J. X. Li, Y. Hong, and K. M. Chan, "Tai chi: Physiological characteristics and beneficial effects on health," *British Journal of Sports Medicine*, vol. 35, no. 3, pp. 148–156, 2001.

[22] A. M. Kuramoto, "Therapeutic benefits of Tai Chi exercise: research review," *Wisconsin Medical Journal*, vol. 105, no. 7, pp. 42–46, 2006.

[23] J. A. Blumenthal, M. A. Babyak, A. Hinderliter et al., "Effects of the DASH diet alone and in combination with exercise and weight loss on blood pressure and cardiovascular biomarkers in men and women with high blood pressure: the ENCORE study," *Archives of Internal Medicine*, vol. 170, no. 2, pp. 126–135, 2010.

[24] D. T. Villareal, M. Banks, D. R. Sinacore, C. Siener, and S. Klein, "Effect of weight loss and exercise on frailty in obese older adults," *Archives of Internal Medicine*, vol. 166, no. 8, pp. 860–866, 2006.

[25] J. J. Avila, J. A. Gutierres, M. E. Sheehy, I. E. Lofgren, and M. J. Delmonico, "Effect of moderate intensity resistance training during weight loss on body composition and physical performance in overweight older adults," *European Journal of Applied Physiology*, vol. 109, no. 3, pp. 517–525, 2010.

[26] L. J. Appel, T. J. Moore, E. Obarzanek et al., "A clinical trial of the effects of dietary patterns on blood pressure. DASH Collaborative Research Group," *The New England Journal of Medicine*, vol. 336, no. 16, pp. 1117–1124, 1997.

[27] J. A. Blumenthal, M. A. Babyak, A. Sherwood et al., "Effects of the dietary approaches to stop hypertension diet alone and in combination with exercise and caloric restriction on insulin sensitivity and lipids," *Hypertension*, vol. 55, no. 5, pp. 1199–1205, 2010.

[28] C. R. Straight, L. R. Dorfman, K. E. Cottell, J. M. Krol, I. E. Lofgren, and M. J. Delmonico, "Effects of resistance training and dietary changes on physical function and body composition in overweight and obese older adults," *Journal of Physical Activity & Health*, vol. 9, no. 6, pp. 875–883, 2012.

[29] F. M. Sacks, L. P. Svetkey, W. M. Vollmer et al., "Effects on blood pressure of reduced dietary sodium and the dietary approaches to stop hypertension (DASH) diet," *The New England Journal of Medicine*, vol. 344, no. 1, pp. 3–10, 2001.

[30] J. C. Whitney, S. R. Lord, and J. C. T. Close, "Streamlining assessment and intervention in a falls clinic using the timed up and go test and physiological profile assessments," *Age and Ageing*, vol. 34, no. 6, pp. 567–571, 2005.

[31] T. M. Gill, "Assessment of function and disability in longitudinal studies," *Journal of the American Geriatrics Society*, vol. 58, pp. S308–S312, 2010.

[32] N. Takeshima, N. L. Rogers, M. E. Rogers, M. M. Islam, D. Koizumi, and S. Lee, "Functional fitness gain varies in older adults depending on exercise mode," *Medicine and Science in Sports and Exercise*, vol. 39, no. 11, pp. 2036–2043, 2007.

[33] V. Mathiowetz, N. Kashman, G. Volland, K. Weber, M. Dowe, and S. Rogers, "Grip and pinch strength: normative data for adults," *Archives of Physical Medicine and Rehabilitation*, vol. 66, no. 2, pp. 69–74, 1985.

[34] J. V. Bellace, D. Healy, M. P. Besser, T. Byron, and L. Hohman, "Validity of the Dexter Evaluation System's Jamar dynamometer attachment for assessment of hand grip strength in a normal population," *Journal of Hand Therapy*, vol. 13, no. 1, pp. 46–51, 2000.

[35] S. C. Cuthbert and G. J. Goodheart Jr., "On the reliability and validity of manual muscle testing: a literature review," *Chiropractic and Osteopathy*, vol. 15, article 4, 2007.

[36] J. D. Ritchie, C. K. Miller, and H. Smiciklas-Wright, "Tanita foot-to-foot bioelectrical impedance analysis system validated in older adults," *Journal of the American Dietetic Association*, vol. 105, no. 10, pp. 1617–1619, 2005.

[37] D. R. Young, S. H. Jee, and L. J. Appel, "A comparison of the Yale Physical Activity Survey with other physical activity measures," *Medicine and Science in Sports and Exercise*, vol. 33, no. 6, pp. 955–961, 2001.

[38] R. L. Bailey, D. C. Mitchell, C. K. Miller et al., "A dietary screening questionnaire identifies dietary patterns in older adults," *Journal of Nutrition*, vol. 137, no. 2, pp. 421–426, 2007.

[39] R. D. Cook and S. Weisberg, *Residuals and Influence in Regression*, Chapman & Hall, New York, NY, USA, 1982.

[40] R. E. Rikli and C. J. Jones, "Development and validation of criterion-referenced clinically relevant fitness standards for maintaining physical independence in later years," *Gerontologist*, vol. 53, no. 2, pp. 255–267, 2013.

[41] Y. Rolland, V. Lauwers-Cances, M. Pahor, J. Fillaux, H. Grandjean, and B. Vellas, "Muscle strength in obese elderly women: effect of recreational physical activity in a cross-sectional study," *The American Journal of Clinical Nutrition*, vol. 79, no. 4, pp. 552–557, 2004.

[42] Y. Hong, J. X. Li, and P. D. Robinson, "Balance control, flexibility, and cardiorespiratory fitness among older Tai Chi practitioners," *British Journal of Sports Medicine*, vol. 34, no. 1, pp. 29–34, 2000.

[43] T. P. Wycherley, M. Noakes, P. M. Clifton, X. Cleanthous, J. B. Keogh, and G. D. Brinkworth, "A high-protein diet with resistance exercise training improves weight loss and body composition in overweight and obese patients with type 2 diabetes," *Diabetes Care*, vol. 33, no. 5, pp. 969–976, 2010.

[44] J. Zhuang, L. Huang, Y. Wu, and Y. Zhang, "The effectiveness of a combined exercise intervention on physical fitness factors related to falls in community-dwelling older adul," *Clinical Interventions in Aging*, vol. 9, pp. 131–140, 2014.

16

Neighborhood Influences on Late Life Cognition in the ACTIVE Study

Shannon M. Sisco and Michael Marsiske

Department of Clinical and Health Psychology, University of Florida, Gainesville, FL 32610, USA

Correspondence should be addressed to Shannon M. Sisco, ssisco@ufl.edu

Academic Editor: Allison A. M. Bielak

Low neighborhood-level socioeconomic status has been associated with poorer health, reduced physical activity, increased psychological stress, and less neighborhood-based social support. These outcomes are correlates of late life cognition, but few studies have specifically investigated the neighborhood as a unique source of explanatory variance in cognitive aging. This study supplemented baseline cognitive data from the ACTIVE (Advanced Cognitive Training for Independent and Vital Elderly) study with neighborhood-level data to investigate (1) whether neighborhood socioeconomic position (SEP) predicts cognitive level, and if so, whether it differentially predicts performance in general and specific domains of cognition and (2) whether neighborhood SEP predicts differences in response to short-term cognitive intervention for memory, reasoning, or processing speed. Neighborhood SEP positively predicted vocabulary, but did not predict other general or specific measures of cognitive level, and did not predict individual differences in response to cognitive intervention.

1. Introduction

The neighborhood has emerged as a prominent level of analysis in studies of contextual influences on health and well-being in human development. This owes to the social organization of life within neighborhoods, and to the availability of data at neighborhood-like levels of analysis (i.e., census tracts). Neighborhood context has also received greater attention due to ecological psychology's conceptualization of human development as the product of a dynamic interaction between the individual and multiple nested environments, of which the neighborhood is one of the most immediate environments [1]. Contemporary scholarship on neighborhood factors has also highlighted the importance of understanding whether neighborhood variables add explanatory variance above and beyond individual differences.

Neighborhood socioeconomic status (SES) is the most consistently reported neighborhood-level predictor of cognitive outcomes—certainly in childhood, and potentially across the life span [2]. SES is also the strongest and most consistently reported neighborhood-level predictor of health outcomes among older adults—a relationship which may have a cumulative effect across the life span [3]. The association of neighborhood-level SES with health is in fact stronger among adults aged 60–69 than among young and middle-aged adults, and during these years its association with health is comparable to or stronger than the relationship of individual SES to health [4]. In addition to predicting poorer physical health, lower neighborhood SES is also associated with reduced rates of physical activity, increased incidence of depression and psychosocial stress, and less neighborhood-based social support and social engagement [3]. Many of these outcomes have also been identified as correlates of late life cognition [5], yet few studies to date have specifically investigated the role of the neighborhood in cognitive aging.

While neighborhood effects on late life cognition have received less attention, neighborhood effects on early-life cognitive development are relatively well documented. Neighborhood SES is positively correlated with cognitive development across the entire spectrum of child development, from the prenatal stages (in the form of reduced rates of congenital anomalies and neural tube defects among higher-SES neighborhoods, presumably due to reduced risk of exposure to environmental toxins; [6, 7]) and preschool years [8, 9] to academic achievement in the school age [10, 11] adolescent, and young adulthood years (e.g., high school graduation rates and college attendance [12]).

Four recent studies explored relationships between late life cognition and the neighborhood context on a broad scale. Wight and colleagues [13] found that after controlling for individual-level education and area-level median household income, elders living in areas with low neighborhood-level educational attainment (defined by census tract area) achieved lower cognitive status scores compared to elders living in areas with high neighborhood-level educational attainment (as assessed using the mini-mental state examination or MMSE [14]). A United Kingdom study [15] reported a clear and significant downward trend in cognitive performance on the MMSE and tests of verbal fluency and memory for older individuals living in neighborhoods with greater deprivation, after controlling for individual-level wealth, income, and education, across all age and gender groups. These effects were also robust after adjusting for the effects of individual systolic blood pressure, history of stroke, and duration of residence in the current neighborhood. Sheffield and Peek [16] moved beyond cross-sectional analysis to examine how neighborhood SES and ethnic composition (proportion Mexican American) predicted 5-year change in MMSE score in a US national sample. Independent of individual-level risk factors, odds and rate of incident cognitive decline increased as a function of lower neighborhood SES and decreased with the proportion of Mexican American neighborhood residents. Finally, recent findings from the Baltimore Memory Study suggest that the relationship between neighborhood and late life cognition may also depend on genotype [17]. Specifically, neighborhood psychosocial hazards were not found to be related worse cognitive performance. However, apolipoprotein E4 genotype was found to interact with high neighborhood psychosocial hazards, resulting in poorer cognitive performance on measures of processing speed and executive functioning after controlling for individual-level covariates. This suggests evidence of a gene-environment interaction in neighborhood's relation to late life cognition.

The existing studies focused on broad differences in late life cognitive *status* (i.e., MMSE score), but did not investigate the effect of neighborhood on different cognitive domains (see recommendations by Cullum et al. [18]). Furthermore, the use of the MMSE in these studies was not an ideal measure of cognition, as they targeted samples of initially healthy, independent elders. The MMSE is not sensitive to differences among healthy older adults, having been designed to screen for dementia [14]. Cognitive aging research has instead focused increasingly on the use of confirmatory factor analysis (CFA) and structural equation modeling (SEM) to explore whether differences in late life cognitive performance are related to general or specific processes. It has also been noted that conceptualizing late life cognition using a single general factor ("*g*") is a simplistic approach to a complex and dynamic cognitive system [19]. This suggests neighborhood influences should be investigated at both general and domain-specific levels. Neighborhood effects may support some dimensions of cognition more strongly than others, in addition to influencing general cognitive status.

The present study aimed to identify whether neighborhood effects on cognition were global, or specifically related to particular cognitive domains such as memory, reasoning, processing speed, everyday cognition, or vocabulary. Another innovation of the present study is the capacity to address whether neighborhood effects might also influence the magnitude of potential benefit from cognitive intervention. No study, in part because of a lack of data availability, has examined this question. Elucidating both the specificity of neighborhood effects on particular domains of cognition and the extent to which neighborhood affects cognitive training response may provide additional hints toward potential mechanisms by which the neighborhood exerts influence. For example, effects on the fluid cognitive abilities such as processing speed, memory, and reasoning (and their response to cognitive training) would suggest a more biologically mediated influence given their sensitivity to brain integrity. In contrast, effects on measures of crystallized cognitive abilities, especially vocabulary, might hint toward a more socioculturally mediated, and possibly lifespan accumulative influence, as crystallized cognitive abilities are developed with the accumulation of verbal knowledge, developed over a lifetime of experience in engaging with culture [20]. As this lifelong accumulation is strongly influenced during childhood, adolescence, and young adulthood, effects of current neighborhood SEP on crystallized abilities may also reflect, in part, effects of early-life neighborhood SEP.

The Advanced Cognitive Training for Independent and Vital Elderly (ACTIVE) study was a randomized, controlled clinical trial examining the effects of three cognitive interventions for community-dwelling older adults [21]. In ACTIVE, older adults from six US catchment areas (Baltimore/coastal Maryland; the metropolitan areas of Birmingham, Boston, Detroit, and Indianapolis; central Pennsylvania) completed a baseline assessment including multiple cognitive measures. Participants were then randomized to one of three ten-session cognitive intervention programs or a no-contact control condition.

The present study sought to examine whether neighborhood socioeconomic position (SEP) shows bivariate relationships with baseline cognitive level and immediate response to cognitive training, beyond individual-level predictors of cognition. If so, we aimed to discern whether neighborhood effects were significant for general cognitive ability ("*g*"), and whether effects were differential for specific cognitive abilities (memory, reasoning, speed, everyday cognition, and vocabulary). We hypothesized that the potential effect of neighborhood SEP may most likely occur by way of sociocultural processes, and therefore would have significant positive associations with general cognitive ability and with crystallized cognitive domains, including vocabulary. Neighborhood SEP was hypothesized to have relatively weaker, if detectable, associations with fluid cognitive domains, including memory, reasoning, speed, and everyday cognition.

2. Method

2.1. Study Design. The primary objective of ACTIVE was to test the effectiveness and durability of three cognitive interventions. The initial trial randomized individuals to one of three 10-session cognitive interventions designed to improve memory, reasoning, or processing speed performance or to a no-contact control condition [21]. Following training there was an immediate posttest and follow-up assessments at 1-, 2-, 3-, and 5-years after intervention. The current study sought to examine only the immediate pretest-posttest data, focusing on the proximal outcome measures used. The initial clinical trial enrolled participants and collected baseline data between 1997 and 2000. Information on potential covariates was collected, including demographic variables, MMSE, recent depressive symptoms, and general health. Testers at all six sites were trained in standardized assessment protocols and quality control by both study investigators, and the coordinating center ensured fidelity to testing procedures.

2.2. Participants. The initial sample of 2,802 participants was recruited through on-site presentations, letters to interested persons, newspaper advertisements, introductory letters, and follow-up telephone calls. Participants were cognitively healthy, community-dwelling older adults aged 65 to 94 years (mean age = 73.6 years, mean years of education = 13.5, mean MMSE = 27, 75.8% female, 72% Caucasian, 26% African American, and 2% other minority groups). The majority of participants (64%) were not married, and most reported good to excellent health (84.3%). Efforts were aimed at recruiting older adults independent of care at enrollment, as well as recruiting a diverse sample especially inclusive of African Americans, who were previously underrepresented in most cognitive training research. Exclusion criteria included (a) being under age 65 at the start of the study, (b) significant functional and/or cognitive decline at enrollment (e.g., impaired activities of daily living, MMSE < 23, and diagnosis of Alzheimer's disease), (c) having a medical condition disposing the participant to imminent cognitive decline or to mortality within the next 2 years, (d) severe sensory or communicative difficulties precluding participation in assessments and training, (e) having had cognitive training, or (f) planning to be unavailable during the testing and training periods of the study.

2.3. Relationship of the Present Study to the Parent Study. ACTIVE included multiple assessments of participants, but the present paper restricted itself to baseline cognitive performance and the immediate post-test. Neighborhood-level socioeconomic data from publicly available geographic datasets were then merged with ACTIVE data at the individual level. ACTIVE did not aim *a priori* to include multiple measures of individual-level socioeconomic position. Education (highest level achieved) was assessed for all participants, but other person-level socioeconomic indices (e.g., income, occupation) were not collected at baseline; occupational status was collected at the second annual follow-up occasion.

2.4. ACTIVE Cognitive Data. The cognitive domains measured in ACTVE included memory, inductive reasoning, processing speed, everyday cognition, and vocabulary; descriptive statistics on the sample performance for measures within each domain are illustrated in Table 1. Memory was measured using the Hopkins Verbal Learning Test (HVLT, [22]), a 12-word list memory task assessing immediate and delayed recall over 3 learning trials, the Rey Auditory Verbal Learning Test (AVLT, [23]), a 15-word list memory task assessing immediate and delayed recall over 5 consecutive learning trials, and the Rivermead Behavioral Memory Test [24], a paragraph recall task assessing immediate verbal episodic memory. Reasoning was measured using letter series [25], a task requiring accurate identification of the next logical letter group in a series of letters (e.g., a m b a n b a o b), letter sets [26], an inductive reasoning task requiring participants to identify which of 4 sets of letters is unrelated to the others (e.g., eef hhi llm ysy), and word series [27], a task requiring accurate identification of the next logical word in a series. Processing speed was measured using the useful field of view test (UFOV, [28]), a computer-administered task measuring visual sustained, selective, and divided attention through four subtasks, and the complex reaction time test [29], a computer-administered task measuring the time taken to perform various motor behaviors and to complete each task. Everyday cognition was measured using the Everyday Problems Test [30], a performance-based test of ability to solve everyday problems including medications, nutrition, phone use, shopping, and management of finances and household, the Observed Tasks of Daily Living (OTDL) [31], a timed task of problem solving in medication use, telephone use, and financial management, and the Timed Instrumental Activities of Daily Living (TIADL) [32], a timed test of ability to complete daily living tasks (e.g, find telephone number, make change, find and read ingredients on a can, find food items on a shelf, read instructions on medicine bottle). Vocabulary was measured using a multiple-choice measure of vocabulary attainment in which the participant is presented with a word and must choose one of four possible synonyms [26].

2.5. Combining ACTIVE and Census Data. Geocoding [33] is a process by which a location (e.g., street address) is assigned Cartesian mathematical coordinates, allowing for other levels of geographic information to be linked with that location. GeoLytics [34], a commercial provider of geocoding services and census demographic data, (1) geocoded the ACTIVE participant addresses, and (2) appended to these addresses data from the 2000 U.S. Census and 2002 Economic Census, creating a dataset that could be used to characterize the neighborhood environment. Following recommendations by prior U.S. neighborhood research [35], ACTIVE participant addresses were geocoded and linked with their associated census tract numbers, which allowed for census tract-level data from the 2000 U.S. Census to be appended to the individual-level ACTIVE data. Geocodes were checked for quality assurance. Participants receiving mail by post office boxes were excluded as such addresses cannot be verified

Table 1: Minimum, maximum, and mean scores (SD: standard deviation) for the ACTIVE sample on measures of baseline cognition.

Measure	Minimum	Maximum	Mean	SD
HVLT total	4	36	26.05	5.50
AVLT total	0	73	48.45	10.63
Rivermead total	0	17.0	6.30	2.76
Word series total correct	0	30	9.45	4.91
Letter series total correct	0	30	9.99	5.55
Letter sets total correct	0	15	5.72	2.80
UFOV task 1	16	500	30.99	40.71
UFOV task 2	16	500	132.86	124.61
UFOV task 3	43	500	321.09	134.12
UFOV task 4	170	500	456.46	68.64
CRT score 1	0.81	17.0	1.85	0.81
CRT score 2	0.91	18.75	2.25	0.87
OTDL total	1	28	17.58	4.34
EPT total	0	28	18.62	5.76
Vocabulary total correct	0	18	12.37	3.95

to represent the participant's actual place of residence. Addresses with invalid house numbers, street names, and ZIP codes were flagged for followup; invalid addresses or poorly matched addresses were dropped from the analysis (93% of the ACTIVE addresses accurately matched to a US Geological Survey (USGS) geocode; final sample size = 2,521).

Census tracts are subdivisions of a county, with an average size of approximately 4,000 residents designed to capture collectively agreed-upon areas approximating neighborhoods. That is, the boundaries of census tracts were agreed upon by local officials knowledgeable of the area and were intended to be homogenous with respect to population characteristics, economic status, and living conditions [35]. Smaller measurement units of area-level SES (e.g., block group) have been shown to correlate highly with census-level measures of SES, and variability in SES among block groups is small relative to variability within their census tract [35]. The association of area-level SES with the cognitive measures was tested at three different levels of area measurement (block group, census tract, and ZIP code), with no significant difference in the strength of associations across levels. Because the census tract has traditionally been the most frequently used and most strongly recommended unit of measurement for area-level effects in health research [36], especially in terms of SEP [3, 35], and because it differed very little in model fit or regression coefficients from the other geographic levels, the census tract level of aggregation was selected for all final analyses involving SEP.

Neighborhood socioeconomic position was measured by creating a socioeconomic position (SEP) index [37]. Because SES variables such as income, education, and occupation are often strongly correlated and have been found to load onto a common factor at the census level [38], census-level data on these variables were combined into a weighted factor score to create a neighborhood SEP index that parsimoniously represented multiple socioeconomic variables.

2.6. Statistical Analysis. The analytical framework for the study involved exploratory and confirmatory factor analysis, structural equation modeling, and repeated measures mixed effects modeling. In keeping with "best practice" in conducting neighborhood research [38], individual- and area-level effects would ideally have been examined using a multilevel modeling (MLM) approach, with samples of individuals clustered in neighborhoods allowing formal assessment of random variation within neighborhoods. However because ACTIVE was not originally designed to sample data stratified by neighborhood but sampled widely across each region, the insufficient sample size within each neighborhood measured precluded the use of MLM. In keeping with recent scholarship, the current study can instead be classified as ecologic, in which neighborhood variables are measured for each person [39]. Statistical Package for the Social Sciences (SPSS) 18.0 and Analysis of Moment Structures (AMOS) 18.0 were used to conduct all statistical analyses. Prior to analysis, all variables were inspected for consistency with the assumption of multivariate normality (to permit maximum likelihood estimation). Where that assumption was not met, Blom transformations [40] were applied to those variables to improve the normality of their distributions. While no data were missing for any neighborhood-level variables, in a few instances data were missing from the ACTIVE dataset's cognitive variables (e.g., due to failure to complete a task or attrition between the baseline and posttraining testing occasions). Models were estimated using full information maximum likelihood (FIML), which uses all available data (thereby not eliminating participants with incomplete data).

Preparatory to examining the relationship of neighborhood SEP to ACTIVE cognitive outcomes, factor analytic constructs representing neighborhood SEP and baseline cognition were developed. Criteria for acceptable model fit indices included root mean square error of approximation (RMSEA) <0.06, comparative fit index (CFI) >0.95, normed fit index (NFI) >0.95, and Tucker-Lewis Index (TLI) >0.95

[41]. Exploratory factor analyses were first conducted on the neighborhood SEP variables, using Promax rotation to allow optimal fit to the data. A weighted composite measure of SEP was then estimated and optimized in AMOS based on a common factor identified in the exploratory factor analysis. The cognitive measurement model for the present study dimensionalized cognition into several domains, for which the ACTIVE dataset was well designed, having captured at least three measures each of specific cognitive domains including memory, reasoning, processing speed, and everyday cognition, or measures of cognition related to everyday abilities. ACTIVE also collected a measure of vocabulary.

As stated in the introduction, cognitive aging research has increasingly emphasized conceptualization of cognition as both a general ability ("*g*"), and a multifaceted system of specific cognitive domains which may respond differently to neighborhood effects. Therefore the model also estimated effects on each of the above cognitive domains, as well as effects on a higher-order factor representing general cognition or "*g*", which captures the shared variance among the five cognitive domains in the measurement model. The SEP and cognition factor models were combined in a structural equation model estimating regression paths from SEP to the each of the cognitive factors. Model covariates included age, quadratic age, years of education, gender, and race (White, African American). Measures of individual wealth and duration of residence in neighborhood were not collected in ACTIVE, and could not be included as covariates.

Neighborhood SEP as a predictor of training gains was estimated as repeated-measures mixed effects models [42] rather than as structural equation models because this provided a more flexible interface for the analysis of training gains, which was operationalized as a two-occasion difference score (and thus would not significantly benefit from a latent variable approach) while still permitting FIML estimation for maximum power in the presence of missing data (i.e., using all available cases). Model covariates included age, years of education, gender, and race. Separate models were estimated for each domain trained (memory, reasoning, or speed) to examine the gains of each training group relative to other participants who did not receive that training (i.e., the other two training groups and the no-contact controls). Each model tested SEP as a continuous predictor and occasion (baseline, posttest) and training group (received training on the ability being examined or not) each as class variables. Each model also tested all possible two-way interactions and the three-way interaction of SEP, occasion, and group. Interactions were estimated as residualized interaction terms to correct for collinearity with the model's main effects.

3. Results

Neighborhood SEP was initially developed using exploratory factor analysis (EFA) to combine 8 indicators of area-level SES: median household income, % households with income ≥ \$150,000, % persons in poverty, % with ≤9th grade education, % with ≤ high school education, % with ≥ Bachelor's degree, % unemployed, and % working in management or higher. The EFA indicated all 8 variables loaded strongly onto one factor (eigenvalue = 5.97), explaining 71% of the variance (factor loadings ranged from 0.71 – 0.94). All indicators were then included in a confirmatory factor analysis, where modification indices (MI) suggested high intercorrelations of error variances among variables (e.g., ranging up to MI = 1325.42). To derive an optimally-fit, parsimonious set of variables capturing the shared variance of characteristics on which SEP is typically based (e.g., income, education, and occupational attainment), redundant variables were progressively removed from the model.

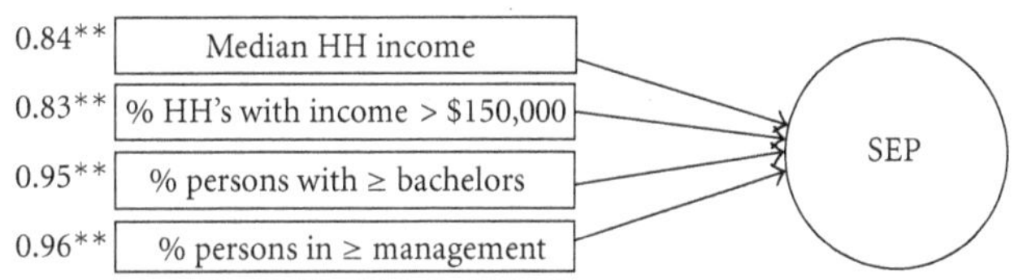

FIGURE 1: SEP factor structure model. Standardized loadings (ß) to the left of each indicator; $^{**}p < 0.001$; HH = household.

The final SEP factor model (Figure 1) consisted of four variables measuring socioeconomic advantage in income, education, and occupation (median household income, % with income ≥ \$150,000, % with ≥ Bachelor's degree, and % in management or higher). As two indices of area-level income would be expected to correlate, a correlation path was estimated between the error variances of median household income and % income ≥ \$150,000 and was retained in all subsequent models. Model fit was good (CFI = 0.999, NFI = 0.999, TLI = 0.996, χ^2/df ratio = 8.23 (p = 0.004), and RMSEA = 0.05 (p = 0.36)). Notably, the variables loading on the latent SEP factor are all indicators of neighborhood affluence or advantage rather than disadvantage; prior neighborhood research has suggested that measures of social advantage, compared to social disadvantage, may be especially important protective factors in neighborhood influences on development [2]. Mean SEP factor scores were found to differ across ACTIVE catchment sites ($F(5, 2515)$ = 184.30, p < .001; Table 2). Reestimating the models with catchment site as an additional covariate did not alter the pattern of effects, but reduced the fit of the model to an unacceptable extent. Thus, ACTIVE catchment site was tested but not retained in the study models as a covariate.

3.1. Measurement Model of Baseline Cognition. The present paper sought to characterize both general and specific domains of late life cognition. The measured variables (Figure 2) related to memory were combined to represent a memory factor; measures of reasoning combined to form a reasoning factor; guided by preliminary exploratory analyses, measures of processing speed optimally first combined into separate factors based on test, which were then combined to form a speed factor, and individual measures of everyday cognition combined on a factor representing everyday cognition. Because these cognitive domains were represented

TABLE 2: Mean, (standard deviation), and range of SEP indicators and factor scores for the overall study sample and by catchment site.

Site	Median household income	% of households with income > $150,000	% with bachelor degree or higher	% in management positions or higher	SEP factor score
All	44,680.96 (22,448.78) 7,610–170,790	5.7 (8.44) 0–54.0	28.45 (21.48) 1.0–90.0	36.19 (16.15) 4.0–84.0	2.91 (0.93) 0.28–5.76
UAB (N = 435)	51,900 (21,214) 7,610–143,968	7.97 (9.18) 0–49.0	37.74 (21.85) 1.0–81.0	42.61 (15.35) 13.0–69.0	3.31 (0.81) 1.04–5.18
IU (N = 450)	45,630 (18,390) 12,154–133,479	5.03 (6.33) 0–42.0	30.6 (19.26) 1.0–75.0	36.18 (14.93) 4.0–69.0	2.94 (0.91) 0.36–5.14
HRCA (N = 346)	62,359.64 (23,438.77) 18,917–148,257	11.46 (10.54) 0–50.0	48.59 (21.93) 5.0–9.0	52.13 (15.49) 6.0–84.0	3.78 (0.74) 0.93–5.76
JHU (N = 415)	32,791.54 (10,699.90) 10,408–84,832	2.0 (2.89) 0–25.0	17.39 (12.38) 2.0–75.0	29.35 (10.4) 10.0–75.0	2.46 (0.64) 0.95–4.59
WSU (N = 459)	48,034.58 (28,051.51) 9,615–170,790	7.28 (10.77) 0–54.0	26.42 (21.27) 1–75.0	34.93 (17.83) 7.0–76.0	2.83 (1.03) 0.28–5.41
PSU (N = 416)	29,345.72 (8,620.85) 10,101–53,096	1.17 (1.01) 0–6.0	12.72 (6.30) 3.0–28.0	24.30 (8.01) 15.0–44.0	2.27 (0.51) 1.35–3.29

Note: UAB: University of Alabama; IU: Indiana University; HRCA: Hebrew Rehabilitation Centre for Aged; JHU: Johns Hopkins University; WSU: Wayne State University; PSU: Pennsylvania State University.

by latent factors (making them "purer" representations of their domains), the vocabulary measure was also represented as a factor by using odd and even scores as indicators loading on a single vocabulary factor; this effectively transforms that factor into a construct representing the odd-even split half reliable variance of the measure. Model covariates included linear age, the quadratic effect of age, years of education, gender, and race. The disturbance terms of all cognitive factors were permitted to correlate with one another. The error variances of the UFOV 2 and 4 subtests, and the Everyday Problems Test and vocabulary were also allowed to correlate in the process of optimizing model fit (Table 3). As the first-order cognitive factors all correlated with one another ($p < 0.001$), and as discussed earlier, the model included a second-order factor, "g", capturing the variance shared by the cognitive factors (Table 4). Model fit was acceptable (CFI = 0.98, NFI = 0.97, RFI = 0.96, TLI = 0.97, RMSEA = 0.046, (p = 1.00), χ^2/df ratio = 6.40, and ($p < 0.001$)).

3.2. Neighborhood SEP Predicting Baseline Cognitive Level. The SEP and cognitive measurement models were combined in a structural equation model (Figure 2) estimating regression paths from neighborhood-level SEP to the cognitive constructs of "g", reasoning, speed, everyday cognition, and vocabulary (a path could not be estimated for SEP or any covariates to memory). Model covariates included linear age, the quadratic effect of age, years of education, gender, and race. Model fit was adequate (CFI = 0.96, NFI = 0.96, TLI = 0.95, χ^2/df ratio = 6.52, ($p < 0.001$), and RMSEA = 0.05 (p = 0.99)). After controlling for individual-level predictors, SEP remained a significant predictor of vocabulary alone ($p < 0.01$; Table 5).

3.3. Response to Cognitive Training. Repeated-measures mixed effects analyses of variance were used to estimate whether neighborhood SEP predicted differences in training-related gains, beyond practice-related gains, on posttraining measures of memory, reasoning, and speed. Three separate models examined the gains of each training group relative to all other participants (control group plus members of other training groups) who did not receive that particular training (i.e., for the reasoning outcome, the reasoning training group was compared to the control plus memory plus speed training groups). Each model tested SEP as a continuous predictor and occasion (baseline, posttest) and training group (received training on the ability being examined or not), all possible two-way interactions, and the three-way interaction of SEP, occasion, and group. Significant effects for occasion, training group, and their interaction were observed as previously reported in the parent study. A main effect was found for SEP, but for SEP to predict differences in response to ACTIVE training the three-way interaction would have to be significant; this was not found for any of the trained abilities (Memory: $F(1, 4594) = 0.66, p = 0.42$; Reasoning: $F(1, 4847) = 0.001$, $p = 0.98$; Speed: $F(1, 4793) = 0.001$, $p = 0.97$).

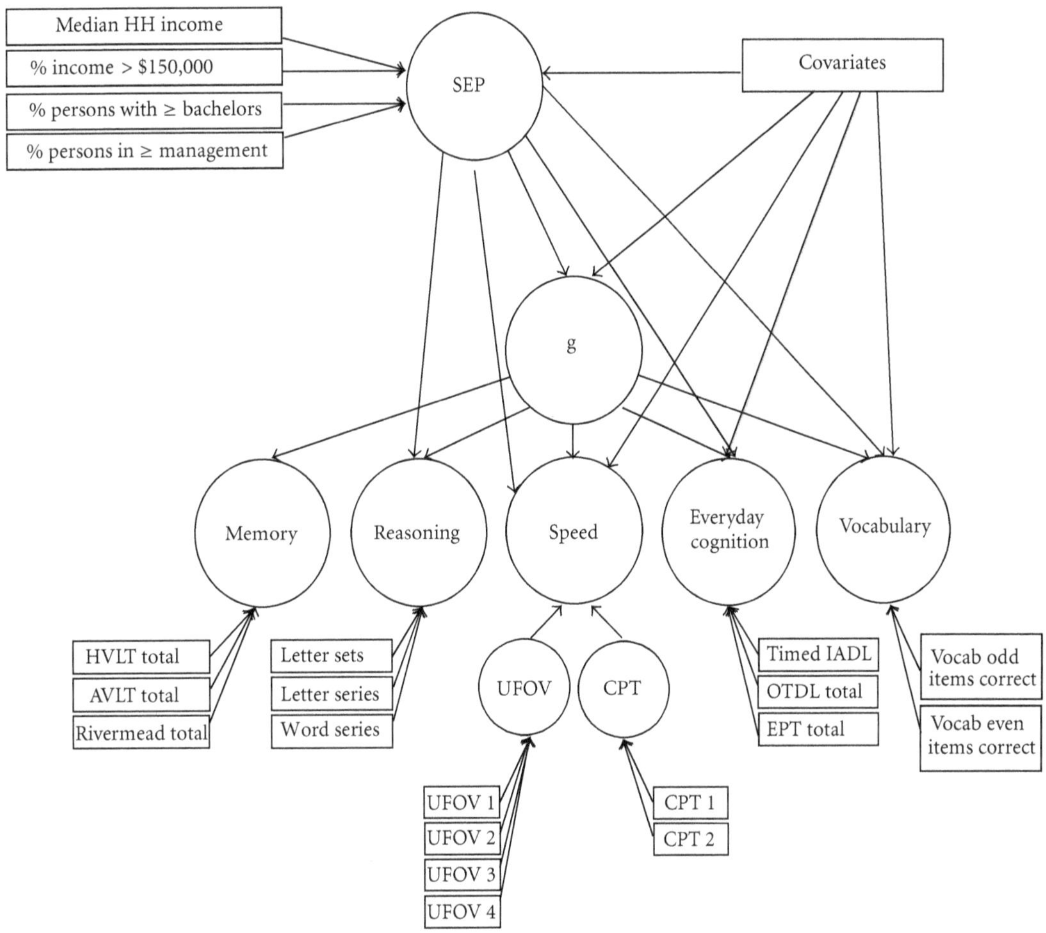

FIGURE 2: Schematic of the predictive model of baseline cognition. Regression paths were estimated from all covariates (gender, age, education, and race) to g, reasoning, speed, everyday cognition, and vocabulary, and could not be estimated for memory. Model covariates included age, quadratic age, education, gender, and race. HH = Household.

4. Discussion

The present study sought to examine the relationship between current neighborhood-level socioeconomic position (SEP) and cognitive level, including several specific cognitive domains in the ACTIVE study, and response to cognitive training. The findings demonstrated that, after controlling for individual-level demographic predictors, census-defined neighborhood socioeconomic position independently predicted differences in late life vocabulary as measured in ACTIVE, but not differences in general cognition ("g"), reasoning, everyday cognition, or speed. These findings differed from the similar prior study by Brandt [22], which found neighborhood SES effects on a composite cognitive measure capturing cognitive status, verbal fluency, verbal learning, and prospective memory. The results also demonstrated that neighborhood SEP does not predict individual differences in the immediate response to cognitive training in memory, reasoning, or processing speed.

The lack of effect for neighborhood SEP on any fluid cognitive ability (memory, reasoning, speed, and everyday cognition) or on cognitive plasticity (i.e., response to training) is somewhat surprising given the extensive research documenting neighborhood effects on factors affecting brain health, such as cardiovascular fitness and chronic diseases (e.g., [43, 44]). It would be reasonable to hypothesize that neighborhood could indirectly affect fluid cognitive abilities and training gains, which are more sensitive to compromised brain health than vocabulary [45], through differences in access to health care, nutrition, and opportunities for exercise; however, results suggest that if these indirect effects are present they may be relatively weak. Given the relatively good health of this cohort at baseline testing, the majority of respondents reported "good" or "excellent" health, and all were independent of care, there also may not have been sufficient variability in baseline fluid cognition scores for neighborhood effects to be detectable.

The specific association of neighborhood SEP with vocabulary suggests neighborhood influences cognition more through sociocultural mechanisms, as vocabulary captures crystallized cognitive abilities, the dimension of cognition related to stored verbal knowledge, developed over a lifetime of engaging with culture [20]. Vocabulary is accumulated socially through acculturation. Crystallized knowledge is also the only domain that continues to improve

TABLE 3: Standardized loadings (β) of cognitive indicators on first-order cognitive factors. $^{**}p < 0.001$.

Indicator variable	Interim factor	Cognitive factor*	β
UFOV1	UFOV		0.53**
UFOV2	UFOV		0.78**
UFOV3	UFOV		0.80**
UFOV4	UFOV		0.65**
CRT1	CRT		0.93**
CRT2	CRT		0.91**
	UFOV	Speed	0.77**
	CRT	Speed	0.77**
AVLT total recall		Memory	0.78**
HVLT total recall		Memory	0.82**
Rivermead total recall		Memory	0.62**
Letter series score		Reasoning	0.92**
Letter sets score		Reasoning	0.70**
Word series score		Reasoning	0.90**
Everyday problems test		Everyday cognition	0.83**
Timed Instrumental Activities of Daily Living (reverse-coded)		Everyday cognition	0.68**
Observed Tasks of Daily Living		Everyday cognition	0.69**
Vocabulary, odd items		Vocabulary	0.83**
Vocabulary, even items		Vocabulary	0.87**

Note: Speed is defined as a second-order factor since better fit was yielded when local associations among UFOV and CRT measures were captured in a first-order factor. These first-order factors were then allowed to load on a second-order speed factor. See Section 2 for full names of tests used.

TABLE 4: Standardized coefficients (β) for loadings of domain-specific cognitive factors on "*g*". $^{**}p < 0.01$.

Cognitive construct	β
Reasoning	0.91**
Speed	−0.85**
Memory	0.79**
Everyday	0.96**
Vocabulary	0.64**

in the presence of advancing age, compared to fluid cognitive abilities which become less efficient with age [46]. A review of vocabulary in aging [20] reported increasing vocabulary scores with advancing age, as well as with higher education (although in the present study neighborhood SEP predicted vocabulary independent of education). Vocabulary measures like the one used in this study, requiring multiple-choice word recognition rather than production of word meanings, are especially robust to the effects of aging [20].

Neighborhood may influence vocabulary by facilitating or constraining one's capacity for, and influencing the results of, sociocultural engagement in the community. It may do so by providing resources or facilities [47] encouraging cultural interaction or by encouraging acculturation through modeling and social comparisons. That is, high-SEP neighborhoods may support vocabulary because more neighbors with high educational and occupational attainment provide more social models of high achievement. This modeling may foster upward social comparisons [48, 49], pressuring or evoking desire in an individual to be more like his or her neighbors, resulting in greater engagement in activities enhancing cognitive skills and abilities. Positive community social processes may also foster sociocultural interaction. Certainly, other researchers have hinted toward social processes (i.e., social norms, interactions and ties, and collective efficacy) as the mechanism linking neighborhoods with developmental outcomes [2, 47].

While vocabulary is related to current neighborhood SEP, it is important to consider that vocabulary is also highly correlated with childhood cognitive level [45]. Vocabulary often reflects both cognitive reserve and premorbid ability level [50], as it is most robust to not only aging but physical insults to the brain, including head trauma, medical conditions, and exposure to neurotoxins [45]. Expressed differently, when cognition is measured in late life, vocabulary is the strongest index of early life cognitive ability [51]. Therefore, the current neighborhood-vocabulary association found in this study may reflect both historical and current relationships between neighborhood context and cognition; the well-established relationship between neighborhood and cognition in childhood supports this hypothesis. Thus, a part of the late life neighborhood effects on cognition observed here may represent an "echo" of this earlier relationship during a critical period of development. There is evidence

TABLE 5: Standardized coefficients (β) for prediction of cognitive domains by SEP and covariates. $^{**}p < 0.01$.

	Cognitive factors				
	"g"	Speed	Reasoning	Everyday cognition	Vocabulary
SEP	0.02	0.02	0.03	−0.02	0.07**
Education	0.37**	0.11**	0.03	0.09**	0.21**
Age	−0.49**	0.14**	0.11**	0.13**	0.36**
Gender	0.34**	0.40**	−0.27**	−0.26**	−0.15**
Race	0.35**	0.02	0.01	0.02	0.13**

Note: Beta weights to general cognition, or *g*, are predicting total variance in that factor. Beta weights to the remaining cognitive factors represent additional significant predictor effects after controlling for *g*.

that early life socioeconomic indicators also predict late life cognitive outcomes. Berkman and Glymour [52] found that the county of residence during primary schooling, by way of the laws guiding educational requirements in that county, predicted individual differences in both educational attainment and late life cognitive performance. Similarly, Wilson and colleagues [53] reported that parental education during childhood independently predicted cognitive activity across the lifespan and into old age. Therefore, it is likely that childhood SEP, had it been collected in ACTIVE, may be associated with both late life vocabulary and late life neighborhood SEP.

Finally, it was reported in the results that there were catchment site-level differences in mean SEP. Clearly, an individual's neighborhood SEP is also part of the general SEP of the region in which that individual lived; the interaction between neighborhood and regional SEP may influence how a neighborhood's SEP relates to cognition. For example, in regions with lower overall SEP, it may be more "normal" to live in a lower-SEP neighborhood; this experience might differ from the experience of living in a low-SEP neighborhood within a high-SEP region, and might differently affect cognition. Such issues have been explored on the level of individual SES-to-neighborhood SES interactions (e.g., low individual education predicts worse cognition for those living in low-education neighborhoods versus high-education neighborhoods, [13]), but neighborhood-region SEP interactions affecting cognition have not been described to our knowledge.

4.1. Study Limitations and Future Directions. This study was limited in several ways due to its nature as a secondary analysis. Several covariates would ideally have been included had they been collected in the parent study, including individual-level income and occupation (although this may later be examined in for the subset present at the 2nd-annual followup) and the length of time lived at current residence. As a consequence, this study included only a single measure of individual-level socioeconomic status. This is an important limitation, as the observed neighborhood association may be attributable, partially or completely, to unmeasured differences in individual-level socioeconomic status. The possibility that the relationship between vocabulary and neighborhood SEP can be explained by childhood neighborhood SEP must also remain speculation, as this data was not originally collected in ACTIVE. This study therefore was unable to examine measures of childhood socioeconomic status (e.g., mother's or father's education and income, neighborhood SEP in childhood). It is likely that childhood SEP is associated with both vocabulary and late life SEP, in which case vocabulary's relationship with current neighborhood SEP would be expected to diminish or disappear if childhood SEP was accounted for in the study.

The cross-sectional nature of effects also limits discussion to relationships among variables at a particular time rather than to causal or temporal relationships between variables. Longitudinal assessment of these relationships is an important next step that will be attempted in future studies. At the time this study was conducted, ACTIVE collected its 10th annual follow-up testing occasion, allowing examination of the interaction between 2000 neighborhood and cognition with 2010 neighborhood and cognition. Future studies will also attempt to examine (a) neighborhood effects on change trajectories, and (b) whether there were neighborhood moves for participants, and whether such moves were associated with functional changes. Furthermore, at this follow-up data was collected documenting participant's county of primary schooling. National historical data will allow investigators to use county information to explore whether and how distal environmental influences (i.e., county-level SEP and educational laws during primary schooling years) might predict contextual neighborhood characteristics and cognitive outcomes later in life.

5. Conclusions

This paper adds to the body of research examining neighborhood-cognition associations in late life, and extends previous findings by looking beyond general cognition or cognitive status to examine effects of neighborhood across specific cognitive domains. The finding that neighborhood SEP predicts crystallized cognitive abilities (specifically, vocabulary) suggests that neighborhood effects may be most related to sociocultural influences on cognitive development. There was a lack of association between neighborhood SEP and fluid cognitive abilities, as well as between neighborhood SEP and immediate cognitive change following training. As discussed above, future research should investigate how associations between early life neighborhood context and cognitive development may influence cognitive function and neighborhood selection in late life.

Acknowledgments

This work was supported by the National Institute on Aging (S.S., T32- AG- 020499 and S.S, and F31 AG034002). The ACTIVE cognitive training trial was supported by Grants from the National Institutes of Health to six field sites and the coordinating center, including Hebrew SeniorLife, Boston (NR04507), the Indiana University School of Medicine (NR04508), the Johns Hopkins University (AG14260), the New England Research Institutes (AG14282), the Pennsylvania State University (AG14263), the University of Alabama at Birmingham (AG14289), and the University of Florida (AG014276). Publication of this article was funded in part by the University of Florida Open-Access Publishing Fund. This work represents part of a doctoral dissertation completed by Ms. Sisco. A portion of this work has been shared in an oral presentation at the 2010 annual meeting of the Gerontological Society of America. Dr. M. Marsiske has received support from Posit Science in the form of site licenses for the Insight program (derived from the ACTIVE useful field of view training) for a different research project. The opinions expressed here are those of the authors and do not necessarily reflect those of the funding agencies, academic, research, governmental institutions, or corporations involved.

References

[1] U. Bronfenbrenner, *The Ecology of Human Development: Experiments by Nature and Design*, Harvard University Press, Cambridge, Mass, USA, 1979.

[2] T. Leventhal and J. Brooks-Gunn, "The neighborhoods they live in: the effects of neighborhood residence on child and adolescent outcomes," *Psychological Bulletin*, vol. 126, no. 2, pp. 309–337, 2000.

[3] I. H. Yen, Y. L. Michael, and L. Perdue, "Neighborhood environment in studies of health of older adults. A systematic review," *American Journal of Preventive Medicine*, vol. 37, no. 5, pp. 455–463, 2009.

[4] S. A. Robert and L. W. Li, "Age variation in the relationship between community socioeconomic status and adult health," *Research on Aging*, vol. 23, no. 2, pp. 233–258, 2001.

[5] C. Hertzog, A. F. Kramer, R. S. Wilson, and U. Lindenberger, "Enrichment effects on adult cognitive development: can the functional capacity of older adults be preserved and enhanced?" *Psychological Science in the Public Interest, Supplement*, vol. 9, no. 1, pp. 1–65, 2008.

[6] C. R. Wasserman, G. M. Shaw, S. Selvin, J. B. Gould, and S. L. Syme, "Socioeconomic status, neighborhood social conditions, and neural tube defects," *American Journal of Public Health*, vol. 88, no. 11, pp. 1674–1680, 1998.

[7] M. Vrijheid, H. Dolk, D. Stone, L. Abramsky, E. Alberman, and J. E. S. Scott, "Socioeconomic inequalities in risk of congenital anomaly," *Archives of Disease in Childhood*, vol. 82, no. 5, pp. 349–352, 2000.

[8] J. Brooks-Gunn and G. J. Duncan, "The effects of poverty on children," *Future of Children*, vol. 7, no. 2, pp. 55–71, 1997.

[9] M. T. Greenberg, L. J. Lengua, J. D. Coie, and E. E. Pinderhughes, "Predicting developmental outcomes at school entry using a multiple-risk model: four American communities. The Conduct Problems Prevention Research Group," *Developmental psychology*, vol. 35, no. 2, pp. 403–417, 1999.

[10] D. R. Entwisle, K. L. Alexander, and L. S. Olson, "The gender gap in math: its possible origins in neighborhood effects," *American Sociological Review*, vol. 59, no. 6, pp. 822–838, 1994.

[11] A. P. Jackson, "The effects of family and neighborhood characteristics on the behavioral and cognitive development of poor black children: a longitudinal study," *American Journal of Community Psychology*, vol. 32, no. 1-2, pp. 175–186, 2003.

[12] R. J. Sampson, S. W. Raudenbush, and F. Earls, "Neighborhoods and violent crime: a multilevel study of collective efficacy," *Science*, vol. 277, no. 5328, pp. 918–924, 1997.

[13] R. G. Wight, C. S. Aneshensel, D. Miller-Martinez et al., "Urban neighborhood context, educational attainment, and cognitive function among older adults," *American Journal of Epidemiology*, vol. 163, no. 12, pp. 1071–1078, 2006.

[14] M. F. Folstein, S. E. Folstein, and P. R. McHugh, ""Mini mental state". A practical method for grading the cognitive state of patients for the clinician," *Journal of Psychiatric Research*, vol. 12, no. 3, pp. 189–198, 1975.

[15] I. A. Lang, D. J. Llewellyn, K. M. Langa, R. B. Wallace, F. A. Huppert, and D. Melzer, "Neighborhood deprivation, individual socioeconomic status, and cognitive function in older people: analyses from the English Longitudinal Study of Ageing," *Journal of the American Geriatric Society*, vol. 56, pp. 191–198, 2008.

[16] K. M. Sheffield and M. K. Peek, "Neighborhood context and cognitive decline in older Mexican Americans: results from the Hispanic established populations for epidemiologic studies of the elderly," *American Journal of Epidemiology*, vol. 169, no. 9, pp. 1092–1101, 2009.

[17] B. K. Lee, T. A. Glass, B. D. James, K. Bandeen-Roche, and B. S. Schwartz, "Neighborhood psychosocial environment, apolipoprotein E genotype, and cognitive function in older adults," *Archives of General Psychiatry*, vol. 68, no. 3, pp. 314–321, 2011.

[18] S. Cullum, F. A. Huppert, M. McGee et al., "Decline across different domains of cognitive function in normal ageing: results of a longitudinal population-based study using CAMCOG," *International Journal of Geriatric Psychiatry*, vol. 15, no. 9, pp. 853–862, 2000.

[19] J. J. McArdle, F. Hamagami, W. Meredith, and K. P. Bradway, "Modeling the dynamic hypotheses of Gf-Gc theory using longitudinal life-span data," *Learning and Individual Differences*, vol. 12, no. 1, pp. 53–79, 2000.

[20] P. Verhaeghen, "Aging and vocabulary scores: a meta-analysis," *Psychology and Aging*, vol. 18, no. 2, pp. 332–339, 2003.

[21] J. B. Jobe, D. M. Smith, K. Ball et al., "Active: a cognitive intervention trial to promote independence in older adults," *Controlled Clinical Trials*, vol. 22, no. 4, pp. 453–479, 2001.

[22] J. Brandt, "The Hopkins Verbal Learning Test: development of a new memory test with six equivalent forms," *Clinical Neuropsychologist*, vol. 5, no. 2, pp. 125–142, 1991.

[23] A. Rey, "L'examen psychologique dans les cas d'encephalopathie tramatique," *Archives de Psychologie*, vol. 28, p. 21, 1941.

[24] B. A. Wilson, J. Cockburn, and A. Baddeley, *The Rivermead Behavioral Memory Test*, Thames Valley Test Company, Reading, UK, 1985.

[25] L. L. Thurstone and T.G. Thurstone, *Examiner Manual for the SRA Primary Mental Abilities Test (Form 10–14)*, Science Research Associates, Chicago, Ill, USA, 1949.

[26] R. B. Ekstrom, J. W. French, H. Harman, and D. Derman, *Kit of Factor-Referenced Cognitive Tests*, Educational Testing Service, Princeton, NJ, USA, 1976.

[27] J. Gonda and K. Schaie, *Schaie-Thurstone Mental Abilities Test: Word Series Test*, Thames Valley Test Company, Reading, UK, 1985.

[28] K. Ball, C. Owsley, M. E. Sloane, D. L. Roenker, and J. R. Bruni, "Visual attention problems as a predictor of vehicle crashes in older drivers," *Investigative Ophthalmology and Visual Science*, vol. 34, no. 11, pp. 3110–3123, 1993.

[29] K. Ball and C. Owsley, "Increasing mobility and reducing accidents in older drivers," in *Societal Impact on Mobility in the Elderly*, K. W. Schaie, Ed., Springer, New York, NY, USA, 2000.

[30] S. Willis and M. Marsiske, *Manual for the Everyday Problems Test*, Pennsylvania State University, University Park, Pa, USA, 1993.

[31] M. Diehl, S. L. Willis, and K. W. Schaie, "Everyday problem solving in older adults: observational assessment and cognitive correlates," *Psychology and Aging*, vol. 10, no. 3, pp. 478–491, 1995.

[32] C. Owsley, M. Sloane, G. McGwin, and K. Ball, "Timed instrumental activities of daily living tasks: relationship to cognitive function and everyday performance assessments in older adults," *Gerontology*, vol. 48, no. 4, pp. 254–265, 2002.

[33] M. Rezaeian, G. Dunn, S. S. Leger, and L. Appleby, "Geographical epidemiology, spatial analysis and geographical information systems: a multidisciplinary glossary," *Journal of Epidemiology and Community Health*, vol. 61, no. 2, pp. 98–102, 2007.

[34] Geolytics, "Incorporated: Demographic data, US Census and GIS Products," 2012, http://geolytics.com/.

[35] N. Krieger, J. T. Chen, P. D. Waterman, D. H. Rehkopf, and S. V. Subramanian, "Race/ethnicity, gender, and monitoring socioeconomic gradients in health: comparison of area-based socioeconomic measures—the public health disparities geocoding project," *American Journal of Public Health*, vol. 93, no. 10, pp. 1655–1671, 2003.

[36] A. V. Diez Roux, "Investigating neighborhood and area effects on health," *American Journal of Public Health*, vol. 91, no. 11, pp. 1783–1789, 2001.

[37] N. Krieger, "A glossary for social epidemiology," *Journal of Epidemiology and Community Health*, vol. 55, no. 10, pp. 693–700, 2001.

[38] A. V. Diez-Roux, C. I. Kiefe, D. R. Jacobs Jr. et al., "Area characteristics and individual-level socioeconomic position indicators in three population-based epidemiologic studies," *Annals of Epidemiology*, vol. 11, no. 6, pp. 395–405, 2001.

[39] A. V. Diez Roux, "Estimating neighborhood health effects: the challenges of causal inference in a complex world," *Social Science and Medicine*, vol. 58, no. 10, pp. 1953–1960, 2004.

[40] G. Blom, *Statistical and Estimates and Transformed Beta-Variables*, Wiley, New York, NY, USA, 1958.

[41] B. G. Tabachnick and L.S. Fidell, *Using Multivariate Statistics*, Pearson Education, 5th edition, 2007.

[42] A. Cnaan, N. M. Laird, Slasor, and P. and, "Tutorial in biostatistics: using the general linear mixed model to analyse unbalanced repeated measures and longitudinal data," *Statistics in Medicine*, vol. 16, pp. 2349–2380, 1997.

[43] C. K. Nordstrom, A. V. Diez Roux, S. A. Jackson, and J. M. Gardin, "The association of personal and neighborhood socioeconomic indicators with subclinical cardiovascular disease in an elderly cohort. The cardiovascular health study," *Social Science and Medicine*, vol. 59, no. 10, pp. 2139–2147, 2004.

[44] A. F. Brown, A. Ang, and A. R. Pebley, "The relationship between neighborhood characteristics and self-rated health for adults with chronic conditions," *American Journal of Public Health*, vol. 97, no. 5, pp. 926–932, 2007.

[45] I. J. Deary and G. D. Batty, "Cognitive epidemiology," *Journal of Epidemiology and Community Health*, vol. 61, no. 5, pp. 378–384, 2007.

[46] D. C. Park and A. H. Gutchess, "Aging, cognition, and culture: a neuroscientific perspective," *Neuroscience and Biobehavioral Reviews*, vol. 26, no. 7, pp. 859–867, 2002.

[47] R. J. Sampson, J. D. Morenoff, and T. Gannon-Rowley, "Assessing "neighborhood effects": social processes and new directions in research," *Annual Review of Sociology*, vol. 28, pp. 443–478, 2002.

[48] L. Festinger, "A theory of social comparison processes," *Human Relations*, vol. 7, no. 2, pp. 117–140, 1954.

[49] M. D. Alicke, F. M. LoSchiavo, J. Zerbst, and S. Zhang, "The person who outperforms me is a genius: maintaining perceived competence in upward social comparison," *Journal of Personality and Social Psychology*, vol. 73, no. 4, pp. 781–789, 1997.

[50] M. Richards and A. Sacker, "Lifetime antecedents of cognitive reserve," *Journal of Clinical and Experimental Neuropsychology*, vol. 25, no. 5, pp. 614–624, 2003.

[51] B. Johnstone, C. D. Callahan, C. J. Kapila, and D. E. Bouman, "The comparability of the WRAT-R reading test and NAART as estimates of premorbid intelligence in neurologically impaired patients," *Archives of Clinical Neuropsychology*, vol. 11, no. 6, pp. 513–519, 1996.

[52] L. F. Berkman and M. M. Glymour, "How society shapes aging: the centrality of variability," *Daedalus*, vol. 135, no. 1, pp. 105–114, 2006.

[53] R. S. Wilson, L. L. Barnes, K. R. Krueger, G. Hoganson, J. L. Bienias, and D. A. Bennett, "Early and late life cognitive activity and cognitive systems in old age," *Journal of the International Neuropsychological Society*, vol. 11, no. 4, pp. 400–407, 2005.

17

Investment Trait, Activity Engagement, and Age: Independent Effects on Cognitive Ability

Sophie von Stumm

Department of Psychology, University of Edinburgh, 7 George Square, EH8 9JZ Edinburgh, UK

Correspondence should be addressed to Sophie von Stumm, svonstum@staffmail.ed.ac.uk

Academic Editor: Allison A. M. Bielak

In cognitive aging research, the "engagement hypothesis" suggests that the participation in cognitively demanding activities helps maintain better cognitive performance in later life. In differential psychology, the "investment" theory proclaims that age differences in cognition are influenced by personality traits that determine when, where, and how people invest their ability. Although both models follow similar theoretical rationales, they differ in their emphasis of behavior (i.e., activity engagement) versus predisposition (i.e., investment trait). The current study compared a cognitive activity engagement scale (i.e., frequency of participation) with an investment trait scale (i.e., need for cognition) and tested their relationship with age differences in cognition in 200 British adults. Age was negatively associated with fluid and positively with crystallized ability but had no relationship with need for cognition and activity engagement. Need for cognition was positively related to activity engagement and cognitive performance; activity engagement, however, was not associated with cognitive ability. Thus, age differences in cognitive ability were largely independent of engagement and investment.

1. Introduction

In cognitive aging research, the "engagement hypothesis" predicts that engagement in physical, social, and intellectual activity contributes to reducing age-related cognitive decline and the risk of neurodegenerative disorders [1, 2]. That is, frequent participation in cognitively demanding activities is thought to "exercise" the brain with more cognitively engaged people having better cognition over time because of practice benefits. Thus, the preservation of cognition is thought to depend on the extent to which "a diverse behavioral repertoire is integrated into daily life" [3, page 487]. In differential psychology, the "investment theory" suggests that age-related changes in cognitive development are influenced by personality traits that determine where, when, and how people apply their mental ability [4, 5]. Thus, investment traits are thought to predispose individuals to seek cognitively stimulating environments that in turn prompt the development, application, and practice of cognitive strategies [3, 5]. That said, investment traits may also lead to approaching even mundane experiences in a cognitively stimulating manner, thereby enhancing intellectual development (cf. [6]).

In spite of their native disciplines' differential emphasis on decline versus growth, the engagement hypothesis and investment theory have a lot in common. First, both models propose that individual differences in intellectual engagement are reflected in lifespan trajectories of cognitive development [1, 5]. Second, both models have received some empirical support (e.g., [7–9]), as well as some rejections (e.g., [10–12]). Third, both are subject to the same criticism that the effects of engagement or investment on cognitive change (i.e., differential preservation) are explained by alternative factors, in particular by prior cognitive ability (i.e., preserved differentiation, cf. [2]). That said, the engagement hypothesis and investment theory also differ in one crucial point: cognitive aging researchers tend to assess differences in engaging in substantively complex environments, while investment theorists measure latent traits of personality that refer to "the tendency to seek out, engage in, enjoy, and continuously pursue opportunities for effortful cognitive activity" [13, page 225]. That is, activity engagement is typically assessed with reference to a specific set of activities or environments, such as going to the theatre, while investment traits refer to the intrinsic motivation to think, and corresponding scales assess, for example, one's preference of complex over simple problems. Despite following different rationales, investment and engagement measures rely equally on self-reports, and neither construct has a gold standard scale or equivalent (cf. [2, 13]). Cognitive aging measures of activity engagement vary in their foci, ranging between the frequency of an activity (e.g., regular versus sporadic; [14]), its intensity (e.g., gentle versus vigorous exercise; [15]), life-stage-specific activities (e.g., educational attainment in young adulthood versus occupational achievements in later life; [16]), and specific activity domains (e.g., social versus physical; [11]). Conversely, theoretical and psychometric definitions of investment range from comparatively narrow investment trait scales (e.g., need for cognition; [17]) to broad trait dimensions (e.g., openness to experience; [18]), to even broader trait complexes [5]. To systematically address the role of engagement and investment for cognitive performance, the current study compares the need for cognition scale and a measure of cognitive activity engagement, as well as their relationship with age differences in cognitive ability.

Two previous studies that assessed a wide range of activities, including, for example, housework and religious service attendance, found little support for the notion that activity engagement mediated the effects of an investment trait on cognitive performance [3, 19], which may have been due to the breadth of the included investment and engagement measures. Here, a narrowly focused scale was developed to assess the frequency of participating in typical cognitive activities (e.g., reading a novel; visiting a museum). To measure individual differences in intellectual investment, the need for cognition scale was selected. It refers to the "tendency to engage in and enjoy thinking" [17, page 116] and is a widely used, well-validated and precise measure of investment (cf. [20–22]). Need for cognition scale items makes no reference to specific cognitive activities or environments but measure the extent to which a person enjoys deliberating, abstract thinking and problem solving [17].

In line with previous research [3, 23], it was hypothesized that need for cognition was not meaningfully associated with age because it is a relatively stable trait dimension. Conversely, the frequency of activity engagements is likely to change according to age. That is, during some life periods that allow for the time and financial resources (e.g., young adulthood or early retirement), activity levels can be expected to be relatively high compared to others that are more restricted (e.g., adolescence and parenthood). It follows that activity engagement may have a nonlinear relationship with age.

With respect to age differences in cognitive ability, the so-called fluid abilities (i.e., reasoning capacity) were expected to be negatively correlated with age, while the crystallized abilities (i.e., vocabulary) were expected to be positively associated with age (cf. [4, 5]). Accordingly, age differences in fluid and crystallized ability may be mediated or moderated by cognitive activity engagement and need for cognition (cf. [24, 25]; Figure 1). In a mediation model, the effect of age on cognition is accounted for by activity engagement, which in turn should be positively associated with need for cognition. Thus, the predisposition to seek cognitively stimulating environments is thought to result in a greater frequency of activity engagement, which explains part of the association between age and cognition. By comparison in a moderation model, strength and direction of the relationship between age and cognition is expected to depend on the level of activity engagement and need for cognition (cf. [24]). Thus, people with high need for cognition and subsequently frequent cognitive activity engagements may show smaller age differences in fluid ability and greater ones in crystallized ability than those with low need for cognition and few activity engagements. Because mediation and moderation models are equally plausible in this research context, the current study explores both alternatives.

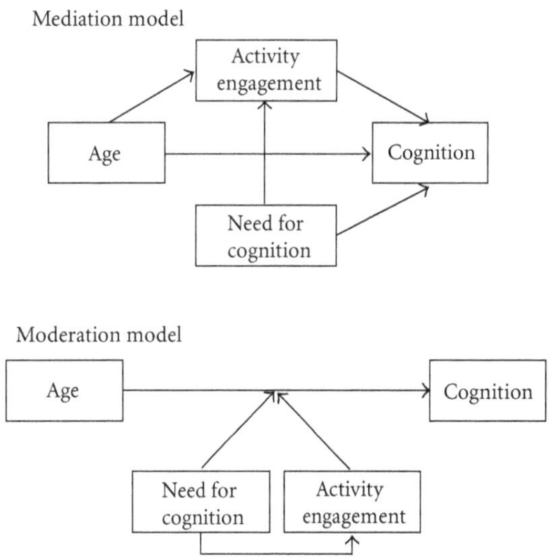

Figure 1: Mediation and moderation models.

2. Methods

2.1. Sample. 200 British adults (97 men) were recruited with an average age of 34.6 years (SD = 11.8; range from 18 to 69 years; two participants did not report their age). As their highest educational qualification, 14% participants had completed general certificates of secondary education (10th grade); 15% A-levels (12th grade); 18% a vocational qualification or equivalent; 33.5% an undergraduate degree, and 19% a postgraduate degree. About half of the sample reported to earn less than £15.000 ($22,500) per annum, while about 8% declared to earn more than £35.000 ($52,000) per annum.

2.2. Measures

Need for Cognition (see [17]). The 18-item scale measures the desire to engage in effortful cognitive activity on a 5-point Likert scale, ranging from strongly disagree, disagree, somewhat agree, agree, to strongly agree. An example item

Table 1: Descriptives of cognitive activity engagement items.

	Item	N	M	SD
1	Read a book?	198	135.13	141.54
2	Read the newspapers?	199	203.59	137.46
3	Attend a music event or concert?	199	29.38	56.88
4	Attend evening classes?	197	18.71	43.91
5	Write for pleasure?	200	63.16	109.54
6	See a play at the theatre?	197	17.76	37.32
7	Go to a museum or gallery?	198	29.45	44.59
8	Attend a public talk or lecture?	196	22.03	50.23
9	Visit the cinema?	199	35.70	64.12
10	Google things?	200	273.56	126.51

Note: activity engagement was recorded on a 5-point scale and recoded in days per annum (i.e., every day = 365; every other day = 182; every week = 52; once or twice a month = 18; never = 0).

reads: "I would prefer difficult to simple problems." Internal consistency typically ranges from .83 to .97 [20].

Cognitive Activity Engagement. Nine items that were most frequently used in previous studies to assess cognitive activity engagement were adapted [7, 14, 26] and complemented by one addressing the use of modern information technology (i.e., google; Table 1). Participants indicated on a Likert-type scale how often they engaged in the activities listed ranging from 1 to 5, including never, once or twice a month, every week, every other day, and every day.

Cognitive Ability. Fluid and crystallized abilities were assessed with three tests each, including Raven's matrices [27] and five other tests [28]. *Fluid ability:* (1) Raven's progressive matrices: 12 items showed grids of 3 rows × 3 columns, each with the lower right-hand entry missing. Participants chose from 8 alternatives the one that completed the 3 × 3 matrix figure. The test was timed at 4 minutes. (2) Lettersets: in 5 sets of 4 letters, participants identified the set that did not fit a rule that explained the composition of the other 4 lettersets. The test had 15 items and was timed at 6 minutes. (3) Nonsense syllogisms: participants judged if a conclusion that followed two preceding statements (premises) showed good (correct) reasoning or not. The test had 15 items and was timed at 4 minutes. *Crystallized ability:* (1) verbal reasoning: participants had to identify the correct pair of words from five options to complete a comparison sentence, whose first and last works were missing. The test had 14 items and was timed at 7 minutes. (2) Vocabulary: participants had to identify the correct synonym for a given word out of five answer options. The test had 18 items and was timed at 4 minutes. (3) Verbal fluency: participants had to write down as many words as possible that started with the prefixes "sub" and "pro." For each prefix, 60 seconds were allowed.

2.3. Procedure. Participants were recruited in London, England, with online and flyer advertisement. Inclusion criteria were as follows: native English speakers; normal or corrected to normal vision, hearing, and motor coordination; having lived in the United Kingdom for at least 10 years. These criteria were self-reported by the participants prior to testing. No university students were recruited. Participants completed a two-hour testing session in groups of up to twenty in designated research laboratories. The ability tests were administered in 40 minutes, then participants completed a range of other measures (not reported here), and finally, they completed the cognitive activity engagement and need for cognition scale, as well as a demographic background questionnaire in their own time (approximately 15 minutes). They received monetary compensation.

2.4. Analysis. The intelligence tests' z-scores were added to form unit-weighted composite scores of fluid and crystallized ability. The cognitive activity responses were weighted on a linear frequency scale of days per annum (i.e., every day = 365; every other day = 182; every week = 52; once or twice a month = 18; never = 0); the psychometric properties of the scale were subsequently analyzed. The study variables were investigated for sex differences in means and variances, and then, their intercorrelations were computed. Next, a series of path models tested if age differences in cognition were mediated or moderated by need for cognition and cognitive activity engagement. To test for mediation, a path model was fitted in line with Figure 1, including fluid and crystallized ability as correlated outcome variables. To test for moderation, all variables were z-transformed. A series of regression models tested two-way interactions (need for cognition × age, activity engagement × age, and need for cognition × activity engagement) and a three-way interaction (age × need for cognition × activity engagement) separately for fluid and crystallized ability. That is, a first set of models (one for fluid, one for crystallized ability) included age and need for cognition in a first step and in a second, their interaction term. A second set of models included age and activity engagement in a first step and then their interaction. A third set of models included first age, activity engagement, and need for cognition, next their two-way interactions, and finally the three-way interaction term.

3. Results

Table 1 shows the descriptives for the cognitive activity engagement items after recoding the Likert scale into days per annum. Item endorsement frequencies did not vary meaningfully with age. A unit-weighted composite score was formed; the corresponding coefficient alpha was .58. The activity engagement score was normally distributed, and so were the test scores of all cognitive ability tests. No meaningful sex differences were observed in the study variables, and thus, data from men and women were analyzed together.

The scatterplot suggested that age was not associated with cognitive activity engagement, neither in a linear nor in a nonlinear fashion. Table 2 shows the descriptives of and correlations between age (in years), need for cognition, activity engagement, and fluid and crystallized ability. Age was significantly negatively associated with fluid and positively with crystallized ability. Furthermore, fluid and crystallized ability were intercorrelated (r = .66), and so were cognitive

TABLE 2: Correlations and descriptives for study variables.

		N	M	SD	1	2	3	4
1	Fluid ability	200	0.00	2.31	—			
2	Crystallized ability	189	−0.01	2.52	.66*	—		
3	Age (years)	198	34.58	11.84	−.14*	.18*	—	
4	Activity engagement	193	830.32	357.84	.08	.10	.00	—
5	Need for cognition	189	3.46	0.60	.34*	.35*	.00	.25*

*$P < .05$.
Note: need for cognition was recorded on a 5-point Likert scale, ranging from strongly disagree, disagree, somewhat agree, agree, to strongly agree. Activity engagement was also recorded on a 5-point scale and recoded in days per annum (i.e., every day = 365; every other day = 182; every week = 52; once or twice a month = 18; never = 0).

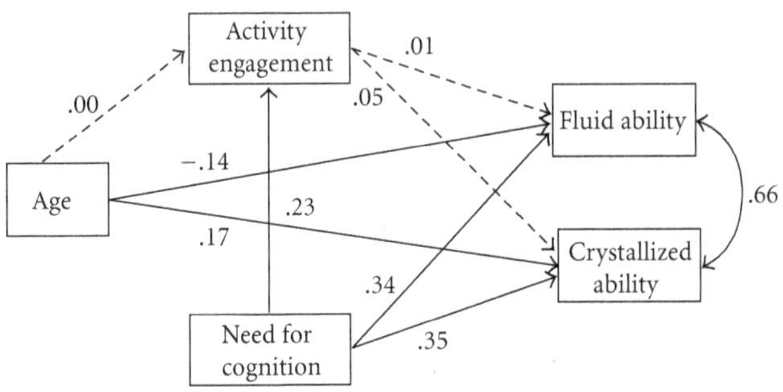

FIGURE 2: Mediation model of age differences in cognitive ability with standardized path parameters. Note: error terms for activity engagement, fluid and crystallized ability have been omitted to sustain graphical clarity. Dashed paths represent nonsignificant pathways ($P > .05$). The double-headed arrow indicates a correlation.

activity engagement and need for cognition, albeit to a much smaller extent ($r = .25$). Cognitive activity engagement was not correlated with age, fluid or crystallized ability, while need for cognition had a significant, positive associations ability but not with age.

Figure 2 shows the mediation model results. As before, age was positively associated with crystallized ability and negatively with fluid intelligence, while need for cognition had positive relationships with activity engagement, fluid and crystallized ability. Activity engagement did not mediate any of the age or need for cognition effects on cognitive ability. Thus, need for cognition and age had only direct effects on fluid and crystallized ability, accounting for 13% and 15% of their total variance, respectively.

Table 3 shows the results of the moderation models. In the first step, age was positively associated with crystallized and negatively with fluid ability, while need for cognition was positively associated with both, and activity engagement was not meaningfully related to ability. Neither two-way nor three-way interaction yielded any significant results. Thus, the level of activity engagement or investment did not interact with age differences in fluid and crystallized abilities. Overall, the results suggest that while investment traits and cognitive activity engagement are moderately associated, neither affects age differences in cognition. That said, need for cognition was significantly correlated with cognitive ability, while activity engagement was not.

4. Discussion

The current study explored the relationship of an investment personality trait (i.e., need for cognition) and a cognitive activity engagement scale with age differences in cognitive performance. In line with earlier research [3, 19], need for cognition and cognitive activity engagement were positively interrelated, albeit weakly so. Therefore, a predisposition to deliberate and think abstractly is somewhat different to actively pursuing cognitively stimulating engagement, such as reading a novel or going to the theatre. Also consistent with previous findings [1, 5], age was negatively associated with fluid and positively with crystallized ability, as well as unrelated to the investment trait need for cognition (cf. [17, 23]). Contradicting the current hypotheses, however, no meaningful age differences were observed in cognitive activity engagement. Thus, while the frequencies of activity engagement were slightly elevated in age groups that are likely to experience the most advantageous conditions for engagement (i.e., financial security and time), these differences were not significant.

Confirming previous research [20, 21, 29], need for cognition was positively associated with both fluid and crystallized ability, while no such association was observed for cognitive activity engagement (cf. [3, 19]). Furthermore, cognitive activity engagement did not mediate the association between age and cognition. That is, age and need for cognition had direct, independent effects on cognition, which were unrelated to cognitive activity engagement. It seems plausible that need for cognition contributes to constructing everyday experiences in an intellectually enriching way, and thus, the effect of need for cognition on cognitive performance is direct and not mediated by engagement (cf. [3, 6]). Future research must establish how need for cognition affects perception and perhaps even intellectual exploitation of daily working and living routines, and how such experiences contribute to cognitive development and aging.

The current study has several limitations. First, the study design was cross-sectional, and all causal inferences are speculative. Second, the recruitment methods of the study may have led to a biased sample composition by attracting

TABLE 3: Standardized regression parameters for two-way and three-way moderation models.

Step	Model 1						Model 2						Model 3					
	Fluid ability			Crystallized ability			Fluid ability			Crystallized ability			Fluid ability			Crystallized ability		
	β	CI (95%)		β	CI (95%)		β	CI (95%)		β	CI (95%)		β	CI (95%)		β	CI (95%)	
1																		
Age	**−.14**	**−0.63**	**−0.01**	**.17**	**0.08**	**0.77**	−.11	−0.59	0.07	**.19**	**0.12**	**0.86**	−.13	−0.63	0.03	**.19**	**0.12**	**0.86**
NFC	**.34**	**0.44**	**1.05**	**.35**	**0.51**	**1.16**	—	—	—	—	—	—	**.32**	**0.39**	**1.02**	**.35**	**0.50**	**1.18**
CAE	—	—	—	—	—	—	.07	−0.18	0.48	.09	−0.13	0.59	.03	−0.27	0.38	.05	−0.22	0.48
2																		
NFC × age	−.03	−0.37	0.24	−.04	−0.41	0.24	—	—	—	—	—	—	−.05	−0.43	0.23	−.01	−0.38	0.32
CAE × age	—	—	—	—	—	—	−.05	−0.43	0.20	−.05	−0.45	0.24	−.05	−0.46	0.23	.01	−0.36	0.39
CAE × NFC	—	—	—	—	—	—	—	—	—	—	—	—	−.09	−0.43	0.10	.00	−0.28	0.29
3																		
CAE × NFC × age	—	—	—	—	—	—	—	—	—	—	—	—	.09	−0.13	0.36	.13	−0.07	0.45

Note: the regressions were stepwise conducted, entering the respective set of independent variables in step 1, and their corresponding interaction terms in step 2 and 3. All models were run separately for fluid and crystallized ability as dependent variables. Model 1 shows the results for the two-way interaction of age and need for cognition; model 2 shows the two-way interaction of age and cognitive activity engagement; model 3 shows the results of testing for the three-way interaction. Significant parameters are shown in bold. Keys: age = age in years; NFC = need for cognition; CAE = cognitive activity engagement.

particularly active or cognitively engaged individuals. Also, the age range of participants (18 to 69 years), about half of whom were aged between 18 and 30 years, is possibly not ideal for detecting age differences in cognition. Indeed, the modesty of the observed associations between age and cognition is likely to be due to the relative youth of the current sample. The latter is unlikely, however, to account for the observed zero-order associations of age with investment and engagement because the sample spanned several life periods. Third, the current study assessed only one dimension of activity engagement (i.e., cognitive), but it may be that other engagement aspects, such as physical or social activity, are more important for age differences in cognition [7]. Also, only the frequency of cognitive activity engagement but not its duration nor the complexity of the activity was assessed here. Finally, the assessment instruments of intellectual investment and cognitive activity both relied on self-reports, which are known to be influenced by social desirability and self-serving bias (cf. [30]).

Notwithstanding these shortcomings, the current study contributes to understanding the role of investment and engagement for age differences in cognition. Echoing previous research (e.g., [7, 9, 11, 12]), it seems as if intellectual engagement—regardless of being assessed in terms of activity participation or trait disposition—has little effect on age differences in cognition. That said, the predisposition to invest (i.e., need for cognition) in one's cognitive competence contributed overall to better cognitive performance and a higher frequency of cognitive activity engagement (cf. [3, 9]). To explain the relationship between investment and cognition, mechanisms other than activity engagement must be explored, for example, individual differences in constructing experiences within daily living routines.

Acknowledgments

The author thanks Eva Zoubek for her indispensable help with the data collection. This work was partially funded by the Central Research Fund of the University of London.

References

[1] T. A. Salthouse, *Theoretical Perspectives on Cognitive Aging*, Erlbaum, Hillsdale, Ind, USA, 1991.

[2] A. A. M. Bielak, "How can we not "lose it" if we still don't understand how to "use it"? unanswered questions about the influence of activity participation on cognitive performance in older age: a mini-review," *Gerontology*, vol. 56, no. 5, pp. 507–519, 2010.

[3] J. M. Parisi, E. A. Stine-Morrow, S. R. Noh, and D. G. Morrow, "Predispositional engagement, activity engagement, and cognition among older adults.," *Aging, Cognition & Neuropsycholog*, vol. 16, no. 4, pp. 485–504, 2009.

[4] R. B. Cattell, "The measurement of adult intelligence," *Psychological Bulletin*, vol. 40, no. 3, pp. 153–193, 1943.

[5] P. L. Ackerman, "A theory of adult intellectual development: process, personality, interests, and knowledge," *Intelligence*, vol. 22, no. 2, pp. 227–257, 1996.

[6] E. A. L. Stine-Morrow, "The dumbledore hypothesis of cognitive aging," *Current Directions in Psychological Science*, vol. 16, no. 6, pp. 295–299, 2007.

[7] A. J. Gow, J. Corley, J. M. Starr, and I. J. Deary, "Reverse causation in activity-cognitive ability associations: the Lothian Birth Cohort 1936," *Psychology and Aging*, vol. 37, pp. 71–89, 2011.

[8] D. F. Hultsch, C. Hertzog, B. J. Small, and R. A. Dixon, "Use it or lose it: Engaged lifestyle as a buffer of cognitive decline in aging?" *Psychology and Aging*, vol. 14, no. 2, pp. 245–263, 1999.

[9] S. von Stumm and I. J. Deary, "Typical intellectual engagement and cognition in the ninth decade of life: the Lothian Birth Cohort 1921," *Psychology and Aging*, vol. 98, pp. 87–91, 2011.

[10] M. J. Aartsen, C. H. M. Smits, T. Van Tilburg, K. C. P. M. Knipscheer, and D. J. H. Deeg, "Activity in older adults: cause or consequence of cognitive functioning? A longitudinal study on everyday activities and cognitive performance in older adults," *Journals of Gerontology B*, vol. 57, no. 2, pp. P153–P162, 2002.

[11] P. Ghisletta, J. F. Bickel, and M. Lövdön, "Does activity engagement protect against cognitive decline in old age? Methodological and analytical considerations," *Journals of Gerontology B*, vol. 61, no. 5, pp. P253–P261, 2006.

[12] A. J. Gow, M. C. Whiteman, A. Pattie, and I. J. Deary, "The personality-intelligence interface: Insights from an ageing cohort," *Personality and Individual Differences*, vol. 39, no. 4, pp. 751–761, 2005.

[13] S. von Stumm, P. L. Ackerman, and T. Chamorro-Premuzic, "Re-visiting intelligence-personality associations: Vindicating intellectual investment," in *Handbook of Individual Differences*, T. Chamorro-Premuzic, S. von Stumm, and A. Furnham, Eds., Wiley-Blackwell, Chichester, UK, 2011.

[14] J. A. Schinka, A. McBride, R. D. Vanderploeg, K. Tennyson, A. R. Borenstein, and J. A. Mortimer, "Florida cognitive activities scale: initial development and validation," *Journal of the International Neuropsychological Society*, vol. 11, no. 1, pp. 108–116, 2005.

[15] Y. E. Geda, R. O. Roberts, D. S. Knopman et al., "Physical exercise, aging, and mild cognitive impairment a population-based study," *Archives of Neurology*, vol. 67, no. 1, pp. 80–86, 2010.

[16] M. J. Valenzuela and P. Sachdev, "Assessment of complex mental activity across the lifespan: Development of the Lifetime of Experiences Questionnaire (LEQ)," *Psychological Medicine*, vol. 37, no. 7, pp. 1015–1025, 2007.

[17] J. T. Cacioppo and R. E. Petty, "The need for cognition," *Journal of Personality and Social Psychology*, vol. 42, no. 1, pp. 116–131, 1982.

[18] P. T. Costa and R. R. McCrae, *Revised NEO Personality Inventory (NEO-PI-R) and NEO Five-Factor Inventory (NEO-FFI): Professional Manual*, Psychological Assessment Resources, Odessa, Fla, USA, 1992.

[19] A. Soubelet and T. A. Salthouse, "The role of activity engagement in the relations between Openness/Intellect and cognition," *Personality and Individual Differences*, vol. 49, no. 8, pp. 896–901, 2010.

[20] J. T. Cacioppo, R. E. Petty, J. Feinstein, and W. B. G. Jarvis, "Dispositional differences in cognitive motivation: The life and times of individuals varying in need for cognition," *Psychological Bulletin*, vol. 119, pp. 197–253, 1996.

[21] P. Mussel, "Epistemic curiosity and related constructs: lacking evidence of discriminant validity," *Personality and Individual Differences*, vol. 49, no. 5, pp. 506–510, 2010.

[22] S. E. Woo, P. D. Harms, and N. R. Kuncel, "Integrating personality and intelligence: Typical intellectual engagement and need for cognition," *Personality and Individual Differences*, vol. 43, no. 6, pp. 1635–1639, 2007.
[23] D. C. Funder, "Personality," *Annual Review of Psychology*, vol. 52, pp. 197–221, 2001.
[24] R. M. Baron and D. A. Kenny, "The moderator-mediator variable distinction in social psychological research: conceptual, strategic, and statistical considerations," *Journal of Personality and Social Psychology*, vol. 51, no. 6, pp. 1173–1182, 1986.
[25] K. J. Preacher and A. F. Hayes, "Asymptotic and resampling strategies for assessing and comparing indirect effects in multiple mediator models," *Behavior Research Methods*, vol. 40, no. 3, pp. 879–891, 2008.
[26] M. Richards, R. Hardy, and M. E. J. Wadsworth, "Does active leisure protect cognition? Evidence from a national birth cohort," *Social Science and Medicine*, vol. 56, no. 4, pp. 785–792, 2003.
[27] J. C. Raven, *Progressive Matrices: A Perceptual Test of Intelligence*, H. K. Lewis, London, UK, 1968.
[28] R. B. Ekstrom, J. W. French, and H. H. Harman, *Manual for Kit of Factor-Referenced Cognitive Tests*, Educational Testing Service, Princeton, NJ, UK, 1976.
[29] M. Fleischhauer, S. Enge, B. Brocke, J. Ullrich, A. Strobel, and A. Strobel, "Same or different? Clarifying the relationship of need for cognition to personality and intelligence," *Personality and Social Psychology Bulletin*, vol. 36, no. 1, pp. 82–96, 2010.
[30] L. R. James, "Measurement of personality via conditional reasoning," *Organizational Research Methods*, vol. 1, no. 2, pp. 131–163, 1998.

18

Active Ageing Level of Older Persons: Regional Comparison in Thailand

Md. Nuruzzaman Haque

Department of Population Science and Human Resource Development, University of Rajshahi, Rajshahi 6205, Bangladesh

Correspondence should be addressed to Md. Nuruzzaman Haque; nzaman_pop@yahoo.com

Academic Editor: Illario Maddalena

Active ageing level and its discrepancy in different regions (Bangkok, Central, North, Northeast, and South) of Thailand have been examined for prioritizing the policy agenda to be implemented. Attempt has been made to test preliminary active ageing models for Thai older persons and hence active ageing index (AAI, ranges from 0 to 1) has been estimated. Using nationally representative data and confirmatory factor analysis approach, this study justified active ageing models for female and male older persons in Thailand. Results revealed that active ageing level of Thai older persons is not high (mean AAIs for female and male older persons are 0.64 and 0.61, resp., and those are significantly different ($p < 0.001$)). Mean AAI in Central region is lower than North, Northeast, and South regions but there is no significant difference in the latter three regions of Thailand. Special emphasis should be given to Central region and policy should be undertaken for increasing active ageing level. Implementation of an Integrated Active Ageing Package (IAAP), containing policies for older persons to improve their health and economic security, to promote participation in social groups and longer working lives, and to arrange learning programs, would be helpful for increasing older persons' active ageing level in Thailand.

1. Introduction

Active ageing (AA) is the global goal of present ageing world for meeting the challenges of older persons and for improving their quality of life. Active ageing can be explained as a concept [1] and Walker (2002) has defined AA as profound strategy to maximize participation and wellbeing as people grow older [1]. World Health Organization (WHO) defined AA as the way of thinking and working on "the process of optimizing opportunities for health, participation and security in order to enhance quality of life as people age" [2]. The concept of AA can be encapsulated as "engaged in life" and it has been recognized as a latent construct which has no specific clear dependent variable to measure it and it may be determined by various latent (unobserved) factors. The AA construct is influenced by several groups of determinants or determinant factors including the cross-cutting determinants (gender and culture) [2]. These determinant factors are unobserved or latent and each of them can be presented by some indicators [2, 3].

The growth of population ageing in Thailand is faster compared to other Asian countries [4]. The pace of recent population ageing in Thailand is faster than other Asian countries and even far more faster than developed countries in the West [4, 5], and proportion of elderly (aged 60 and over) is projected to reach more than 30% within the next three decades in Thailand [6]. Thailand has become an ageing society and is going to increase its older population. A rapid proceeding pace of population ageing, along with demographic changes in Thailand, is posing critical challenges for Thai government to maintain economic growth, social stability, and living standard of people in the nation.

All determinant factors of AA with their indicators (hence active ageing level, AAL) need to be better understood for developing policies and programs focused on active ageing in an ageing society. Moreover, comparison of AAL regarding cross-cutting determinants of AA, gender and culture, should be unveiled for better policy implications for the older persons and for the nation as a whole. Using exploratory factor analysis, one study by Haque et al. found

TABLE 1: Selected indicator variables for validating active ageing determinant factors model in Thailand.

Variables	Coding
Age	1: 60–69 years; 2: 70–79 years; 3: 80+ years
Happiness level[a]	1: 1–6; 2: 7-8; 3: 9; 4: 10
Psychological distress status	1: very high; 2: high; 3: moderate; 4: poor or nearly never
Smoking	0: yes; 1: no
Drinking alcohol	0: yes; 1: no
Basic ADL (activities of daily living) index	0: severe; 1: moderately severe; 2: moderate; 3: independent
Subjective health	0: poor; 1: moderate; 2: good
Illness	0: two and/more chronic illnesses; 1: one chronic illness; 2: none
Visibility	0: no or not clear; 1: clear
Hearing	0: no or not clear; 1: clear
Education	0: no or less than primary; 1: primary; 2: secondary and/or higher
Community participation	0: no; 1: yes
Participation in elderly group	0: no; 1: yes
Work	0: no; 1: yes
Income[a]	1: no or <20000 Baht; 2: 20000–40000 Baht; 3: 40000–60000 Baht; 4: 60000+ Baht
Sufficiency of income	0: not sufficient; 1: sufficient
Savings	0: no; 1: yes

[a]Quartiles.

active ageing determinant factors models with six determinant factors for female and male older persons in Thailand [3]. But the study did not validate the models (i.e., how does the model fit with the sample data?). Along with the lack of model validation, the study by Haque et al. (or any other study so far in knowledge) did not compare AAL for culture of different regions in Thailand. Culture, defined as people's behavior, attitude, or way of life, varies depending on region of residence (e.g., urban or rural, different region of a country) of individuals. Therefore, people's behavior, attitude, or way of life depends on the place or region of society where the society is situated. Though Thailand is perceived as Southeast Asia's most ethnically homogeneous nation state and strong unity of Thai culture, Thailand government's use of regional terms (Central, North, Northeast, and South) indicates some regional cultural diversity in Thailand [7]. Despite the important strength and unity of Thai culture, each region in Thailand has its own unique cultural features [8]. So, doing research or formulating policies on active ageing in Thailand, the variations of active ageing depending on region of residence (Central, North, Northeast, and South) should be considered or should be borne in mind. Hence active ageing level should be compared in different regions of Thailand.

The objective of this study was to gain empirical knowledge on active ageing determinant factors model for Thai older persons including their active ageing level. The main specific objectives of this study are (i) to test the validity of active ageing determinant factors model for Thai older persons and (ii) to test the similarity of active ageing level for various regions (Bangkok, Central (excluding Bangkok), North, Northeast, and South) in Thailand.

2. Materials and Methods

2.1. Data. The data for this study come from a nationally representative sample from the 2011 Survey of Older Persons in Thailand (SOPT). The SOPT was conducted by Thailand's National Statistical Office (NSO). The sample of SOPT consists of 62,840 persons aged 50 years and over, 54% of whom were 60 years and older. The data have been collected in SOPT by using stratified two-stage sampling method. The primary sampling units were villages for nonmunicipal areas and blocks for municipal areas. The secondary sampling units were private dwellings selected by random sampling from the list of all enumerated households in each village or block of the first sampling units. The 2011 SOPT is a nationally representative survey which covers data for population subgroups or geographic subareas (e.g., regions and urban-rural areas). Further details of the methodology, including sampling strategy, for SOPT are available at NSO's "report on the 2011 Survey of Older Persons in Thailand" [9]. This study included individuals (same as in Haque et al. study [3]) aged 60 years and over (n = 23,801; female = 14,369 and male = 9,432).

2.2. Variables. For validating the active ageing determinant factors structure in Thailand (suggested by Haque et al.) [3], the variables used for this study in confirmatory factor analysis (CFA) are provided in Table 1.

2.3. Hypothesized Active Ageing Determinant Factors Model. The study by Haque et al., a pioneer study for finding a model for active ageing determinants, suggested two separate determinant factor structures for each gender [3]. Using the

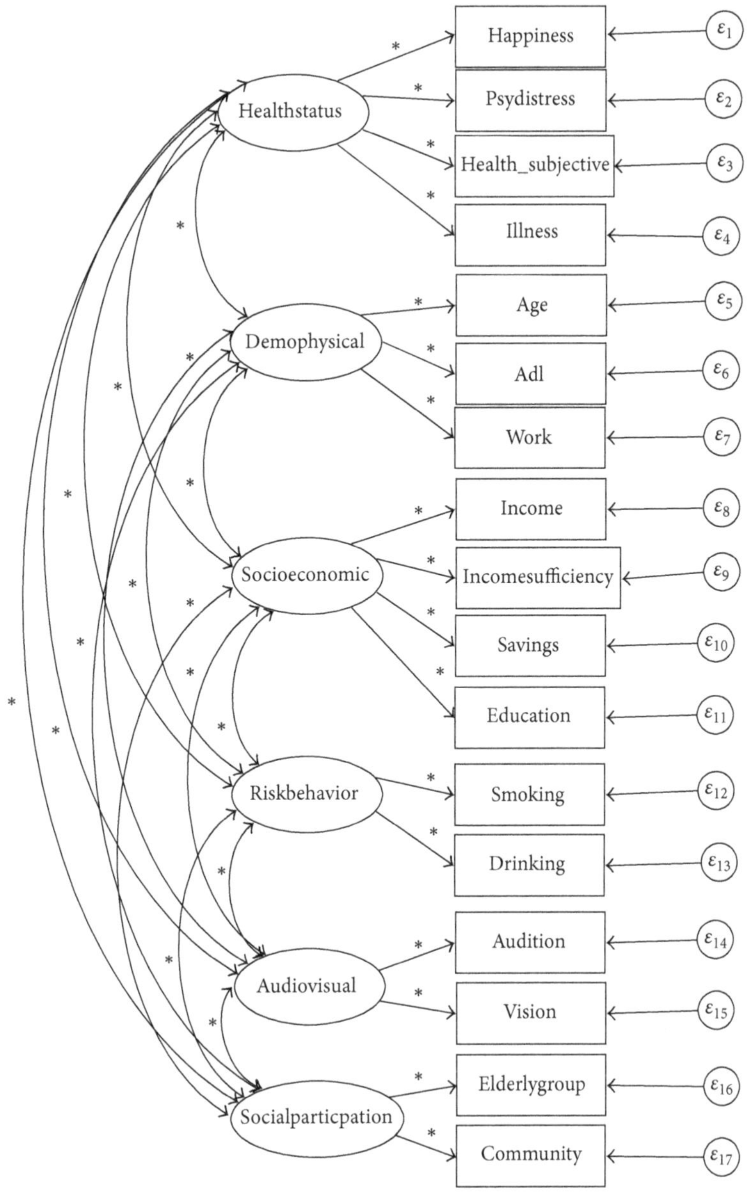

FIGURE 1: Hypothesized active ageing determinant factors model for female older persons in Thailand.

indicator variables, listed in Table 1, the suggested active ageing determinant factors models of female and male older persons [3] are provided in Figures 1 and 2, respectively.

2.4. Description of Hypothesized Models Presented in Diagrams. In the hypothesized models in Figures 1 and 2, the factors are represented in ovals and indicator variables are represented in rectangles. The error terms of indicator variables are indicated by ε. The asterisks indicate parameters (regression coefficient (standardized), covariances of independent variables in the model) to be estimated. Meanwhile, error terms in CFA are considered as independent variables and their variances should be estimated [10]. Unidirectional arrows in the hypothesized models indicate directional linear influences (i.e., linear effect of one variable on another), and both-way directional arrows indicate correlation between connected variables but no directional influence of one on others is hypothesized.

2.5. Model Evaluation. Parameters of each of the hypothesized models can be estimated in CFA framework which was done using STATA 12 (model fit statistics, in CFA, are available after estimation of parameters). Maximum likelihood (ML) estimation method is currently one of the most used methods for parameter estimation [10]. Details of parameter estimation procedure in CFA are available elsewhere [10–12]. As this paper has no aim to estimate the parameters of those models (but has aim to evaluate those models), the parameter estimation results are not shown. Any estimated model should be tested for how well the model fits

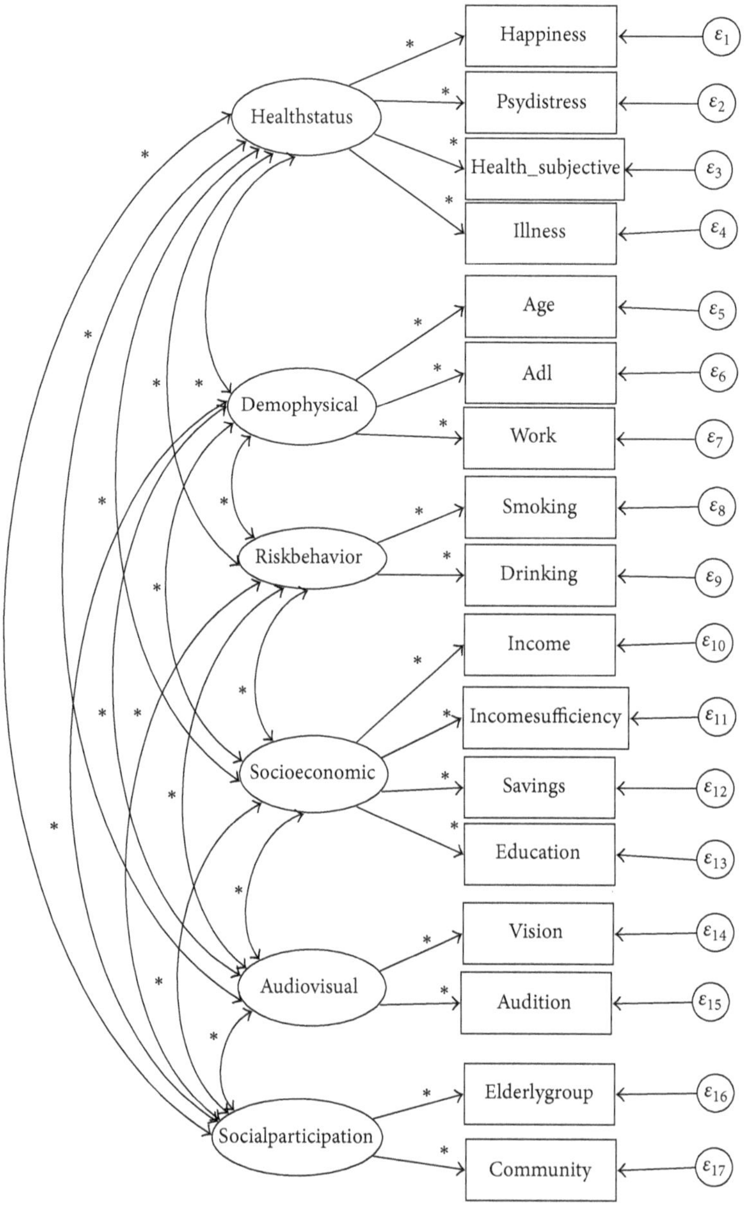

FIGURE 2: Hypothesized active ageing determinant factors model for male older persons in Thailand.

to the sample data. There are many fit indices for evaluating models in CFA framework. This study used Chi-square (χ^2), Root Mean Squared Error of Approximation (RMSEA), Comparative Fit Index (CFI), and Standardized Root Mean Squared Residual (SRMR). The χ^2 is a traditional measure of overall model fit (it assesses the magnitude of differences between sample and estimated covariance matrices) [13]. That is, the null hypothesis for model evaluation is as H_0: there is no difference between sample covariance and estimated covariance; that is, the model fits well to the data. The threshold values of the above fit statistics are provided in Table 2.

2.6. Estimation of Active Ageing Level. Active ageing level can be exhibited by computing the active ageing index (AAI) of older persons [3]. The AAI ranges from 0 to 1 and a higher value of AAI indicates higher active ageing level. The study by Haque et al. (2016) has suggested that AAI should be calculated separately for female and male older persons in Thailand. Using nationally representative sample and exploratory factor analysis (EFA), Haque et al. calculated the AA level for female and male older persons in Thailand [3]. The weakness of results from a model constructed from EFA is that there is no scope to test the model fit. Haque and colleagues study used only EFA and the model (from which AAI has been obtained) was not validated. For overcoming the weakness in EFA, this study used confirmatory factor analysis (CFA). The CFA framework facilitates testing how well the model fits to the sample data. The study by Haque and his colleagues used EFA in Thai national data for establishing

TABLE 2: Some selected model fit indices and their cut-off points (limits).

Fit index	Acceptable threshold levels
Chi-square (χ^2) (df, p value)	Low χ^2 relative to degrees of freedom (df) with an insignificant p value ($p > 0.05$)
Root Mean Squared Error of Approximation (RMSEA)	Values less than 0.07
Comparative Fit Index (CFI)	Closer to 1 is better but ≥0.90 indicates good fit
Standardized Root Mean Squared Residual (SRMR)	<0.05

the preliminary active ageing model of older persons and the study has identified six determinant factors for each gender [3]. Using the same factors (with their corresponding indicator variables) as in Haque et al.'s study, this study runs the model in CFA framework (in STATA 12) which provides the predicted factor scores of each factor. From the predicted factor score, the factor index for each factor has been estimated using the following formula:

Index of F_i:

$$f_i = \frac{[\text{Score of } F_i - \min(\text{Score of } F_i)]}{[\max(\text{Score of } F_i) - \min(\text{Score of } F_i)]}, \quad (1)$$

where F_i is the ith factor.

Score of F_i for every individual has been produced during CFA running in STATA. The theoretical maximum value of any factor index is 1. Then an AAI was calculated by using factor specific indices. Calculation of the AAI, from CFA, used the following formula:

$$\text{AAI} = \frac{\sum_{i=1}^{n=6} f_i}{6}, \quad (2)$$

where f_i is the index of factor i ($n = 6$, because there were 6 factors).

It should be noted here that the AAI has been calculated for every individual. Then an overall average AAI has been calculated using all values of AAI for all individuals. For simplicity, the AAI is a composite index which combines a number of factor indices.

2.7. Active Ageing Level Comparison Depending on Region of Residence. Because of social change over time and of cultural diversities in different places, possible changes may occur in individual AAL over time, as has occurred in other aspects of individual or population in Thailand; for example, between 1994 and 2007 Thailand experienced rapid social changes (population ageing, socioeconomic development, health policies, etc.) and these changes affect health across groups (rural-urban) and overall [15]. As has been stated in Introduction, there exists cultural variability in Thailand depending on region of residence (Bangkok, Central, North, Northeast, and South). It also may be hypothesized that under the circumstances of cultural diversities in different cultural settings, there would be variability of AA level in various cultural contexts, that is, in various regions within a country.

AA level quartiles would be the one method of comparing changes in the AAL at a community over time or for comparing it in different places or for groups. AA level quartiles can be calculated by ranking individuals from lowest AAI to the highest value and then dividing list into four groups or quartiles. Each quartile for individuals, in whole Thailand, for instance, contains 25% of individuals (along with specific mean level of AAI). Then we may compare those distributions of quartiles (percentage distribution) for individuals overall (national) with different places (e.g., Bangkok, Central, North, Northeast, and South). This quartile method of comparison will provide only the overview of difference(s) but is unable to test the significance of the differences. Similarity with significance of AA levels in different regions could be tested by using one-way analysis of variance (ANOVA). One-way ANOVA is appropriate for one categorical variable with k levels (e.g., region of residence with 5 levels in this study) or k groups and there should be a population of interest for which there is a quantitative variable for each of the k levels of the categorical variable (e.g., AAI in this study). The AAIs for each group have mean parameters (population means) that we may label as μ_1 through μ_k. The number of individuals (older persons) in group i ($1 \le i \le k$) is defined as n_i and $n = \sum_{i=1}^{k} n_i$ is the total sample size. The null hypothesis to be tested in one-way ANOVA states that all the population means are equal; that is, H_0: $\mu_1 = \mu_2 = \mu_3 = \mu_4 = \mu_5$ (for 5 regions of this study). The ANOVA technique can identify significant differences (if there were any) but is unable to specify where the significant differences exist. So, post hoc comparisons using a built-in test in STATA (e.g., Bonferroni test) were conducted.

3. Results and Discussion

3.1. Results

3.1.1. Model Fit Statistics. It has been stated, in Materials and Methods, that the model fit statistics can be obtained after the model estimation in CFA. The hypothesized models have been run in CFA in STATA 12 and the obtained model fit indices are summarized in Table 3.

The Chi-square (χ^2) statistics for two models are very high and indicated that none of the models fits well to the sample data. But the χ^2 statistic is very sensitive to sample size; usually for large sample (which is the case for two models) it shows significant result which rejects the null hypothesis (H_0: there is no difference between sample covariance and estimated covariance; i.e., the model fits well to the data). For correcting the sensitivity of χ^2 statistic to large sample (i.e., tendency to reject the null hypothesis), there are other test statistics which are most widely used (e.g., Root Mean Squared Error of Approximation (RMSEA),

Table 3: Goodness of model fit indices for confirmatory factor analysis for models of active ageing for older persons in Thailand.

Fit index	Female	Male
Chi-square (χ^2) (df, p value)	3548.33 (104, 0.00)	3131.96 (104, 0.00)
Root Mean Squared Error of Approximation (RMSEA)	0.048	0.056
Comparative Fit Index (CFI)	0.867	0.839
Standardized Root Mean Squared Residual (SRMR)	0.035	0.043

Table 4: Mean level of active ageing of older persons in Thailand.

	Mean of AAI	
	Female	Male
Lowest group	0.49	0.46
Medium lowest	0.61	0.58
Medium highest	0.69	0.66
Highest group	0.77	0.74
Overall mean AAI	0.64	0.61

$t = 21.554$, $p < 0.001$.

Comparative Fit Index (CFI), and Standardized Root Mean Squared Residual (SRMR)). However, comparing the estimated RMSEA, CFI, and SRMR fit indices presented in Table 3 with the threshold values of those indices presented in Table 2 suggests that both the estimated models seemed to fit well to the data. That is, active ageing determinant factors model for each gender can be adequately described by those six respective (to each model) correlated factors.

3.1.2. Active Ageing Level for Female and Male Older Persons. As, in the Haque et al. study, relationships of indicator variables with determinant factors of active ageing (factor structure of active ageing, i.e., the active ageing determinant factors model) are different for female and male older persons [3], separate active ageing index has been estimated for female and male older persons. The calculated mean AAIs for female and male older persons are 0.64 and 0.61, respectively. Comparing these mean AAIs with UNDP's Human Development Index (HDI), female and male older persons in Thailand had moderate level mean AAI [16].

Female and male older persons have been divided into four groups according to their mean AAI (i.e., they are divided according to quartiles of mean AAI); mean AAI for each group has been presented in Table 4.

An independent-samples t-test was run to determine if there were differences in mean AAI of female and male older persons. This study found that active ageing level of female is bit higher than active ageing level of male older persons. The calculated statistic, $t(23799) = 21.554$ with $p < 0.001$, indicates a statistical significant difference of two populations' mean level of active ageing (may reject the null hypothesis that there is no difference between the mean of AAI of female and male older population). It implies that mean active ageing levels of female older population and male older population, in Thailand, are significantly different.

3.1.3. Active Ageing Level Comparison Depending on Region of Residence. The calculated average active ageing levels of female and male older persons for every five regions (Bangkok, Central, North, Northeast, and South) have been portrayed in Figure 3. Region-wise mean active ageing level of older persons represented in Figure 3 shows the glimpse of situation only. But distribution of older persons according to AAI quartiles and region of residence enables showing the apparent disparities of AAL in different regions. Distribution of older persons according to AAI quartiles and region of residence is provided in Tables 5 and 7.

The results in Table 5 exhibited that highest proportion of female older persons in Bangkok was the lowest group of mean AAI whereas in North and Northeast region highest proportion was in medium highest group of mean AAI. The highest percentage of female older persons in South region was in highest group of mean AAI. Female older persons from the North and Northeast region had equal mean AAI and higher mean AAI than other regions. Comparing with UNDP's HDI, overall mean AAIs of female elderly in all five regions were in moderate level [16].

A one-way ANOVA between female elderly persons was conducted to compare the mean AAI for regions (Bangkok, Central, North, Northeast, and South). There was a significant difference of mean AAI at the $p < 0.001$ level for the five regions [$F(4, 14364) = 56.79$; $p = 0.00$]. The results of ANOVA found significant differences but could not specify where the significant differences exist. So, post hoc comparisons using Bonferroni test were conducted and the results are presented in Table 6.

Post hoc comparisons by Bonferroni test indicated that the mean AAI of female older persons is significantly lower in Bangkok than all other regions. Mean AAI of female older persons is significantly higher in Central region than Bangkok but the first two regions are lower than the other three regions (North, Northeast, and South). There is no significant difference in female elderly's mean AAI in North, Northeast, and South of Thailand.

The results in Table 7 revealed that highest proportion of male older persons in Bangkok and in Central region were in the lowest group of mean AAI whereas in North region highest proportion were in medium highest group of mean AAI. The highest percentage of male older persons in Northeast and in South region was in highest group of mean AAI. Overall, it can be mentioned from the sample results that male older persons from Northeast and South region had equal mean AAI and higher mean AAI than that of other regions. Comparing with UNDP's HDI, overall mean AAI male older persons in all five regions were in moderate level [16].

A one-way ANOVA between male elderly persons was conducted to compare the mean AAI for regions (Bangkok,

TABLE 5: Distribution of female older persons according to quartiles of mean active ageing level and region.

Region	Bangkok	Central*	North	Northeast	South	Total
Total cases	*652*	*4,706*	*3,560*	*3,496*	*1,955*	*14,369*
Lowest group	43.56	28.58	21.15	19.94	26.29	25.00
Medium lowest	30.98	25.18	24.02	25.69	23.12	25.00
Medium highest	09.05	22.16	29.80	28.86	21.48	25.00
Highest group	16.41	24.08	25.03	25.51	29.10	25.00
Overall mean AAI	0.59	0.63	0.65	0.65	0.64	0.64

*Excluding Bangkok, F-statistic = 56.59, $p < 0.001$.

TABLE 6: Comparison of mean AAI of female older persons by region (Bonferroni test).

Row mean-col. mean	Bangkok	Central	North	Northeast
Central	0.04 (0.00)			
North	0.06 (0.00)	0.02 (0.00)		
Northeast	0.06 (0.00)	0.02 (0.00)	0.00 (1.00)	
South	0.05 (0.00)	0.01 (0.001)	−0.01 (0.291)	−0.01 (0.044)

Note. Numbers within bracket indicate the level of significance (the test is considered significant at <0.01).

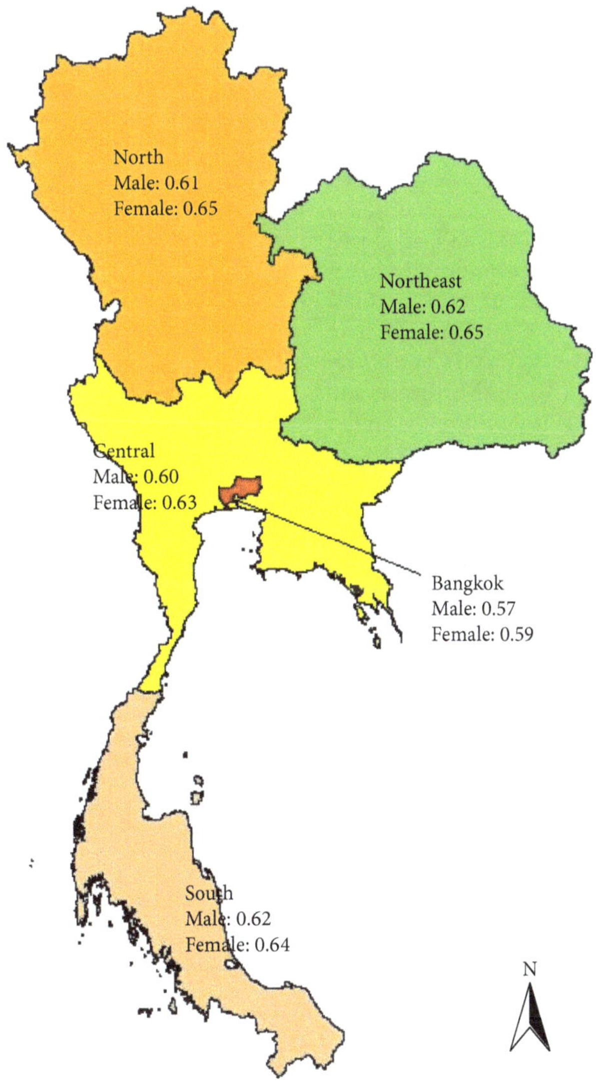

FIGURE 3: Map of Thailand with region-wise mean active ageing index value of female and male older persons.

TABLE 7: Distribution of male older persons according to quartiles of mean active ageing level and region.

Region	Bangkok	Central*	North	Northeast	South	Total
Total cases	*394*	*2,914*	*2,558*	*2,206*	*1,360*	*9,432*
Lowest group	40.10	29.72	22.91	19.63	23.16	25.00
Medium lowest	29.95	24.09	23.18	28.42	23.38	25.00
Medium highest	14.21	22.82	29.52	25.43	23.60	25.00
Highest group	15.74	23.37	24.39	26.52	29.85	25.00
Overall AAI	0.57	0.60	0.61	0.62	0.62	0.61

Note. F-statistic = 28.58; $p < 0.001$; *excluding Bangkok.

TABLE 8: Comparison of mean AAI of male elderly by region (Bonferroni).

Row mean-col. mean	Bangkok	Central	North	Northeast
Central	0.03 (0.00)			
North	0.04 (0.00)	0.01 (0.00)		
Northeast	0.05 (0.00)	0.02 (0.00)	0.01 (1.00)	
South	0.05 (0.00)	0.02 (0.00)	0.01 (1.00)	0.00 (1.00)

Note. Numbers within bracket indicate the level of significance (the test is considered significant at <0.01).

Central, North, Northeast, and South). There was a significant difference of mean AAI at the $p < 0.001$ level for the five regions [$F(4, 9427) = 28.58$; $p = 0.00$]. The results of ANOVA found significant differences but could not specify where the significant differences exist. So, post hoc comparisons using Bonferroni test were conducted and the results are presented in Table 8.

Post hoc comparisons by Bonferroni test indicated that the mean AAI of male older persons is significantly lower in Bangkok than all other regions. Mean AAI of male older persons is significantly higher in Central region than Bangkok but the first two regions (Bangkok and Central) are lower than the other three regions (North, Northeast, and South). Male older persons' mean AAI is significantly similar in North, Northeast, and South region.

3.2. Discussion. As it has been stated and also proved that active ageing determinant factors model varies for female and male older persons, their active ageing level also varies; for instance, results revealed that the overall mean AAI for female and male older persons was revealed as 0.64 and 0.61, respectively. These estimates proved the hypothesis regarding the one cross-cutting determinant, gender, (i.e., active ageing determinant factors model and active ageing level vary depending on gender in Thailand) as true. The numerical values of AAI for both female and male older persons must aim for further improvement. Because active ageing index shows that even top performing female older persons still fall short by almost 36% to the highest desired status possible (i.e., the goalpost of AAI is equal to 1).

If we look at region-wise active ageing level, then it is evident that active ageing level of older persons in Central region is comparatively lower than other regions. Results for comparing active ageing level in different regions revealed that there were disparities in mean AAI for female older population. Female older persons from Bangkok region had the lowest level of mean AAI among the five regions. Even though mean AAI of female older persons in the three regions (North, Northeast, and South) seemed significantly the same, female older persons in Central region had significantly lower mean AAI than the North, Northeast, and South region. On the other hand, as stated earlier that overall estimated mean AAI of male older persons is lower than female older persons, it also revealed from the results that the above is also true for every five regions. Also, the test results for regional differences for mean AAI of male older persons follow the same pattern as for female older persons.

As active ageing level in Thailand is not high (evidenced as far behind the goal), so, for promoting active ageing, focus should be given to the identified determinant factors of active ageing. As determinant factors are latent, hence focus should be given to their corresponding indicator variables (i.e., measured variables) aiming to promote active ageing. To make results more understandable, relation of directly measured variables with active ageing level should be interpreted which may be helpful for other researchers and policy makers. Using measured variables for each model, correlations between AAI and measured variables could be estimated. Correlation coefficient between measured variables and AAI for older persons has been calculated in the study by Haque et al. (2016). As data are the same for this study and Haque et al.'s study, so recommendations depending on the results regarding correlation coefficients (as in Haque et al.'s study) [3] could be appropriate for this study also. Haque et al.'s study urged that good health condition, opportunities of longer working lives, continuous income, participation in social group(s), and lifelong learning influence active ageing among the Thai older persons [3]. So, an Integrated Active Ageing Package (IAAP) would be helpful for increasing older persons' active ageing level. The IAAP should include policies for older persons to improve their health and economic security, to promote participation in social groups and longer working lives, and to arrange learning programs.

4. Conclusions

As active ageing level of older persons in Thailand is not high, so, some policy recommendations should be considered to increase the active ageing level of future older persons. The Thai government's national policy on the elderly (NPE) should include a new strategy on increasing active ageing level of elderly. Special emphasis should be given to Central region, as older persons in Central region are lower in respect to active ageing level compared to other regions. Policy should be focused for older persons on improving health and economic security, on promoting participation in social groups and longer working lives, and on arranging education (e.g., lifelong learning) programs for increasing their active ageing level. All the above policies should be integrated into one package as Integrated Active Ageing Package (IAAP). Along with the policy for extension of compulsory retirement age, incentives for elderly workers, and incentives for employers (who employed older persons), the IAAP should include some programs. The IAAP programs may include health programs—curative care for illness and continuous mental health care, easy access for assistive devices (e.g., walker/mover, eye glasses), and preventive and promotive health measures such as exercise and annual health checkup; community and elderly group participation programs; tobacco cessation counseling program; special knowledge and information for quality of life development program for elderly; and vocational training (including occupational retraining) program.

The proposed strategy, for NPE, on increasing active ageing level of older persons can be fulfilled by implementing the IAAP. The Ministry of Social Development and Human Security (MoSDHS), Thailand, may lead the implementation of IAAP. The MoSDHS may collaborate with the Ministry of Health and the Department of Non-Formal Education for full implementation of those programs. Implementation of IAAP would be helpful for increasing active ageing level of older persons which, in turn, is helpful for prolonging good health and independent living of older persons, that is, for increasing the quality of older persons' lives.

Competing Interests

The author declares that there are no competing interests regarding the publication of this paper.

Acknowledgments

The author expressed his deep sense of gratitude to his honorable Ph.D. principal advisor Dr. Kusol Soonthorndhada who died after seven days of the submission. Thanks are due to her for her contribution in looking through the draft of the paper.

References

[1] A. Walker, "A strategy for active ageing," *International Social Security Review*, vol. 55, no. 1, pp. 121–139, 2002.

[2] World Health Organization, Active ageing. A policy framework, a contribution of the World Health Organization (WHO) to the second United Nations World Assembly on Ageing, http://whqlibdoc.who.int/hq/2002/WHO_NMH_NPH_02.8.pdf.

[3] Md. N. Haque, K. Soonthorndhada, P. Hunchangsith, and M. Kanchanachitra, "Active ageing level in Thailand: a comparison between female and male elderly," *Journal of Health Research*, vol. 30, no. 2, pp. 99–107, 2016.

[4] United Nations, *World Population Aging and Development*, United Nations, New York, NY, USA, 2012.

[5] J. Knodel and N. Chayovan, "Older persons in Thailand: a demographic, social and economic profile," *Ageing International*, vol. 33, no. 1, pp. 3–14, 2008.

[6] J. Knodel, V. Prachuabmoh, and N. Chayovan, *The Changing Well-Being of Thai Elderly: An Update from the 2011 Survey of Older Persons in Thailand Populations Studies Center Research Report 13-793*, Institute for Social Research, University of Michigan, 2013.

[7] P. Jory, "Multiculturalism in Thailand: cultural and regional resurgence in a diverse kingdom," *Harvard Asia Pacific Review*, vol. 4, no. 1, pp. 18–22, 2000.

[8] Reach to Teach, Country Guides, Thailand Country Guide, Culture in Thailand, 2015.

[9] National Statistical Office (NSO), *Survey of Older Persons in Thailand, 2011*, National Statistical Office, Bangkok, Thailand, 2012 (Thai).

[10] J. B. Ullman, "Structural equation modeling: reviewing the basics and moving forward," *Journal of Personality Assessment*, vol. 87, no. 1, pp. 35–50, 2006.

[11] K. A. Bollen, *Structural Equations with Latent Variables*, John Wiley & Sons, New York, NY, USA, 1989.

[12] A. P. Field, *Discovering Statistics Using SPSS*, Sage, London, UK, 2nd edition, 2005.

[13] L.-T. Hu and P. M. Bentler, "Cutoff criteria for fit indexes in covariance structure analysis: conventional criteria versus new alternatives," *Structural Equation Modeling*, vol. 6, no. 1, pp. 1–55, 1999.

[14] D. Hopper, J. Coughlan, and M. R. Mullen, "Structural equation modeling: guidelines for determining model fit," *The Electronic Journal of Business Research Methods*, vol. 6, no. 1, pp. 53–60, 2008.

[15] Z. Zimmer and V. Prachuabmoh, "Comparing the socioeconomic status—health gradient among adults 50 and older across rural and urban areas of Thailand in 1994 and 2007," *Social Science and Medicine*, vol. 74, no. 12, pp. 1921–1928, 2012.

[16] United Nations Development Programme (UNDP), *Human Development Report 2014*, United Nations Development Programme (UNDP), New York, NY, USA, 2014.

19

Everyday Health among Older People: A Comparison between Two Countries with Variant Life Conditions

Cecilia Fagerström,[1,2] Lena Sandin Wranker,[3] Zarina Nahar Kabir,[4] and Ola Sternäng[5,6]

[1] *Blekinge Center of Competence, Karlskrona, Sweden*
[2] *Department of Health and Caring Sciences, Linnaeus University, 391 82 Kalmar, Sweden*
[3] *Department of Health Sciences, Division of Geriatric Medicine, Lund University, Lund, Sweden*
[4] *Division of Nursing, NVS, Karolinska Institute, Stockholm, Sweden*
[5] *Institute of Gerontology, School of Health and Welfare, Ageing Research Network-Jönköping (ARN-J), Jönköping University, Jönköping, Sweden*
[6] *Stockholm Centre for Health and Social Change (SCOHOST), Södertörn University, Huddinge, Sweden*

Correspondence should be addressed to Cecilia Fagerström; cecilia.fagerstrom@ltblekinge.se

Academic Editor: F. R. Ferraro

This study described health factors of importance for everyday health, such as pain, tiredness, and sleeping problems, in a cross-national context. Data for persons 60+ years were obtained from the Poverty and Health in Aging study, Bangladesh, and the Swedish National Study on Aging and Care-Blekinge. The strongest associations with everyday health in Sweden were found for pain and tiredness, while in Bangladesh they were financial status, tiredness, and sleeping problems. As similarities were found regarding the associations of tiredness on everyday health, tiredness may be a universal predictor of everyday health in older adults irrespective of country context.

1. Introduction

Health and health related quality of life (HRQoL) are concepts that are frequently used in research on older people (persons aged 60 years or more) to increase the understanding of their well-being, although the topics studied and the instruments used vary [1–3]. HRQoL instruments are often limited in their ability to perform contextual comparisons in nations where life circumstances differ, since they are mainly focused on individual's physical and mental health and less on the individual's life situation. An indicator of health that is suitable for most contexts would be valuable and useful. Such an indicator should reflect how older people perceive their current life situation and should be highly affected by their health [4]. Thus, in cross-national studies of high- and low-income nations, a composite variable of health in everyday life might provide an appropriate way of assessing the health situation in advanced age.

Our intention was to develop a short subjective assessment of health and life situation which could be used in countries that vary greatly in economic development. In order to identify common patterns, data were accessed from two population studies, one in Bangladesh and one in Sweden, to compare the results of two contrasting settings in which living conditions are highly different.

Focusing on health and ill health, rather than the diagnoses per se, is rational as older people feel more hindered by their symptoms than by their diseases [5]. Pain and sleeping problems are common symptoms in advanced age. However, although knowledge about pain in the aging population has improved during the last two decades [6, 7], little evidence has been published about how pain and sleeping problems affect an older person's perceptions of current life and whether this relationship differs between countries. Prevalence of sleeping problems and pain vary by disease, clinical setting, gender, age, and country of residence. Pain [8] and impaired sleep [9, 10] are both related to advanced age [8] and general health [8, 10].

Pain is an unpleasant sensory and/or emotional experience [11], but the factors underlying individual differences in pain response are not yet fully understood [12]. The prevalence of pain is however high among older persons, especially women [13, 14]. Normal aging does not necessarily influence perceived health in everyday life in a negative way [15]. The experience of pain is affected by biological, social, or cultural factors [16, 17]. From a contextual perspective, it is interesting to note that pain is more commonly reported and of a greater severity among Bangladeshis than Caucasians living in the United Kingdom [18]. However, the authors of the study did not find evidence of differences between ethnic groups in the impact of pain on perceived health.

Significant variations by ethnicity in sleep characteristics of older men have been observed [19]. Older people appear to have an increased risk of reporting both sleep complaints and low perceived health (low HRQoL), particularly if they live with a high degree of comorbidity [20]. Among older people in rural Bangladesh, the prevalence of multimorbidity is high (53.8%), especially among women [21]. Razzaque and his colleagues [22] investigated the health of older people in Bangladesh and found that individuals who suffered from illness and were in the greatest need of support were older, single women with low education levels and economically disadvantaged. These conditions can also be translated to the Swedish context. It can, therefore, be assumed that pain and insomnia are common conditions in both Bangladesh and Sweden and may be factors that influence everyday health.

Older people, especially in rural areas, are vulnerable in health status and access to health services (Elnitsky and Alexy, 2010). In different settings, the financial status influences the use of healthcare as well as the life situation. In Sweden, income differentials in healthcare-seeking behaviours that favour higher-income groups have been observed among men irrespective of age and among older women [23]. For instance, people with a higher income made almost 50% more healthcare visits than those with lower incomes [23]. Furthermore, perceived illness and financial access to health services are both factors that are known to contribute to accessing treatment in Bangladesh [24]. In summary, people in Bangladesh and Sweden, two countries that differ greatly in living conditions, may have different views of their health in everyday life. The aim of this study was to examine health factors of importance for everyday health in a cross-national context. The two factors comprising everyday health in this study, that is, people's life situation and perceived health, have previously been mentioned as components of self-reported good life in older people [25]. Associations between everyday health and pain, tiredness, and sleeping problems in persons 60 years and older in Bangladesh and Sweden were studied.

2. Methods

2.1. Sample. Data were collected from two population-based studies. The cross-sectional "Poverty and Health in Aging" (PHA) study was conducted in 2003, and the participants were aged 60 years and above and resided in a rural region, MATLAB, situated approximately 60 km southeast of the capital Dhaka in Bangladesh. The participants were randomly drawn from a demographic register and after they agreed to participate, they first completed a home interview and then had medical and cognitive examinations performed at a nearby health clinic. A total of 625 persons participated in home interviews. For information about dropouts, see Kabir et al. [26]. Approximately 60% of the participants were illiterate. Among the literate, the mean years of education were 4.8, SD 2.8. No one reported that they lived alone and half of the sample (56.7%) was married. Trained interviewers completed the questionnaires based on the responses from the participants.

The baseline sample of the longitudinal Swedish National Study on Aging and Care-Blekinge (SNAC-B) was collected from 2001 to 2003 and comprised 1,402 individuals aged 60 to 96 years. The study population consisted of randomly selected residents living in the Karlskrona municipality, which is situated in southeast Sweden (with approximately 60,600 inhabitants). The participants came from both urban and rural areas and lived both at home and in special housing. The response rate was 61%. Potential participants were sent a letter inviting them to participate in the study. Informed consent was obtained. The examination and testing by research personnel were conducted in two sessions, each lasting about two hours. Data were collected through medical examination, structured interviews, and questionnaires. Those who agreed to participate but were unable to travel to the research center were assessed in their homes. Approximately 70% had primary school education and the rest of the sample had education higher than primary school. Half of the sample was married and lived together with someone (54.5% and 51.6%, resp.). Further information about the protocols of the SNAC-B study can be found elsewhere [27].

In Sweden, 6% of the sample was estimated to have severe cognitive impairment (MMSE scale < 17) and 4% were diagnosed with dementia according to DSM IV in Bangladesh. For participants with cognitive impairment, questionnaires were completed by proxies in order to increase the reliability. Ethical approvals were obtained from the Regional Research Ethics Committees at the Karolinska Institute (Dnr 264/03), the Centre for Population and Health Research at the International Centre for Diarrhoeal Disease Research, Bangladesh (number 2003-025), and Lund University (Dnr LU 128-00, LU 604-00). For characteristics of the participants in the present study, see Table 1.

2.2. Measures. The variables were reviewed to ensure that the questions from the two databases (PHA and SNAC-B) were the same. Two other criteria taken into consideration were that the response options were adjusted to be equal and that the correlations between everyday health and the main variables were similar on an overall level in the two countries. The everyday health variable was constructed as the sum of the responses to two questions: "(A) How is your life situation?" with the response options of very poor (1), poor (2), rather good (3), or very good (4) and "(B) Compared to other people of your age, how do you feel your health is?" with not as good as others (1), as good as others (2), or better than others (3), as the possible responses.

The everyday health variable had six categories (2–7) ranging from a very poorly rated life situation and health (2) to a very highly rated life situation and health (7). The

Table 1: Description of the participants from the PHA (n = 625) and the SNAC-B (n = 1402) studies.

Variables	PHA	%	SNAC-B	%	p value
Age mean (SD)	69.6 (7.1)		76.7 (10.2)		<0.001
Women (n)	345	55	795	58	n.s.
Worried about money (n)	447	72	77	6	<0.001
Have not cash (n)	383	61	232	19	<0.001
Problems bending (n)	234	37	128	10	<0.001
Sometimes have pain (n)	246	39	800	66	
Often or always have pain (n)	252	40	69	6	<0.001
Feel tired (n)	196	31	158	13	<0.001
Problems sleeping (n)	175	28	376	30	n.s.
Life situation mean (SD)	2.9 (0.5)		3.2 (0.5)		<0.001
Health compared to others mean (SD)	1.8 (0.6)		2.4 (0.6)		<0.001
Everyday health mean (SD)	4.7 (0.9)		5.6 (0.8)		<0.001

Note. Differences between the two samples were tested for significance with t-tests (for means) or Chi square tests (for percentages). PHA = Poverty and Health in Aging in Bangladesh. SNAC-B = Swedish National Study on Aging and Care-Blekinge.

correlation between the two questions (A, B) was 0.33 ($p < 0.001$) in the PHA study and 0.19 ($p < 0.001$) in the SNAC-B study.

2.2.1. Age and Gender. Age and gender were included as demographic variables. In Bangladesh, birth certificates did not exist for all in the age group in the study; in such cases, age was determined based on relevant biological and historical events in the person's life. This method of determining age in low-income countries is well established [28, 29].

2.2.2. Worried about Money. This variable was based on the question "Are you worried about having enough money for the household?" with the alternatives yes (1) and no (2).

2.2.3. Have Cash. This variable was related to the participant's financial situation and was based on the question "Do you always have some cash?" The response options for this variable were no (1) and yes (2).

2.2.4. Problem in Bending. This was assessed with the question "Do you have any problem bending forward?" with the two alternatives yes (1) and no (2).

2.2.5. Pain. The question "Do you suffer from bodily pain?" was asked with three options: yes (1), sometimes (2), and no (3).

2.2.6. Feel Tired. Tiredness was based on the question "Do you usually feel tired?" with the response alternatives yes (1) and no (2).

2.2.7. Problem Sleeping. The question "Do you have trouble sleeping?" was used. This question had two response options: yes (1) and no (2).

2.3. Statistical Analysis. The analyses were conducted in SPSS version 22 (SPSS Inc., Chicago, IL, USA). Alpha levels were set at 0.05. Age, gender and financial situation, tiredness, problem sleeping, pain, and the outcome variable of everyday health were presented with their descriptive statistics for each country (see Table 1). Spearman's rho (r_s) was used to calculate the correlations between the independent variables and everyday health. A hierarchical regression model was performed on the total sample (see Table 2). In the first step, the background variables of age, gender, worrying about money, and having no cash were entered into the model as control. In the second step, the potential predictors of problem bending, pain, feeling tired, and problem sleeping were included. In the third step, the country variable was entered, and finally, interactions between country and each of the independent variables were entered. Everyday health was the outcome variable. Regression models were also performed separately for the two countries.

3. Results

The total sample included 2,027 participants; 1,402 (69%) were drawn from the Swedish study SNAC-B. Participants from Bangladesh were younger, had less financial resources, felt more frequently tired, and experienced pain and mobility problems more often (p values < 0.001). Approximately 70% of the sample in Bangladesh stated that that they did not have enough money. The corresponding proportion in Sweden was 6%.

The distribution of the everyday health variable is presented in Figure 1. Approximately 40% of the sample reported that they had good everyday health (score 5), and one-tenth rated their everyday health as very good (score 7). Higher percentages of older persons in Sweden reported better everyday health compared to their counterparts in Bangladesh. In the total sample, the relationships between everyday health and life situation, everyday health and health compared to others, and life situation and health compared to others were r_s = .875, r_s = .740, and r_s = .315, respectively. When the country samples were separated, the significant relationships between the variables remained, but

TABLE 2: Everyday health and its associations with the background and predictor variables in the total sample.

	β	p value	Cumulated R^2
Step 1			0.23
Age	.066	0.003	
Gender (reference: women)	−.078	<0.001	
Worried about money	−.349	<0.001	
Having no cash	−.162	<0.001	
Step 2			0.31
Problems bending	−.063	0.012	
Pain	−.198	<0.001	
Feeling tired	−.111	<0.001	
Problems sleeping	−.069	0.001	
Step 3			0.32
Country	.208	<0.001	
Step 4			0.35
Age × country	.008	0.711	
Gender × country	−.029	0.175	
Worried about money × country	−.048	0.159	
Having no cash × country	−.102	<0.001	
Problems bending × country	−.009	0.759	
Pain × country	−.149	<0.001	
Feeling tired × country	−.022	0.390	
Problems sleeping × country	−.037	0.083	

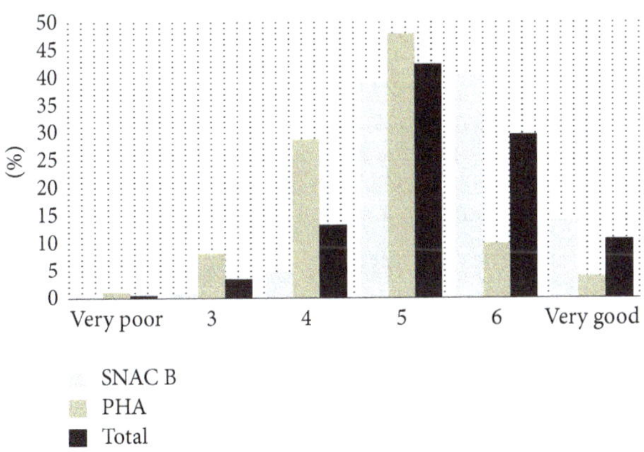

FIGURE 1: The distribution of the everyday health variable. Note: the everyday health variable was constructed as the sum of two questions: "How is your life situation?" (with the response alternatives very poor to very good (1–4)) and "Compared to other people your age, how do you feel your health is?" (with not as good as others, as good as others, or better than others as the possible responses (1–3)). The resulting variable "everyday health" had six categories (2–7) ranging from a very poorly rated life situation and health (2; very poor) to a very highly rated life situation and health (7; very good). PHA = Poverty and Health in Aging in Bangladesh, SNAC-B = Swedish National Study on Aging and Care-Blekinge.

the relationships were found to be slightly weaker in the Swedish sample.

3.1. Associations of Everyday Health with Pain and Sleeping Problems in the Total Sample. A hierarchical model was first performed for the total sample to examine the predictors of everyday health. After controlling for age, gender, and financial situation, the variables entered in step 2 (problem bending, pain, feeling tired, and problem sleeping) increased the explained variance (R^2) in everyday health by .08 (from .23 to .31) (see Table 2). Entered variables in steps one and two were significant. When the country of residence was included in the model (step 3), R^2 increased only slightly. In the last step (step 4), the eight two-way interactions between country of residence and each independent variable increased the explained variance by .03 to a total R^2 = .35. Two significant interaction effects were detected: pain × country (β = −.149) and having no cash × country (β = −.102). Age, gender, worrying about money, pain, feeling tired, problems sleeping, and country of residence remained significant in the final model.

3.2. Associations of Everyday Health with Pain and Sleeping Problems by Country of Residence. The data was also analysed through a hierarchical regression model for each country to establish whether there were any country-specific predictors of everyday health. This model consisted of two steps (see Table 3). In the first step, gender was significant in SNAC-B (β = −0.071), and gender (β = −0.123), worrying about money (β = −0.221), and having no cash (β = −0.227) were significant in PHA. The second step, in which the predictive variables were included, increased the explained variance (R^2) in everyday health by .11 for participants in SNAC-B and by .07 for participants in PHA. After controlling for background variables in SNAC-B, pain (β = −.306) and feeling tired (β = −.076) were significant predictors of

TABLE 3: Everyday health and its association with the background and predictor variables in the two samples from Sweden and Bangladesh.

	SNAC-B (n = 1,402)			PHA (n = 625)		
	β	p value	Cumulated R^2	β	p value	Cumulated R^2
Step 1			.01			.15
Age	.052	0.103		.017	0.651	
Gender (women reference)	−.071	0.026		−.123	0.002	
Worried about money	−.056	0.089		−.221	<0.001	
Having no cash	−.012	0.709		−.227	<0.001	
Step 2			.12			.22
Problems bending	−.032	0.302		−.080	0.068	
Pain	−.306	<0.001		−.047	0.268	
Feeling tired	−.076	0.014		−.155	<0.001	
Problems sleeping	−.054	0.086		−.127	0.001	

Note. Hierarchical regression on data from the two databases SNAC and PHA. PHA = Poverty and Health in Aging in Bangladesh; SNAC-B = Swedish National Study on Aging and Care-Blekinge.

everyday health. Corresponding figures in PHA were feeling tired (β = −.155) and problem sleeping (β = −.127).

4. Discussion

A composite variable of health and life situation that generates a subjective assessment of everyday health may provide us with new knowledge. This study of older people is the first to include the concept of everyday health. We assessed everyday health of older people's perceptions of their health compared with peers in a high- and in a low-income country. The purpose of the study was to examine the associations between everyday health and potential predictor variables such as pain, tiredness, and sleeping problems as well as any country-specific association between these variables. Low perceived everyday health was reported most commonly by women. The results indicated that older people's perceptions of everyday health can be explained by pain, sleeping problems, and the sociodemographic variables assessed in this study. Health problems and sociodemographic variables explained 35% of the variance in everyday health, but country-specific patterns still existed.

The concept of everyday health is focused on a person's present situation and reflects how older people perceive their current health and life. The present study confirmed that health issues are central but do not equate to people's perception of their life situation. This distinction justifies our choice to combine the two measures of HRQoL into a composite variable.

The differences between the two countries in this study were that pain and tiredness had the greatest impact on everyday health in Sweden, while financial status, tiredness, and sleeping problems had the highest impact on everyday health of older people in Bangladesh. A notable finding was that pain was associated with everyday health in Sweden only and was the main factor affecting their everyday health. Those with pain had a considerably higher probability of impaired everyday health compared to their counterparts with no pain. This pattern is consistent with a recent study of the same sample from SNAC-B, in which pain was found to be strongly associated with low HRQoL [30]. However, in that study, this relationship was significant only in women. Similarly, Hawkins and colleagues [31] found that pain was strongly associated with low HRQoL among older adults after controlling for demographic, socioeconomic, and health status characteristics. In the present study, pain was not a predictor of everyday health in Bangladesh despite the fact that pain was reported more often than in Sweden. One possible explanation could be that financial survival in a low-income country such as Bangladesh may be overriding physical problems, whereas in a high-income country such as Sweden where financial worries are not predominant, the focus is on physical discomfort. It is notable that pain treatment has a low priority among Bangladeshis [cf. [32]], whereas people in Sweden may assume that pain treatment, or at least pain relief, is included in the standard treatment.

As similarities between the two countries were found regarding the effects of tiredness on perceptions of everyday health, tiredness may be considered as a universal factor of everyday health irrespective of country context. However, significant between-country differences were also found. Having sleeping problems influenced a person's everyday health only in Bangladesh, and feeling tired influenced everyday health in both countries. Impaired sleep was commonly reported in both countries, which is supported by other studies on older adults [9, 10]. In old age, sleep is often experienced as normal by an older person even if the sleep is impaired. For instance, it has been stressed that while their sleeping patterns could be irregular [33], older people tend to adapt to age to variations in their sleeping patterns. However, as sleeping problems are associated with everyday health and are commonly reported in the population, irrespective of country, this needs to be considered further.

In the analyses, country-specific factors on everyday health were identified. The differences in results may be dependent on the sociocultural factors in the investigated country. For example, financial status may universally influence the perceptions of everyday health, but its meaning differs between high- and low-income contexts. Financial situation significantly affected older people's everyday health in Bangladesh but not in the Swedish population. Also, Diener [34] stressed that the factors influencing people's perception of HRQoL may vary in different societies. However, these results require further attention as the majority of the population in Bangladesh reported a poor financial situation compared with approximately only 6% of the population in Sweden. It could be assumed that this difference between the two countries depends on the infrastructure of the societies, for example, each country's pension system, which may in turn influence the residents' perceptions of their current life situation more than their health conditions. The differences may also be explained by other sociodemographic characteristics, such as marital status, income, and leisure activities, which have a significant impact on older people's life situations [22, 35]. Finally, in-country geographical area may also play a role in the proportion of people in poor financial situations, as the sample in Bangladesh lived in a rural area, whereas the Swedish sample lived in both urban and rural areas.

While sleeping problems and pain [36] as well as economic situation [37] were expected to be closely associated with each other, it is still not clear whether these findings indicate that the symptoms are equally prominent in different countries. Having a low perceived everyday health was most commonly reported among women. As older women in general have fewer material resources than men [38], it can be assumed that it is not being a woman that influences everyday health but rather the financial situations of women compared with men. In future studies, it would be useful to investigate health problems with a particular focus on different types of pain and sleep problems and, if possible, how poor financial situations influence everyday health among older persons.

The collection of data in different contexts increases the risk of bias [39], but the benefits may exceed the disadvantages. For example, the same question might not necessarily have the same meaning in different cultures [40]. The outcome variable everyday health was based on three criteria (see Methods) to minimize this cultural difference. The benefit is the validation of results when data are collected in a similar way in different contexts and a similar phenomenon is described; this increases the opportunity to generalise results [41]. More information related to the participants' everyday health, for instance, sociodemographic factors, mood and depression symptoms, morbidity pattern, and healthcare utilization, may be important to include to verify subjective health information and to describe country-wise differences. Not including such additional health data can be seen as a limitation of the study, but no such comparative data were available in the two data bases. Although much of this type of information exists in the two databases, these variables were measured differently in the two countries. Since the focus of the present study was on comparisons between the two samples in Sweden and Bangladesh, we refrained from including these variables in the analyses. Furthermore, to control for unique and country-specific variations in background variables, the final models were constructed separately for each country in addition to the combined model. Anyhow, the results must be carefully interpreted. Further analyses are of interest to gain a deeper understanding of the relationship between everyday health and the commonly used HRQoL as well as QoL.

5. Conclusions

We suggest that the everyday health variable can be applied in countries that vary greatly in economic development as a subjective assessment of a person's health and life conditions. There were similarities between the countries regarding the factors associated with everyday health. The difference between the two countries was that pain and tiredness had the greatest impact on everyday health in Sweden, whilst financial status, tiredness, and sleeping problems had the highest impact in Bangladesh. The results of the study can help community health providers and administrators strategically plan to meet older people with health problems at risk for decreased everyday health and to meet their healthcare needs in different country contexts.

Conflicts of Interest

The authors declare that there are no conflicts of interest regarding the publication of this paper.

Acknowledgments

The Swedish National Study on Aging and Care, SNAC (https://www.snac.org), is financially supported by the Ministry of Health and Social Affairs, Sweden, and the participating county councils, municipalities, and university departments. The Poverty and Health in Ageing (PHA) was funded by Department for International Development (DfID), UK and Swedish Agency for Research Cooperation/Swedish International Development Agency, and the Swedish Research Council. We acknowledge Professor Åke Wahlin, Jönköping University, for constructive feedback on the manuscript. The authors also acknowledge the participants, the participating counties, and municipalities in the SNAC project and PHA project.

References

[1] Y. Yamada, L. Merz, and H. Kisvetrova, "Quality of life and comorbidity among older home care clients: role of positive attitudes toward aging," *Quality of Life Research*, vol. 24, no. 7, pp. 1661–1667, 2014.

[2] J. Halpern, M. Cohen, G. Kennedy, J. Reece, C. Cahan, and A. Baharav, "Yoga for improving sleep quality and quality of life for older adults," *Alternative Therapies in Health and Medicine*, vol. 20, no. 3, pp. 37–46, 2014.

[3] C. Fagerström and G. Borglin, "Mobility, functional ability and health-related quality of life among people of 60 years or older," *Aging Clinical and Experimental Research*, vol. 22, no. 5-6, pp. 387–394, 2010.

[4] J. P. Serrano, J. M. Latorre, and M. Gatz, "Spain: Promoting the welfare of older adults in the context of population aging," *Gerontologist*, vol. 54, no. 5, pp. 733–740, 2014.

[5] C. Fagerström, G. Holst, and I. R. Hallberg, "Feeling hindered by health problems and functional capacity at 60 years and

above," *Archives of Gerontology and Geriatrics*, vol. 44, no. 2, pp. 181–201, 2007.

[6] K. Herr, M. G. Titler, M. L. Schilling et al., "Evidence-based assessment of acute pain in older adults: Current nursing practices and perceived barriers," *Clinical Journal of Pain*, vol. 20, no. 5, pp. 331–340, 2004.

[7] A. L. Van Ojik, P. A. Jansen, J. R. Brouwers, and E. N. Van Roon, "Treatment of chronic pain in older people: Evidence-based choice of strong-acting opioids," *Drugs and Aging*, vol. 29, no. 8, pp. 615–625, 2012.

[8] C. Luthy, C. Cedraschi, A.-F. Allaz, F. R. Herrmann, and C. Ludwig, "Health status and quality of life: results from a national survey in a community-dwelling sample of elderly people," *Quality of Life Research*, vol. 24, no. 7, pp. 1687–1696, 2014.

[9] S. Ancoli-Israel, "Insomnia in the elderly: a review for the primary care practitioner," *Sleep*, vol. 23, no. 1, pp. 23–30, 2000.

[10] J. R. Cooke and S. Ancoli-Israel, "Normal and abnormal sleep in the elderly," *Handbook of Clinical Neurology*, vol. 98, no. C, pp. 653–665, 2011.

[11] H. Merskey and N. Bogduk, "Classification of Chronic Pain," in *IASP Task force on Taxonomy. Part III: Pain Terms, A current list with definitions and notes on usage*, pp. 209–214, IASP Press, Seattle, 1994.

[12] M. S. Angst, N. G. Phillips, D. R. Drover et al., "Pain sensitivity and opioid analgesia: A pharmacogenomic twin study," *Pain*, vol. 153, no. 7, pp. 1397–1409, 2012.

[13] A. Tsang, M. Von Korff, S. Lee et al., "Common chronic pain conditions in developed and developing countries: gender and age differences and comorbidity with depression-anxiety disorders," *Journal of Pain*, vol. 9, no. 10, pp. 883–891, 2008.

[14] E. Webb, D. Blane, A. McMunn, and G. Netuveli, "Proximal predictors of change in quality of life at older ages," *Journal of Epidemiology and Community Health*, vol. 65, no. 6, pp. 542–547, 2011.

[15] G. Netuveli and D. Blane, "Quality of life in older ages," *British Medical Bulletin*, vol. 85, no. 1, pp. 113–126, 2008.

[16] I. N. Ackerman, K. L. Bennell, and R. H. Osborne, "Decline in Health-Related Quality of Life reported by more than half of those waiting for joint replacement surgery: A prospective cohort study," *BMC Musculoskeletal Disorders*, vol. 12, article no. 108, 2011.

[17] C. Bilotta, A. Bowling, P. Nicolini, A. Casè, and C. Vergani, "Quality of life in older outpatients living alone in the community in Italy," *Health and Social Care in the Community*, vol. 20, no. 1, pp. 32–41, 2012.

[18] Y. Choudhury, S. A. Bremner, A. Ali et al., "Prevalence and impact of chronic widespread pain in the Bangladeshi and White populations of Tower Hamlets, East London," *Clinical Rheumatology*, vol. 32, no. 9, pp. 1375–1382, 2013.

[19] Y. Song, S. Ancoli-Israel, C. E. Lewis, S. Redline, S. L. Harrison, and K. L. Stone, "The association of race/ethnicity with objectively measured sleep characteristics in older men," *Behavioral Sleep Medicine*, vol. 10, no. 1, pp. 54–69, 2011.

[20] C. Fagerström and A. Hellström, "Sleep complaints and their association with comorbidity and health-related quality of life in an older population in Sweden," *Aging and Mental Health*, vol. 15, no. 2, pp. 204–213, 2011.

[21] M. A. Khanam, P. K. Streatfield, Z. N. Kabir, C. Qiu, C. Cornelius, and Å. Wahlin, "Prevalence and patterns of multimorbidity among elderly people in rural Bangladesh: a cross-sectional study," *Journal of Health, Population and Nutrition*, vol. 29, no. 4, pp. 406–414, 2011.

[22] A. Razzaque, L. Nahar, M. Akter Khanam, and P. Kim Streatfield, "Socio-demographic differentials of adult health indicators in Matlab, Bangladesh: self-rated health, health state, quality of life and disability level," *Global Health Action*, vol. 3, no. 1, p. 4618, 2010.

[23] J. Agerholm, D. Bruce, B. BurstrÃm, and A. Ponce Leon, "Socioeconomic differences in healthcare utilization, with and without adjustment for need: An example from Stockholm, Sweden," *Scandinavian Journal of Public Health*, vol. 41, no. 3, pp. 318–325, 2013.

[24] J. Uddin, M. Hossin, F. Mahbub, and M. Hossain, "Healthcare-seeking behavior among the chakma ethnic group in bangladesh: Can accessibility and cultural beliefs shape healthcare utilization?" *International Quarterly of Community Health Education*, vol. 33, no. 4, pp. 375–389, 2012.

[25] S. Lyubomirsky and H. S. Lepper, "A measure of subjective happiness: preliminary reliability and construct validation," *Social Indicators Research*, vol. 46, no. 2, pp. 137–155, 1999.

[26] Z. N. Kabir, T. Ferdous, T. Cederholm, M. A. Khanam, K. Streatfied, and Å. Wahlin, "Mini nutritional assessment of rural elderly people in Bangladesh: The impact of demographic, socio-economic and health factors," *Public Health Nutrition*, vol. 9, no. 8, pp. 968–974, 2006.

[27] M. Lagergren, B.-M. Sjölund, C. Fagerström et al., "Horizontal and vertical target efficiency - A comparison between users and non-users of public long-term care in Sweden," *Ageing and Society*, vol. 34, no. 4, pp. 700–719, 2014.

[28] T. J. Allain, A. O. Wilson, Z. A. R. Gomo et al., "Morbidity and disability in elderly Zimbabweans," *Age and Ageing*, vol. 26, no. 2, pp. 115–121, 1997.

[29] O. Sternäng, Z. N. Kabir, J. D. Hamadani, and Å. Wahlin, "A cross-cultural perspective on aging and memory: Comparisons between Bangladesh and Sweden," *PsyCh Journal*, vol. 1, no. 2, pp. 69–81, 2012.

[30] L. S. Wranker, M. Rennemark, J. Berglund, and S. Elmståhl, "Relationship between pain and Quality of Life-Findings from the Swedish National Study on Aging and Care-Blekinge study," *Scandinavian Journal of Pain*, vol. 5, no. 4, pp. 270–275, 2014.

[31] K. Hawkins, S. Musich, F. G. Bottone Jr. et al., "The impact of pain on physical and mantal quality of life in adults 65 and older," *Journal of Gerontological Nursing*, vol. 39, no. 6, pp. 32–44, 2013.

[32] R. Vijayan, "Managing acute pain in the developing world," *Pain. Clinical updates*, vol. 3, 2011.

[33] S. C. Bolge, J. F. Doan, H. Kannan, and R. W. Baran, "Association of insomnia with quality of life, work productivity, and activity impairment," *Quality of Life Research*, vol. 18, no. 4, pp. 415–422, 2009.

[34] E. Diener, "Subjective well-being: the science of happiness and a proposal for a national index," *American Psychologist*, vol. 55, no. 1, pp. 34–43, 2000.

[35] T. da Silva Alexandre, R. C. Cordeiro, and L. R. Ramos, "Factors associated to quality of life in active elderly," *Revista de Saude Publica*, vol. 43, no. 4, pp. 613–621, 2009.

[36] J. McBeth, R. Wilkie, J. Bedson, C. Chew-Graham, and R. J. Lacey, "Sleep Disturbance and Chronic Widespread Pain," *Current Rheumatology Reports*, vol. 17, no. 1, 2015.

[37] M. A. Grandner, N. P. Patel, P. R. Gehrman et al., "Who gets the best sleep? Ethnic and socioeconomic factors related to sleep complaints," *Sleep Medicine*, vol. 11, no. 5, pp. 470–478, 2010.

[38] V. Burholt and G. Windle, *The material resources and well-being of older people*, vol. 54, University of Wales Bangor, 2006.

[39] F. van de Vijver and K. Leung, *Methods and Data Analysis for Cross-Cultural Research*, Sage Publications, Thousand Oaks, 1997.

[40] M. Bullinger, R. Anderson, D. Cella, and N. Aaronson, "Developing and evaluating cross-cultural instruments from minimum requirements to optimal models," *Quality of Life Research*, vol. 2, no. 6, pp. 451–459, 1993.

[41] J. Vitterso, E. Roysamb, and E. Diener, "The concept of life satisfaction across cultures: exploring its diverse meaning and relation to economic wealth," in *The Universality of subjective wellbeing indicators a multi-disciplinary and multi-national perspective (Volume 16)*, E. Gullone and R. A. Cummins, Eds., pp. 81–103, Kluwer Academic Publishers, Dordrecht, 2002.

20

Risk Factors for Six Types of Disability among the Older People in Thailand in 2002, 2007, and 2011

Pattaraporn Khongboon,[1,2] Sathirakorn Pongpanich,[1] and Robert S. Chapman[1]

[1] *College of Public Health Sciences, Chulalongkorn University, Pathumwan, Bangkok 10330, Thailand*
[2] *Prince Mahidol Award Foundation under the Royal Patronage, Faculty of Medicine, Siriraj Hospital, Bangkoknoi, Bangkok 10700, Thailand*

Correspondence should be addressed to Sathirakorn Pongpanich; sathirakorn.p@chula.ac.th

Academic Editor: Arshad Jahangir

Background. There is an important need to characterize risk factors for disability in Thailand, in order to inform effective prevention and control strategies. This study investigated factors associated with risk of 6 types of disability in Thailand's ageing population in 2002, 2007, and 2011. *Methods.* Data came from the Cross-Sectional National Surveys of Older Persons in Thailand conducted by the National Statistical Office (NSO) in 2002, 2007, and 2011. Stratified two-stage sampling was employed. Interviews of 24,835, 30,427, and 34,173 elderly people aged 60 and above were conducted in the respective study years. Prevalence of disabilities was measured, and factors associated with disability risk were assessed with probability-weighted multiple logistic regression. *Results.* Disability prevalence decreased slightly over the study period. The characteristics with greatest positive impact on disability prevalence were not working over the past week (average impact: 61.2%), age (53.7% per decade), and suffering from one or more chronic illnesses (46.3%). *Conclusions.* The strong observed positive impact of not working on disability prevalence suggests that raising the mandatory retirement age might result in some reduction of disability risk. Also, the observed positive impact of living with others (versus alone) on disability risk was somewhat unexpected.

1. Introduction

The population of old people is rising exponentially in Thailand. According to The Foundation of Thai Gerontology Research and Development Institute, TGRI (2013) [1], the country has the second highest population of elderly folk in southeast Asia. The aged population includes persons who have lived for 60 years or more. It is projected that the aged population in Thailand will significantly rise to approximately 22 million by 2040. In 25 years, 33.5% of the entire Thailand population will be old people. People in this age group usually have the highest rate of disability and are often the most dependent.

In spite of the efforts made by the Thai government to enhance the quality of healthcare services for the older population, the prevalence of disparate access to services, inadequate quantity of healthcare resources (such as equipment, personnel, and finance), and lack of interinstitutional and intrainstitutional coordination among healthcare institutions still persists. In a bid to counter these problems, the Thai government commissioned a working group to make changes to the country's National Plan on Older Persons in 2009. The working group drew inspiration from the findings of an evaluation of this plan that had been previously conducted and recommended for the establishment of community-based long-term care institutions for the elderly. These institutions would offer medical and social care for the elderly in the comfort of their homes.

In the past, ADL scale was basically constructed for individuals suffering from stroke and has two items pertaining to climbing stairs and continence. A combination scale that assesses ADL, social involvement, and communication is known as the functional independence measure. An earlier step in disability intensity may be recognized as a limitation in instrumental activities of daily living (IADL). Such activities essentially involve cognitive functions and other basic actions such as shopping, telephoning, shifting from one place to another, and dealing with medicines and funds.

These days ADL and IADL are often used for measuring health in both clinical studies and community-based surveys of older group [2, 3]. The calculations regarding IADLs are asymmetrical across diverse cultures, even if the evaluations of ADLs have been normally regular among various countries and in varying time frame. All of those activities that are auxiliary in everyday life are different for every country as seen in the national surveys, due to cultural, geographical, and temporal deviations [4–8].

So, the Barthel Index has been modified for assessment of activity in daily living in Thai older people [9]. This ADL instrument comprises eating, grooming, transferring in house, toileting, walking, climbing stairs, dressing, bathing, control of urination, and control of defecation. In addition, Chula ADL Index (CAI) has been modified for assessment of instrumental activity in daily living, which includes walking outdoors, cleaning house, public transportation, cooking, and money exchange [9].

Also, the documents that reported the prevalence of disability in Thailand are rare. A study conducted by village health communicators in 1989 in a rural northern Thai community found that the overall prevalence rate of the disabled aged population was 6.3/1000 [10]. A study conducted in 1997 reported that 19% of participants aged 60 years and over have a long-term disability [11]. Later, the study in 2001 found that the prevalence rates of disability in females were higher than that of males among the elderly living in Central region [12].

With respect to international comparison, the occurrence of the ADL disability in a population aged 60 years and above was as much as 25.7% in Lebanon [13]. However, more recent studies carried out after 2008 showed that the ADL disability is not as widely prevalent, with a population comprising 65-year-old and older population in China showing a prevalence of around 14.9% [14], whereas in the United States it was about 18.4% [15].

Much effort has been invested in identifying the risk factors associated with how disability sets in, and the corresponding model proposed by Nagi (1976) [16] is a major source of input in this regard, constituting components related to pathology, functional impairments, functional limitations, and disability. Beyond any doubt factors like age and gender are linked with the functional limitation and complexity with ADLs and IADLs. People who are over 70 years of age are more prone to these problems in contrast to the individuals in their 60s [17]. Moreover, it was clearly expressed that females tend to show more difficulties than men when they are asked to perform a similar task [18–20]. Area of residence does not play a predominant role in alteration of function but it is generally believed that older people or rural areas show less functional restrictions than the residents of urban areas [21]. Therefore, it is demonstrated in the literature review that there are several elderly people suffering from functional disability, with an annual increase in this dependency rate.

Down the line, disabled individuals could be expected to require a certain amount of LTC services in formal or informal settings, within an institution, in the community or at home [22].

It is important to understand that the elderly have lots of different needs which are not adequately met, thereby forcing many of them to go about their daily lives with these additional challenges. Likewise, it is expected that the risks involving disability and long-term illnesses on the part of the elderly will see a steady and sharp rise because of the increase in people's longevity.

Nonetheless, no current studies have been conducted to look into the disability risk factors throughout the country beginning from the year 2002 to 2011.

In view of this, the study sought to determine the disability risk factors of six disabilities (eating, dressing, squatting, lifting a 5 kg object, ease of stair use, and being able to travel by bus) among Thai aged population in 2002, 2007, and 2011. For each of the disability items the question was phrased as "can you perform these activities by yourself?" with response categories "no, not all," "yes, with aid," or "yes, without aid."

In so doing, the disability items were transformed prior to merging three datasets; then we defined disability as "older people who could not do the task" or "older people who could do it only with help." In addition, we excluded the urination and defecation continence from our analysis, since it was considered as physical health in the survey.

2. Materials and Methods

2.1. Data Source and Sampling. The National Statistical Office (NSO) had conducted four cross-sectional surveys in 1994, 2002, 2007, and 2011. Unfortunately, the NSO does not allow using 1994 dataset, so there are three datasets. The prime goal of this survey is to form a database of demographic, socioeconomic, and health characteristics and living arrangements of people aged 50 years and over in Thailand can be represented nationally.

To obtain this goal, a stratified multistage sampling technique was done by the National Statistical Office in all 76 provinces of Thailand which were further classified based on administered classification into urban and rural areas. The blocks for municipal areas and villages for nonmunicipal areas were the main sampling units. The probability of selection depends on the number of households existing in a block or village. A total of 5,796 blocks/villages were chosen in 2002 and 2011, while 5,793 blocks/villages were chosen in 2007.

Secondly, the private households were sampled. There were 15 households including a person aged 50 years or older chosen systematically from each chosen block and for the nonmunicipal area; 12 households were chosen systematically from each village. In 2002 and 2011, 79,560 households were chosen for final sample and, in 2007, 79,542 households were chosen for final sample.

In this study we selected only people aged 60 and above so the interviews were conducted with 24,835, 30,427, and 34,173 people in the 2002, 2007, and 2011 surveys of elderly Thai people, respectively. It was covered by the survey of the elderly in Thailand with a variety of demographic, socioeconomic, and health characteristics and management of people. Disability indicator in old age was the capability of doing activities on daily basis which is associated with the need for personal assistance.

Since the surveys have almost the identical questions on doing activities, then the availability of three cross-sectional datasets potentially presents the capability to quantify the differences of disability between three points of time while caution will require to be exercised.

2.2. Data Management. Data management will be undertaken to ensure database integrity and confidentiality. The following were approached.

2.2.1. Data Cleaning. This part deals with detecting and removing errors and inconsistencies from data in order to improve the quality of data. Also, missing data were coded as system-missing in SPSS.

2.2.2. Data Extraction. This part was employed in order to determine whether the formatting of the variables needs to be changed. Consistency in setting up response category values such as yes and no is one way to make the dataset more user friendly. The original response category values of variables of each study are shown in Table 1.

2.2.3. Data Transformation. The variables were recoded to make the data fit with the purpose of the study. To do so we identified variables that were present in three datasets and recoded them. The identifier variable assures that the values of the same individual are on the same line. At this step, the dependent variables were recoded to dummy variable (see the new variables list in Table 2).

Persons who could do the task without help were considered not to have the disability. Persons who could not do the task or could do it only with help were considered to have the disability.

2.2.4. Data Combination. The purpose is to have a longitudinal file which allows the understanding of changes, so we combined files from different years in order to run a regression utilizing year indicators.

2.3. Study Variables

2.3.1. Dependent Variables. In the 2002 survey, eight items related to self-care were questioned (feeding, dressing, bathing plus toileting, squatting, lifting 5 kg objects, walking 1 kilometer, stair climbing: 2-3 steps, and transferring by bus or boat alone). In 2007 survey, nine items related to self-ability were questioned including eating, dressing, bathing/toileting/toothbrushing, squatting, lifting 5 kg object, walking 200–300 meters, stair climbing: 2-3 steps, getting out by bus or boat alone, and money management. In 2011 survey, fourteen items were queried (feeding, putting on clothes, taking a bath, washing face/brushing teeth, toileting/cleaning oneself after urinating/defecating, shaving/combing, putting on shoes, squatting, lifting 5 kg object, walking 200–300 meters, stair climbing: 2-3 steps, taking a bus or boat alone, money management, and taking medicine correctly).

Since three surveys have six identical questions on doing activities, there are six activities in this study that determine disability status: eating, dressing, squatting, lifting a 5 kg object, ease of stair use, and being able to travel by bus or boat. Survey participants in all three years (2002, 2007, and 2011) specified for each task whether they

(1) could not do the task at all;

(2) could do the task with help;

(3) could do the task without help.

Before merging the data, we recoded these 3 responses into a dummy variable. Persons who could do the task without help were considered not to have the disability. Persons who could not do the task or could do it only with help were considered to have the disability.

2.3.2. Independent Variables. The following sixteen independent variables were transformed to dummy variables and considered in multiple logistic regression analysis as follows: (1) age in years, (2) gender, (3) education, (4) income, (5) married but not living as a couple (unmarried is reference), (6) married and living as a couple (unmarried is reference), (7) working status in the past 7 days, (8) any of five chronic diseases, (9) area (0 = urban; 1 = rural), (10) year 2007 (year 2002 is reference), (11) year 2011 (year 2002 is reference), (12) living in Bangkok, (13) the Central region (excluding Bangkok), (14) the Northeast region, (15) the North region (the South region is reference for all regions), and (16) living arrangements were self-reported during an interview according to living alone = 0 and living with others = 1.

2.4. Data Analysis. Descriptive statistics were used to summarize characteristics of study participants. Logistic regression analysis was used to assess the extent to which the selected independent variables explain the disability of the elderly in Thailand. Confidence intervals (CIs) were calculated at the 95% level to estimate statistical significance. Sample probability weights were applied to data for each year. Statistical analysis was conducted using IBM-SPSS version 18.

In addition to odds ratios, the modeled absolute prevalence of each disability was calculated with and without each independent variable, at the mean values of all other independent variables. For each independent variable, the resulting difference in modeled prevalence was calculated as a proportion of weighted prevalence of that disability. This procedure gave a measure of the impact of each independent variable on each disability (e.g., the modeled prevalence of difficulty lifting 5 kg, in persons who had and had not worked during the past 7 days, and at the mean levels of all other independent variables was 32.8% and 15.6%, respectively, for a modeled prevalence difference of 17.2%. This difference constituted a proportion of 0.560 of the weighted lifting disability prevalence of 30.7% (0.172/0.307 = 0.560)). Then, for each independent variable, these proportions were averaged over all 6 disabilities. To enable comparison of the relative impacts of the independent variables, proportions for the independent variables were arranged in descending order of this average proportion. (This approach is somewhat similar to calculating and comparing modeled population-attributable risk fractions for the independent variables,

TABLE 1: The original values of each study variable from each dataset (original variable names are given in bold type).

Dataset		2002	2007	2011
Study year		**Yr**	**Yr**	**Yr**
Age		**A2**	**A2**	**A5**
Marital status		**A5**	**A4**	**A10**
	Original value labels	1 = single 2 = married and living together in household 3 = married but not living together in household 4 = widowed 5 = divorced 6 = separated	1 = single 2 = married and living together in household 3 = married but not living together in household 4 = widowed 5 = divorced 6 = separated	1 = single 2 = married and living together in household 3 = married but not living together in household 4 = widowed 5 = divorced 6 = separated
Region		**REG**	**REG**	**REG**
	Original value label	1 = Bangkok 2 = Central (excluding Bangkok) 3 = North 4 = Northeast 5 = South	1 = Bangkok 2 = Central (excluding Bangkok) 3 = North 4 = Northeast 5 = South	1 = Bangkok 2 = Central (excluding Bangkok) 3 = North 4 = Northeast 5 = South
Area		**Area**	**Area**	**Area**
	Original value label	1 = municipal 2 = nonmunicipal	1 = municipal 2 = nonmunicipal	1 = municipal 2 = nonmunicipal
Living status		**B12**	**Members**	**Members**
	Original value label	1 = living alone 2 = living with others	1 = living alone 2 = living with others	1 = living alone 2 = living with others
Working status		**C1**	**A52**	**OP14**
	Original value label	1 = working 2 = not working	1 = working 2 = not working	1 = working 2 = not working
Income		**C25**	**A80**	**OP41**
	Original value label	0 = no income 1 = inadequate 2 = adequate 3 = more than adequate 9 = not known	1 = more than adequate 2 = adequate 3 = somewhat adequate 4 = inadequate	1 = more than adequate 2 = adequate 3 = somewhat adequate 4 = inadequate
Hypertension Diabetes Heart disease Cancer Stroke		**G16** **G18** **G19** **G21** **G26/27**	**B22** **B23** **B24** **B25** **B26**	**Op96_1** **Op96_2** **Op96_3** **Op96_5** **Op96_13**
	Original value labels	0 = no 1 = yes 2 = not known	0 = no 1 = yes 2 = not known	0 = no 1 = yes 2 = not known
Eating Dressing Squatting Lifting 5 kg Stairs: 2-3 steps Bus/boat alone		**G33** **G34** **G36** **G37** **G39** **G40**	**B28** **B29** **B31** **B32** **B34** **B35**	**Op104** **Op105** **Op111** **Op112** **Op114** **Op115**
	Original value label	0 = no, cannot do 1 = yes, can do 9 = not known (considered cannot do)	0 = no 1 = can do with aid 2 = can do without aid	1 = no 2 = yes, with aid 3 = yes, without aid

TABLE 2: New study variables.

Variables	New value label
Eating	0 = no, can do; 1 = yes, cannot do
Dressing	0 = no, can do; 1 = yes, cannot do
Squatting	0 = no, can do; 1 = yes, cannot do
Lifting 5 kg	0 = no, can do; 1 = yes, cannot do
Stairs: 2-3 steps	0 = no, can do; 1 = yes, cannot do
Bus/boat alone	0 = no, can do; 1 = yes, cannot do
Age (years)	Continuous
Chronic disease	0 = no; 1 = presenting at least one of five chronic diseases (hypertension, diabetes, cancer, stroke, heart)
Education	0 = any education; 1 = no education
Female	0 = no; 1 = yes
Income	0 = adequacy; 1 = inadequacy
Living arrangement	0 = living alone; 1 = living with others
Marital status	0 = never married (reference) 1 = married, living as couple 2 = married, not living as couple
Working status	0 = working; 1 = not working
Rural	0 = no; 1 = yes
Bangkok	0 = no; 1 = yes
Central (excluding Bangkok)	0 = no; 1 = yes
North	0 = no; 1 = yes
Northeast	0 = no; 1 = yes
South	0 = no; 1 = yes (reference)
Year 2002	0 = no; 1 = yes (reference)
Year 2007	0 = no; 1 = yes
Year 2011	0 = no; 1 = yes

except that it does not take their prevalence into account. Thus this approach may be viewed as an assessment of "absolute impact" of the risk factors, regardless of their frequency in the study population.) Also, this approach adds the benefit of considering absolute prevalence differences associated with risk factors and not merely odds ratios, which differ substantially at different baseline prevalence rates of studied outcomes and which can therefore be misleading.

2.5. Ethics Statement. As indicated above, the analyses reported here employed secondary data, which were originally collected by Thailand's National Statistical Office (NSO) in its nationwide surveys of 2002, 2007, and 2011. The NSO obtained written consent from all participants in these surveys. Completed consent forms are on file at the NSO. Additionally, the analyses reported here were approved by the Ethics Review Committee for Research Involving Human Research Subjects, Health Sciences Group, Chulalongkorn University, Certificate of Approval number 031/2015.

3. Results

3.1. Characteristics of the Study Population. The total numbers of the elderly with the people aged 60 and above were about 5,969,030 people in 2002, 7,020,959 people in 2007, and 8,266,304 people in 2011. The mean age of all participants was 68.6, 69.0, and 69.2 years in the 2002, 2007, and 2011 surveys, respectively. Females represented the majority of the population in all three surveys. More than 90% of the elderly in the samples lived with others, decreasing slightly but continually from 93.7 in 2002 to 92.3 in 2007 and to 91.4 in 2011. The percentage of elderly people who had at least one chronic disease increased from 29.6 in 2002 to 40.3 in 2007 and to 43.8 in 2011 (Table 3).

The number of elderly people who had not attended school decreased from 20.6 in 2002 to 16.4 in 2007 and to 11.8 in 2011. Approximately 30% lived in the Northeast region, which had the highest proportion of elderly people of all regions in Thailand.

3.2. Prevalence of Disabilities in the Three Study Years. Figure 1 and Table 3 show the prevalence of the six limiting activities by years. It was found that the prevalence of difficulty in lifting 5 kg decreased from 37.4% in 2002 to 27.0% in 2007 and increased slightly to 29.2% in 2011. Prevalence of difficulty in transportation declined somewhat, from 30.5% in 2002 to 25.8% and 24.0% in 2007 and 2011, respectively. The percentage of the elderly in 2002 that reported difficulty to step up 2-3 stairs was 10.1% which was increased to 13.6% in 2007 and it witnessed a bit decrease to 11.9% in 2011. For difficulty in squatting, the prevalence was 6.5%, 12.4%, and 12.7% in 2002, 2007, and 2011, respectively. The prevalence of the elderly who reported being difficulty in dressing was 2.1%

TABLE 3: Characteristics of study population and unadjusted prevalence of disability, by year, weighted by probability weight.

	2002 N (%)	2007 N (%)	2011 N (%)	Total N (%)
N	24,835	30,427	34,173	89,435
Demographic				
Mean age	68.61 ± 7.2	69.03 ± 7.4	69.24 ± 7.5	68.96 (7.3)
Female	13,480 (54.3)	16,859 (55.4)	19,119 (55.9)	49,938 (55.7)
No education	5,113 (20.6)	5,002 (16.4)	4,030 (11.8)	14,145 (16.26)
Low income	8,548 (34.4)	12,751 (41.9)	13,149 (38.6)	34,448 (38.3)
Did not work	16,848 (67.8)	19,552 (64.3)	21,077 (61.7)	57,477 (64.6)
Marital status				
Married not together	7,732 (35.2)	10,592 (34.8)	12,352 (36.1)	22,944 (35.4)
Married couple	13,677 (62.2)	19,001 (62.4)	20,494 (60.0)	53,172 (61.5)
Never married	584 (2.7)	834 (2.7)	1,325 (3.9)	2,743 (3.1)
Living arrangement				
Living alone	1,554 (6.3)	2,332 (7.7)	2,933 (8.6)	6,819 (7.5)
Living with another	23,281 (93.7)	28,095 (92.3)	31,240 (91.4)	82,616 (92.5)
Chronic disease				
Absent	17,482 (70.4)	18,176 (59.7)	19,210 (56.2)	54,868 (62.1)
At least one chronic disease	7,353 (29.6)	12,251 (40.3)	14,963 (43.8)	34,567 (37.9)
Geographic				
Rural	17,130 (69.0)	21,737 (71.4)	22,728 (66.5)	61,595 (68.9)
Bangkok	2,577 (10.4)	2,806 (9.2)	3,366 (9.9)	8,749 (9.8)
Central (excluding Bangkok)	6,373 (25.7)	7,166 (23.6)	7,918 (23.2)	21,457 (24.2)
North	5,230 (21.1)	6,360 (20.9)	6,948 (20.3)	18,538 (20.8)
Northeast	7,591 (30.6)	10,224 (33.6)	11,647 (34.1)	29,462 (32.8)
South	3,063 (12.3)	3,872 (12.7)	4,293 (12.6)	11,228 (12.5)
Prevalence				
Lifting 5 kg	9,067 (37.3)	8,147 (26.9)	9,970 (29.2)	26,730 (30.7)
Travelling alone	7,019 (30.4)	7,792 (25.8)	8,207 (24.0)	23,018 (26.3)
Climbing 2-3 steps	2,326 (10.1)	4,103 (13.6)	4,066 (11.9)	10,495 (12.0)
Squatting	1,514 (6.5)	3,738 (12.4)	4,325 (12.7)	9,577 (10.9)
Dressing	593 (2.1)	915 (3.0)	926 (2.7)	2,334 (2.7)
Eating	274 (1.2)	684 (2.3)	738 (2.2)	1,696 (1.9)
Number of disabilities				
1-2	9,410 (40.7)	8,299 (27.4)	10,154 (29.7)	27,863 (31.8)
≥3	967 (4.2)	2,339 (7.7)	2,313 (6.8)	5,619 (6.4)
Any disability	10,377 (44.9)	10,638 (35.2)	12,467 (36.5)	33,482 (38.4)

in 2002 which increased to 3.0% in 2007 and then slightly decreased to 2.7% in 2011. The prevalence of elderly persons who had eating limitation was 1.2% in 2002, 2.3% in 2007, and 2.2% in 2011. Overall, prevalence of lifting-related and travel-related disabilities was high, prevalence of squatting- and stair climbing-related disabilities was intermediate, and prevalence of dressing- and eating-related disabilities was low.

Over all three surveys, the disability with highest prevalence activity that was most difficult for the sample population was lifting 5 kg (30.7), followed by traveling alone by bus or boat (26.4). Twelve percent of elderly people had difficulty climbing 2-3 stairs, a proportion slightly higher than that for squatting (10.9).

3.3. Logistic Regression of Risk Factors over All Three Survey Years. Table 4 demonstrated the associations of subject characteristics with disability risk. As expected, age indicated the highest risk for difficulty with dressing (OR = 1.09, 95% CI: 1.09–1.10), eating (OR = 1.09, 95% CI: 1.08–1.10), using stairs (OR = 1.10, 95% CI: 1.09–1.10), traveling alone (OR = 1.12, 95% CI: 1.12–1.13), lifting 5 kg (OR = 1.10, 95% CI: 1.09–1.10), squatting (OR = 1.08, 95% CI: 1.08–1.09), and any disability (OR = 1.11, 95% CI: 1.10–1.11) at $p < 0.001$.

For education level, no education indicated highest risk for difficulty with dressing (OR = 1.34, 95% CI: 1.20–1.49), eating (OR = 1.59, 95% CI: 1.41–1.79), using stairs (OR = 1.21, 95% CI: 1.14–1.28), traveling alone (OR = 1.42, 95% CI: 1.36–1.49), lifting 5 kg (OR = 1.27, 95% CI: 1.21–1.33), squatting

Table 4: Logistic regression over all three years (sample probability weights).

(a)

Independent variable	Any disabilities			Eating		
	Coefficient	Odds ratio (95% CI)	*p* value	Coefficient	Odds ratio (95% CI)	*p* value
Age (years)	0.11	1.11 (1.10–1.11)	<0.001	0.09	1.09 (1.08–1.10)	<0.001
Female versus male	0.63	1.88 (1.81–1.94)	<0.001	−0.30	0.74 (0.66–0.83)	<0.001
No education versus any education	0.33	1.39 (1.32–1.45)	<0.001	0.46	1.59 (1.41–1.79)	<0.001
Inadequate versus adequate income	0.18	1.20 (1.16–1.24)	<0.001	0.26	1.29 (1.16–1.43)	<0.001
Married (couple) versus unmarried	−0.21	0.81 (0.74–0.89)	<0.001	−0.60	0.55 (0.42–0.72)	<0.001
Married (not together) versus unmarried	−0.07	0.93 (0.85–1.02)	0.146	−0.53	0.59 (0.45–0.77)	<0.001
Living with others versus alone	0.11	1.12 (1.05–1.19)	<0.001	0.68	1.96 (1.54–2.51)	<0.001
Did not work in the past 7 days	0.97	2.64 (2.54–2.75)	<0.001	1.64	5.15 (4.10–6.47)	<0.001
Any chronic disease*	0.57	1.77 (1.71–1.83)	<0.001	1.16	3.19 (2.85–3.56)	<0.001
Rural versus urban	0.02	1.02 (0.98–1.06)	0.316	−0.26	0.77 (0.69–0.87)	<0.001
Bangkok versus South	0.21	1.23 (1.14–1.33)	<0.001	−0.04	0.96 (0.79–1.18)	0.719
Central versus South	0.13	1.14 (1.08–1.21)	<0.001	−0.01	0.99 (0.84–1.16)	0.896
North versus South	0.33	1.39 (1.31–1.48)	<0.001	−0.58	0.56 (0.46–0.67)	<0.001
Northeast versus South	0.34	1.40 (1.32–1.48)	<0.001	−0.27	0.76 (0.64–0.90)	0.002
Year 2007 versus 2002	−0.58	0.56 (0.54–0.58)	<0.001	0.66	1.93 (1.65–2.25)	<0.001
Year 2011 versus 2002	−0.52	0.60 (0.57–0.62)	<0.001	0.56	1.75 (1.50–2.04)	<0.001
Constant	−8.99		<0.001	−12.47		<0.001

(b)

Independent variable	Dressing			Squatting		
	Coefficient	Odds ratio (95% CI)	*p* value	Coefficient	Odds ratio (95% CI)	*p* value
Age (years)	0.09	1.09 (1.09–1.10)	<0.001	0.08	1.08 (1.08–1.09)	<0.001
Female versus male	−0.28	0.76 (0.68–0.83)	<0.001	0.30	1.36 (1.29–1.43)	<0.001
No education versus any education	0.29	1.34 (1.20–1.49)	<0.001	0.12	1.13 (1.06–1.20)	<0.001
Inadequate versus adequate income	0.34	1.41 (1.29–1.54)	<0.001	0.23	1.26 (1.20–1.32)	<0.001
Married (couple) versus unmarried	−0.72	0.49 (0.39–0.62)	<0.001	−0.16	0.85 (0.74–0.97)	0.015
Married (not together) versus unmarried	−0.48	0.62 (0.49–0.78)	<0.001	−0.09	0.92 (0.80–1.05)	0.196
Living with others versus alone	1.03	2.79 (2.21–3.52)	<0.001	0.37	1.45 (1.32–1.59)	<0.001
Did not work in the past 7 days	1.80	6.03 (4.88–7.45)	<0.001	0.96	2.61 (2.44–2.80)	<0.001
Any chronic disease*	1.23	3.41 (3.10–3.76)	<0.001	0.73	2.07 (1.97–2.17)	<0.001
Rural versus urban	−0.18	0.83 (0.75–0.93)	0.001	−0.18	0.84 (0.79–0.88)	<0.001
Bangkok versus South	−0.01	0.99 (0.83–1.18)	0.887	0.05	1.05 (0.95–1.16)	0.360
Central versus South	−0.04	0.97 (0.84–1.11)	0.633	0.02	1.02 (0.94–1.10)	0.645
North versus South	−0.34	0.71 (0.61–0.83)	<0.001	−0.06	0.94 (0.87–1.02)	0.165
Northeast versus South	−0.34	0.71 (0.61–0.83)	<0.001	−0.38	0.69 (0.63–0.74)	<0.001
Year 2007 versus 2002	0.33	1.38 (1.28–1.57)	<0.001	0.73	2.07 (1.93–2.22)	<0.001
Year 2011 versus 2002	0.14	1.15 (1.02–1.30)	0.023	0.72	2.05 (1.91–2.19)	<0.001
Constant	−12.53		<0.001	−9.65		<0.001

(c)

Independent variable	Lifting 5 kg			Climbing 2-3 steps		
	Coefficient	Odds ratio (95% CI)	*p* value	Coefficient	Odds ratio (95% CI)	*p* value
Age (years)	0.09	1.10 (1.09–1.10)	<0.001	0.10	1.10 (1.09–1.10)	<0.001
Female versus male	0.62	1.85 (1.79–1.92)	<0.001	0.22	1.25 (1.19–1.32)	<0.001
No education versus any education	0.24	1.27 (1.21–1.33)	<0.001	0.19	1.21 (1.14–1.28)	<0.001
Inadequate versus adequate income	0.09	1.09 (1.05–1.13)	<0.001	0.30	1.35 (1.29–1.41)	<0.001
Married (couple) versus unmarried	−0.08	0.93 (0.84–1.02)	0.115	−0.41	0.66 (0.58–0.76)	<0.001
Married (not together) versus unmarried	0.06	1.06 (0.97–1.17)	0.214	−0.24	0.79 (0.69–0.89)	<0.001
Living with others versus alone	0.09	1.10 (1.03–1.17)	0.004	0.32	1.38 (1.27–1.51)	<0.001

(c) Continued.

Independent variable	Lifting 5 kg			Climbing 2-3 steps		
	Coefficient	Odds ratio (95% CI)	*p* value	Coefficient	Odds ratio (95% CI)	*p* value
Did not work in the past 7 days	0.97	2.64 (2.53–2.76)	<0.001	1.39	4.04 (3.73–4.37)	<0.001
Any chronic disease*	0.53	1.70 (1.64–1.76)	<0.001	0.77	2.16 (2.06–2.26)	<0.001
Rural versus urban	−0.08	0.92 (0.89–0.96)	<0.001	−0.04	0.96 (0.91–1.01)	0.126
Bangkok versus South	0.30	1.35 (1.25–1.45)	<0.001	−0.25	0.78 (0.70–0.86)	<0.001
Central versus South	0.05	1.05 (0.99–1.11)	0.138	−0.19	0.83 (0.77–0.89)	<0.001
North versus South	0.35	1.42 (1.33–1.51)	<0.001	−0.42	0.66 (0.61–0.72)	<0.001
Northeast versus South	0.35	1.42 (1.34–1.51)	<0.001	−0.16	0.85 (0.79–0.92)	<0.001
Year 2007 versus 2002	−0.64	0.53 (0.50–0.55)	<0.001	0.31	1.37 (1.28–1.45)	<0.001
Year 2011 versus 2002	−0.53	0.59 (0.57–0.62)	<0.001	0.09	1.09 (1.02–1.16)	0.007
Constant	−8.62		<0.001	−10.50		<0.001

(d)

Independent variable	Travelling alone		
	Coefficient	Odds ratio (95% CI)	*p* value
Age (years)	0.12	1.12 (1.12–1.13)	<0.001
Female versus male	0.49	1.64 (1.57–1.71)	<0.001
No education versus any education	0.35	1.42 (1.36–1.49)	<0.001
Inadequate versus adequate income	0.25	1.28 (1.23–1.33)	<0.001
Married (couple) versus unmarried	−0.33	0.72 (0.65–0.80)	<0.001
Married (not together) versus unmarried	−0.18	0.83 (0.75–0.92)	<0.001
Living with others versus alone	0.16	1.18 (1.10–1.26)	<0.001
Did not work in the past 7 days	1.19	3.28 (3.12–3.44)	<0.001
Any chronic disease*	0.61	1.85 (1.78–1.92)	<0.001
Rural versus urban	0.12	1.13 (1.08–1.18)	<0.001
Bangkok versus South	0.10	1.11 (1.02–1.21)	0.014
Central versus South	0.08	1.08 (1.01–1.15)	0.019
North versus South	0.08	1.08 (1.01–1.15)	0.020
Northeast versus South	0.20	1.22 (1.15–1.30)	<0.001
Year 2007 versus 2002	−0.37	0.69 (0.66–0.72)	<0.001
Year 2011 versus 2002	−0.51	0.60 (0.57–0.63)	<0.001
Constant	−10.51		<0.001

*Any chronic disease includes heart problems, hypertension, diabetes, cancer, and stroke.

(OR = 1.13, 95% CI: 1.06–1.20), and any disability (OR = 1.39, 95% CI: 1.32–1.45) at $p < 0.001$. Income inadequacy showed highest risk for difficulty with dressing (OR = 1.14, 95% CI: 1.29–1.54), eating (OR = 1.29, 95% CI: 1.16–1.43), using stairs (OR = 1.35, 95% CI: 1.29–1.41), traveling alone (OR = 1.28, 95% CI: 1.23-1.33), lifting 5 kg (OR = 1.09, 95% CI: 1.05–1.13), squatting (OR = 1.26, 95% CI: 1.20–1.32), and any disability (OR = 1.20, 95% CI: 1.16–1.40) at $p < 0.001$. Living with others indicated highest risk for difficulty with dressing (OR = 2.79, 95% CI: 2.21–3.52), eating (OR = 1.96, 95% CI: 1.54–2.51), using stairs (OR = 1.38, 95% CI: 1.27–1.51), traveling alone (OR = 1.18, 95% CI: 1.10–1.26), lifting 5 kg (OR = 1.10, 95% CI: 1.03–1.17), squatting (OR = 1.45, 95% CI: 1.32–1.59), and any disability (OR = 1.12, 95% CI: 1.05–1.19) at $p < 0.001$.

Having at least one chronic disease (heart problems, diabetes, hypertension, cancer, or stroke) had a highly significant association with dressing (OR = 3.41, 95% CI: 3.10–3.76), eating (OR = 3.19, 95% CI: 2.85–3.56), using stairs (OR = 2.16, 95% CI: 2.06–2.26), traveling alone (OR = 1.85, 95% CI: 1.78–1.92), lifting 5 kg (OR = 1.70, 95% CI: 1.64–1.76), squatting (OR = 2.07, 95% CI: 1.97–2.17), and any disability (OR = 1.77, 95% CI: 1.71–1.83) at $p < 0.001$. Being female had a negative association with difficulty in eating and dressing and a positive association with squatting, lifting 5 kg, using stairs, traveling by bus, and any disability. In terms of marital status, those who were married and lived with a spouse showed better ability to perform daily activities than their counterparts who were not married (divorced, widowed, and separated). Those who lived in a rural residence had a higher likelihood of having difficulty performing with any disability and traveling alone by bus/boat than those in an urban residence, but they were less likely to have difficulty eating, dressing, squatting, lifting 5 kg, and using stairs.

Interestingly, being unemployed seven days prior to interview indicated the highest risk for difficulty with dressing (OR = 6.03, 95% CI: 4.88–7.45), eating (OR = 5.15, 95%

TABLE 5: Proportional impacts of independent variables on prevalence of six disabilities in the elderly in Thailand in 2002, 2007, and 2011.

Independent variable	Having difficulty with indicated activity						Overall average
	Lifting 5 kg	Traveling by oneself	Climbing stairs	Squatting	Dressing	Eating	
Did not work for 7 days	0.560	0.647	0.685	0.545	0.600	0.574	0.602
Age 65 to 75	0.608	0.739	0.586	0.532	0.374	0.384	0.537
Any of 5 chronic diseases*	0.338	0.383	0.462	0.489	0.559	0.546	0.463
Lives with others versus lives alone	0.057	0.094	0.160	0.202	0.264	0.205	0.164
No formal education versus any education	0.154	0.227	0.111	0.077	0.122	0.215	0.151
Lower versus higher income	0.053	0.149	0.170	0.148	0.135	0.104	0.126
Female versus male	0.376	0.292	0.122	0.187	−0.108	−0.122	0.125
Year 2007 versus 2002	−0.380	−0.216	0.179	0.501	0.129	0.290	0.084
Year 2011 versus 2002	−0.318	−0.298	0.048	0.480	0.055	0.237	0.034
Bangkok versus South	0.195	0.064	−0.127	0.029	−0.005	−0.014	0.024
Central versus South	0.029	0.046	−0.101	0.011	−0.013	−0.004	−0.005
Northeast versus South	0.224	0.124	−0.087	−0.224	−0.121	−0.103	−0.031
North versus South	0.227	0.047	−0.207	−0.035	−0.116	−0.198	−0.047
Rural versus urban	−0.049	0.071	−0.024	−0.116	−0.071	−0.107	−0.050
Married, not living as couple, versus unmarried	0.038	−0.109	−0.129	−0.053	−0.171	−0.197	−0.104
Married, living as couple, versus unmarried	−0.049	−0.204	−0.237	−0.105	−0.300	−0.260	−0.192

* Any chronic diseaseincludes heart problems, hypertension, diabetes, cancer, and stroke.

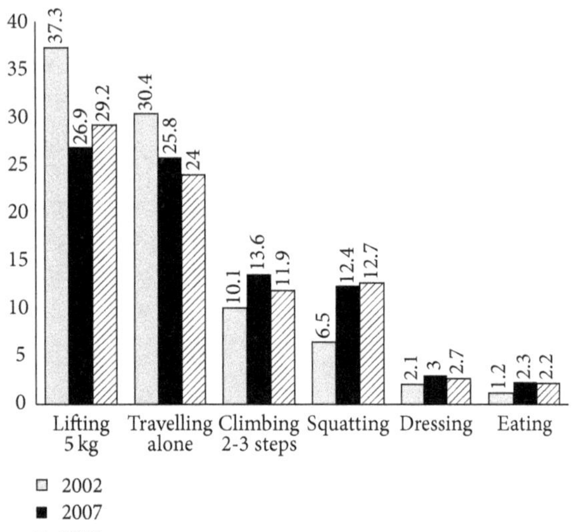

FIGURE 1: Weighted prevalence (percent) of the six studied disabilities by year.

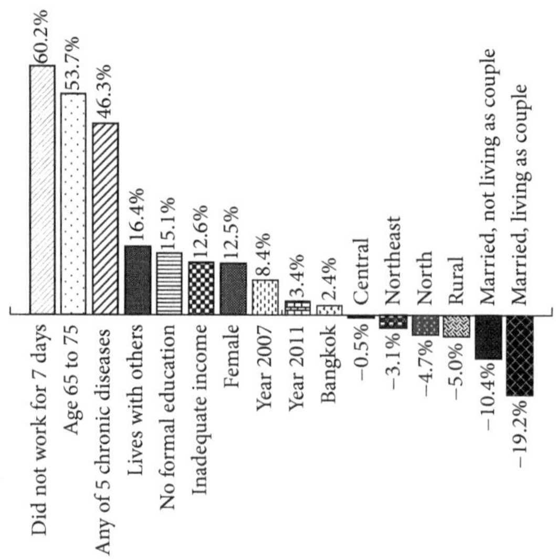

FIGURE 2: Proportional impacts of modeled independent variables on prevalence of the 6 disabilities studied.

CI: 4.10–6.47), using stairs (OR = 4.04, 95% CI: 3.73–4.37), traveling alone by bus (OR = 3.28, 95% CI: 3.12–3.44), lifting 5 kg (OR = 2.64, 95% CI: 2.53–2.76), having any disability (OR = 2.64, 95% CI: 2.54–2.75), and squatting (OR = 2.61, 95% CI: 2.44–2.80) at $p < 0.001$.

Proportional impacts of independent variables on disability prevalence are presented in Figure 2 and Table 5. On average, the characteristics with the greatest adverse impact on disability prevalence were not working in the past 7 days (average impact: 61.2%), age per 10 years (53.7%), and presence of one or more chronic diseases (46.3%). Living with others, lack of education, and lower income were associated with moderate positive proportional impacts on disability prevalence (average impacts: 16.4%, 15.1%, and 12.6%, resp.). Female gender was associated with an overall positive impact but exhibited considerable variability across disabilities (average 12.5%, range 37.6% to −12.2%). Proportional impacts of study year varied widely across disabilities. Impacts of region were generally modest; there was appreciable variability across disabilities. Living in a rural area was generally associated with lower disability risk than living in an urban area. Being married was consistently associated with lower risk than being unmarried, especially for married participants who lived together as couples.

4. Discussion

4.1. Main Results. The levels of difficulty experienced by those surveyed decreased between the 2002 and 2007 surveys. The sole category in which the level of difficulty decreased between 2002 and 2007 and increased between 2007 and 2011 was the ability to travel alone by bus or boat. In one to two disabilities, the level of difficulty was reported to decline in 2007 and increase mildly in 2011. In more than three disabilities, the opposite was the case, with the level of difficulty rising in 2007 and dropping in 2011. Across all six activities, the overall level of difficulty decreased slightly. As it is not necessarily the case that all surveys were completed by the concerned parties themselves, there may be slight inconsistencies found with regard to the levels of difficulty observed in the results. The reasons for these trends are complex and include shifts in socioeconomic status of the elder population, in the distribution of underlying conditions and limitations in capacity that may be related to use of medical treatments, and in the uptake of assistive and other convenience technologies.

This study has shown that the factors most associated with disability are old age, being female, lack of education, low income, cohabitation, unemployment seven days prior to interview, having at least one chronic disease (hypertension, heart problems, diabetes, strokes, or cancer), and living in a rural setting. It has already been demonstrated in past studies that categories such as age, gender, and socioeconomic status may be linked to physical disability in the elderly [23, 24]. This study connects the factors of age, income, and marital status to the issue. Age is the most commonly noted associative factor with physical disability.

4.2. Relation to Other Research Findings. There are variations in occurrence of the ADL disability in different studies. It is not easy to compare the different studies because a variety of the ADL measurements and age groups have been used. In Malaysia, people over 60 had an ADL disability prevalence of 10.6% [25]. The uniqueness of the studies lies in the fact that the sample used in Malaysia was younger (mean age: 69.0) than that of the U.S. and Chinese population samples (74.5 and 75.1). Ofstedal et al. (2007) [26] show that prevalence of ADL and IADL limitations varies across Asian countries and trend was increasing. The prevalence of ADL disability in Singapore was 3.9% (1999), in Beijing it was 4.7% (1997), in Indonesia it was 6.5% (1997), in Taiwan it was 9.2%, and in Philippines it was 14.7% (2000). IADL restrictions in Singapore were 17.2% (1999), in Beijing they were 17.7% (1997), and they were 25.1% in Taiwan and 27.7% in Philippines (2000).

At present, there is a higher burden of dependency in Sub-Saharan African region, which has the dependency region of almost 20%. It is expected that there will be a high increase in this ratio in Sub-Saharan Africa, Latin America, and Asia. It was estimated in this study that there will be a higher increase in the dependency ratio in China (16%) and India (14%) in the next few years, along with the population increase. The study ended on the note that several countries are going to face the burden of rising number of dependent people and a lot more significance needs to be awarded to disability prevention [27].

The physical and mental health issues of the elderly population living in a rural region of Sepand in Malaysia were examined in a cross-sectional study. The random sampling technique was used to choose 5 out of 9 villages. There were 223 participants in the study aged more than 60 years. Prestructured questionnaires were used for interviewing the elderly in the villages, including geriatric depression scale, Barthel's Index, and elderly cognitive assessment questionnaire. The existence of physical health problems like chronic illness and functional dependence was found to be 60.1% and 17.5%. It was further found that the existence of physical reliance in at least one ADL was 17.5% and it was 17.1% for one or more ADLs. The most dependent activities for these people were bathing and toileting [28].

Basic ADL disability and functional restrictive rates among elderly population in America were examined in a study spanning from 2000 to 2005 so as to ascertain if there was an increase or decrease in the percentages of basic ADL disabilities and functional restrictions among the community residents and the institutionalized elderly. The yearly percentages of prevalence of basic ADL disabilities and functional restrictions were computed using data from American Community Survey and National Nursing Home Survey. This data was then used in regression lines to evaluate the changing trends with time. It was observed that there was a 9% increase in the percentages of basic activities of daily living (BADL) disabilities among the elderly in the community aged 65 and over. The institutionalized elderly ADL disability rates were found to be consistent among males but showed an increase for females in the years 2000 to 2005. It was henceforth deduced in this study that this growth in ADL disability with time among the elderly population greatly affects the healthcare mechanism [29].

Even if there is a huge range of disparity in the way surveys have questions regarding ADL functioning, there is some agreement among all of these surveys related to what activities of everyday life should be incorporated. According to Guralnik et al. [30], the calculations might differ merely due to the reason that the participants have a different understanding of the question seeing as the self-report instruments do not include distinct meaning for the calculated activity or plausible answer categories. As stated by M. W. Linn and B. S. Linn [31], the criteria of evaluation of disability by individuals can be affected by language, education, and culture. The factors like time period of disability, the kind of help that was given, and what range of complexity they experience while performing every ADL vary in surveys. Result of our study cannot be straight compared with these results but we can generalize that any disability is elevated along with the Thai elderly.

In terms of gender, ADL disability variations that indicate disability prevalence are more common among females compared to males [25, 32]. A study undertaken in Lebanon revealed that higher disability existed in elderly women

(31.3%) than among elderly men (18.7%) [13]. Another study in Spain on people aged 65 indicated that the ADL disability prevalence among females was 15.8% and for males it was 10.6% [32]. Such differences may be attributed partially to a higher mortality rate among males and a higher ADL disability prevalence in females [33].

Few studies have examined differences in health and ADL disability based on residence (urban versus rural). Most studies emanate from Asia. The studies have indicated that greater ADL disability prevalence and poor health are found among aged rural dwellers [34, 35]. Another study in Australia and Canada established that 18-year-old adults from rural areas had poor health. It was discovered that a correlation existed between the health of over 18-year-old adults and living in rural areas, particularly with regard to poor health [36]. Another study in Finland found similar outcomes for 52-year-old adults [37]. Additionally, adults living in rural areas exhibited an unhealthy way of life, for instance, smoking, overweight, unhealthy eating habits, and less physical activity.

With regard to disability, income, rather than education, appeared related in the current study. Some past studies corroborate the finding [24, 38], whereas others state that income has no role in the elderly disability [39]. However, low-income individuals are not likely to seek proper healthcare.

Interestingly, this study found that aged individuals living with others had a higher risk of disability, an outcome that is consistent with Tsai et al.'s study [40]. It is possible that individuals living alone must complete chores on their own whereas those who live with others have assistance as aged couples assist each other when functional ability wanes. The study may not confirm the relation between living together and disability. The older people might invite another person to come and stay with them when they become disabled. Further research should be undertaken to explain this finding, even though many studies indicate that low economic status and loneliness increase the risk of disability among the older people.

The reason for the strong association between the risk of disability and the status of not working in seven days before the interview is not clear. The high probability may be due to the difficulty of defining unemployment, as it may include people who are not working because of a disability, those who are looking for work or are on temporary sick leave, the retired, home makers, and people whose spouse and/or children do not allow them to work. Thus, this issue must be further explored in depth.

4.3. Strengths and Weaknesses. The main strength point of the study is to provide description of aged individuals and to create a framework of forming practices that offer a better insight on Thai ageing. Different disability limitations and risks in Thailand in 2002, 2007, and 2011 are examined thoroughly in the study and the findings can be applied to the broader Thai population.

This study did not cover all disabilities. Moreover, the surveys depended on the respondents' personal description of circumstances. Thus, the possibility of inaccurate data could not be ruled out, particularly if a family member or friend participated in the reporting.

This study did not consider health behaviour variables, such as drinking clean water, smoking, and exercise, because these behaviours were not queried consistently in the 3 survey years. However, evidence from literature reveals that exercise and physical activities positively affect ADL and physical functioning among the aged. This may reduce the risk of facing an ADL disability. A study in the U.S. found a relationship between lower incidents of disability and higher rates of physical activity [41]. The current study omitted self-rated health as an independent variable because many individuals can rate their health basing on their past health. Finally, since the study was cross-sectional with regard to design, it is possible that determining the causality was not achieved.

4.4. Policy Recommendations. Because chronic illnesses relate strongly to disability, health prevention mechanisms of reducing later life disability should be promoted. Another option for reducing later life disability may entail creating awareness. Lack of work had a strong link with a disability, though the causality factor cannot be dismissed because an increase in working opportunities can reduce disability among aged individuals.

Effects of risk factors over time are often influenced by effects of age, period (time of data collection), and/or birth cohort. The modeled effects of putative risk factors presented in this report were adjusted for age and period (year of data collection). Strictly speaking, it is not possible to model age, period, and cohort simultaneously [42], because these three characteristics are a linear combination of each other (cohort + age = period). To address this issue, we chose to construct separate models (not shown), adjusting for age and birth cohort. In these, modeled effects of factors other than age, period, and cohort were similar to those in the models reported here. Thus, the effects analyzed were robust with different model specifications. This observation increases confidence that the findings reported here are valid.

5. Conclusions

Although overall prevalence has dropped, the absolute number of disabled people continues to increase in Thailand. Thus, the healthcare system and individuals themselves are faced with an increased trouble of disability and new challenges. Since older people who did not work had higher risk for disability in our study, so extending the default retirement age of 60 in Thailand and increasing the work opportunity in older people may reduce the risk of disability although the causality is not clear. In view of the fact that people living alone had a lower risk for disability in our study, so we suppose that older people living alone may be at a lower risk for disability in the future compared to those living with others. However, this needs to be confirmed in future studies.

Competing Interests

The authors declare no potential conflict of interests with

respect to the research, authorship, and/or publication of this article.

Acknowledgments

The authors would like to acknowledge the National Statistical Office of Thailand for providing the dataset. This work was supported by the Ratchadaphisek Sompoch Endowment Fund (2014), Chulalongkorn University [CU-57-069-AS], and The 90th Anniversary of Chulalongkorn University Fund (Ratchadaphisek Sompoch Endowment Fund).

References

[1] Foundation of Thai Gerontology Research and Development Institute, *Report Older Situation*, Foundation of Thai Gerontology Research and Development Institute (TGRI), Bangkok, Thailand, 2013.

[2] V. A. Freedman, E. M. Agree, L. G. Martin, and J. C. Cornman, "Trends in the use of assistive technology and personal care for late-life disability, 1992–2001," *The Gerontologist*, vol. 46, no. 1, pp. 124–127, 2006.

[3] V. A. Freedman, L. G. Martin, and R. F. Schoeni, "Recent trends in disability and functioning among older adults in the United States," *The Journal of the American Medical Association*, vol. 288, no. 24, pp. 3137–3146, 2002.

[4] K.-L. Chou and J. C. B. Leung, "Disability trends in Hong Kong community-dwelling Chinese older adults: 1996, 2000, and 2004," *Journal of Aging and Health*, vol. 20, no. 4, pp. 385–404, 2008.

[5] D. Acosta, R. Rottbeck, G. Rodríguez, C. P. Ferri, and M. J. Prince, "The epidemiology of dependency among urban-dwelling older people in the Dominican Republic; a cross-sectional survey," *BMC Public Health*, vol. 8, article 285, 2008.

[6] K. S. Chan, J. D. Kasper, J. Brandt, and L. E. Pezzin, "Measurement equivalence in ADL and IADL difficulty across international surveys of aging: findings from the HRS, SHARE, and ELSA," *Journals of Gerontology—Series B: Psychological Sciences and Social Sciences*, vol. 67, no. 1, pp. 121–132, 2012.

[7] P. Chen, E. S. H. Yu, M. Zhang, W. T. Liu, R. Hill, and R. Katzman, "ADL dependence and medical conditions in Chinese older persons: a population-based survey in Shanghai, China," *Journal of the American Geriatrics Society*, vol. 43, no. 4, pp. 378–383, 1995.

[8] M. A. Khoei, M. E. Akbari, F. Sharifi, H. Fakhrzadeh, and B. Larijani, "Translation and validation of the activities of daily living scale with iranian elderly cancer patients treated in an oncology unit," *Asian Pacific Journal of Cancer Prevention*, vol. 14, no. 5, pp. 2731–2737, 2013.

[9] S. Jitapunkul, P. Kamolratanakul, and S. Ebrahim, "The meaning of activities of daily living in a Thai elderly population: development of a new index," *Age and Ageing*, vol. 23, no. 2, pp. 97–101, 1994.

[10] W. Swaddiwudhipong, V. Amaritchavarn, and S. Boonyabuncha, "Prevalence of disabling conditions in a rural northern Thai community: a survey conducted by village health communicators," *The Southeast Asian Journal of Tropical Medicine and Public Health*, vol. 25, no. 1, pp. 45–49, 1994.

[11] S. Jitapunkul, C. Kunanusont, W. Phoolcharoen, P. Suriyawongpaisal, and S. Ebrahim, "Determining public health priorities for an ageing population: the value of a disability survey," *Southeast Asian Journal of Tropical Medicine and Public Health*, vol. 34, no. 4, pp. 929–936, 2003.

[12] S. Jitapunkul, N. Krungkraipetch, P. Kamolratanakul, and B. Dhanamun, "Dependence and active life expectancy of the elderly population living in the central region of Thailand," *Journal of the Medical Association of Thailand*, vol. 84, no. 3, pp. 349–356, 2001.

[13] A. Z. Al Hazzouri, A. M. Sibai, M. Chaaya, Z. Mahfoud, and K. M. Yount, "Gender differences in physical disability among older adults in underprivileged communities in Lebanon," *Journal of Aging and Health*, vol. 23, no. 2, pp. 367–382, 2011.

[14] Q. Feng, Z. Zhen, D. Gu, B. Wu, P. W. Duncan, and J. L. Purser, "Trends in ADL and IADL disability in community-dwelling older adults in Shanghai, China, 1998–2008," *The Journals of Gerontology, Series B: Psychological Sciences and Social Sciences*, vol. 68, no. 3, pp. 476–485, 2013.

[15] W. W. Hung, J. S. Ross, K. S. Boockvar, and A. L. Siu, "Recent trends in chronic disease, impairment and disability among older adults in the United States," *BMC Geriatrics*, vol. 11, no. 1, article 47, 2011.

[16] S. Z. Nagi, "An epidemiology of disability among adults in the United States.," *Milbank Memorial Fund Quarterly, Health and Society*, vol. 54, no. 4, pp. 439–467, 1976.

[17] E. Heikkinen, "What are the main risk factors for disability in old age and how can disability be prevented?" WHO regional office for Europe's health evidence network synthesis report, 2003.

[18] Ü. Taş, E. W. Steyerberg, S. M. A. Bierma-Zeinstra, A. Hofman, B. W. Koes, and A. P. Verhagen, "Age, gender and disability predict future disability in older people: the Rotterdam Study," *BMC Geriatrics*, vol. 11, article 22, 2011.

[19] P. Schon, M. G. Parker, I. Kareholt, and M. Thorslund, "Gender differences in associations between ADL and other health indicators in 1992 and 2002," *Aging Clinical and Experimental Research*, vol. 23, no. 2, pp. 91–98, 2011.

[20] S. E. Hardy, H. G. Allore, Z. Guo, and T. M. Gill, "Explaining the effect of gender on functional transitions in older persons," *Gerontology*, vol. 54, no. 2, pp. 79–86, 2008.

[21] L. I. Iezzoni, M. B. Killeen, and B. L. O'Day, "Rural residents with disabilities confront substantial barriers to obtaining primary care," *Health Services Research*, vol. 41, no. 4, part 1, pp. 1258–1275, 2006.

[22] J. M. Wiener, R. J. Hanley, R. Clark, and J. F. Van Nostrand, "Measuring the activities of daily living: comparisons across national surveys," *Journal of Gerontology*, vol. 45, no. 6, pp. S229–S237, 1990.

[23] N. Hoeymans, E. J. M. Feskens, D. Kromhoup, and G. A. M. van den Bos, "Ageing and the relationship between functional status and self-rated health in elderly men," *Social Science and Medicine*, vol. 45, no. 10, pp. 1527–1536, 1997.

[24] Z. Zimmer and J. S. House, "Education, income, and functional limitation transitions among American adults: contrasting onset and progression," *International Journal of Epidemiology*, vol. 32, no. 6, pp. 1089–1097, 2003.

[25] N. N. Hairi, A. Bulgiba, R. G. Cumming, V. Naganathan, and I. Mudla, "Prevalence and correlates of physical disability and functional limitation among community dwelling older people in rural Malaysia, a middle income country," *BMC Public Health*, vol. 10, article 492, 2010.

[26] M. B. Ofstedal, Z. Zimmer, A. I. Hermalin et al., "Short-term trends in functional limitation and disability among older

Asians: a comparison of five Asian settings," *Journal of Cross-Cultural Gerontology*, vol. 22, no. 3, pp. 243–261, 2007.

[27] R. H. Harwood, A. A. Sayer, and M. Hirschfeld, "Current and future worldwide prevalence of dependency, its relationship to total population, and dependency ratios," *Bulletin of the World Health Organization*, vol. 82, no. 4, pp. 251–258, 2004.

[28] S. M. Sidik, L. Rampal, and M. Afifi, "Physical and mental health problems of the elderly in a rural community of Sepang, Selangor," *Malaysian Journal of Medical Sciences*, vol. 11, no. 1, pp. 52–59, 2004.

[29] E. Fuller-Thomson, B. Yu, A. Nuru-Jeter, J. M. Guralnik, and M. Minkler, "Basic ADL disability and functional limitation rates among older Americans from 2000–2005: the end of the decline?" *The Journals of Gerontology, Series A: Biological Sciences and Medical Sciences*, vol. 64, no. 12, pp. 1333–1336, 2009.

[30] J. M. Guralnik, L. P. Fried, and M. E. Salive, "Disability as a public health outcome in the aging population," *Annual Review of Public Health*, vol. 17, no. 1, pp. 25–46, 1996.

[31] M. W. Linn and B. S. Linn, "Self-evaluation of life function (self) scale: a short, comprehensive self-report of health for elderly adults," *Journals of Gerontology*, vol. 39, no. 5, pp. 603–612, 1984.

[32] D. Palacios-Ceña, R. Jiménez-García, V. Hernández-Barrera, C. Alonso-Blanco, P. Carrasco-Garrido, and C. Fernández-de-las-Peñas, "Has the prevalence of disability increased over the past decade (2000–2007) in elderly people? A Spanish population-based survey," *Journal of the American Medical Directors Association*, vol. 13, no. 2, pp. 136–142, 2012.

[33] T. M. Gill, T. E. Murphy, E. A. Gahbauer, and H. G. Allore, "Association of injurious falls with disability outcomes and nursing home admissions in community-living older persons," *American Journal of Epidemiology*, vol. 178, no. 3, pp. 418–425, 2013.

[34] S.-Y. Tsai, L.-Y. Chi, L.-S. Lee, and P. Chou, "Health-related quality of life among urban, rural, and island community elderly in Taiwan," *Journal of the Formosan Medical Association*, vol. 103, no. 3, pp. 196–204, 2004.

[35] Z. Liu, E. Albanese, S. Li et al., "Chronic disease prevalence and care among the elderly in urban and rural Beijing, China—a 10/66 Dementia Research Group cross-sectional survey," *BMC Public Health*, vol. 9, no. 1, article 394, 2009.

[36] M. R. Lavergne and G. Kephart, "Examining variations in health within rural Canada," *Rural and Remote Health*, vol. 12, article 1848, 2012.

[37] M. Fogelholm, R. Valve, P. Absetz et al., "Rural-urban differences in health and health behaviour: a baseline description of a community health-promotion programme for the elderly," *Scandinavian Journal of Public Health*, vol. 34, no. 6, pp. 632–640, 2006.

[38] G. L. Maddox, D. O. Clark, and K. Steinhauser, "Dynamics of functional impairment in late adulthood," *Social Science and Medicine*, vol. 38, no. 7, pp. 925–936, 1994.

[39] C. Boult, R. L. Kane, T. A. Louis, L. Boult, and D. McCaffrey, "Chronic conditions that lead to functional limitation in the elderly," *Journal of Gerontology*, vol. 49, no. 1, pp. M28–M36, 1994.

[40] L.-T. Tsai, M. Rantakokko, E. Portegijs et al., "Environmental mobility barriers and walking for errands among older people who live alone vs. with others," *BMC Public Health*, vol. 13, no. 1, article 1054, 2013.

[41] R. C. Shah, A. S. Buchman, S. Leurgans, P. A. Boyle, and D. A. Bennett, "Association of total daily physical activity with disability in community-dwelling older persons: a prospective cohort study," *BMC Geriatrics*, vol. 12, article 63, 2012.

[42] A. Bell and K. Jones, "The impossibility of separating age, period and cohort effects," *Social Science & Medicine*, vol. 93, pp. 163–165, 2013.

21

Novel Combined Training Approach Improves Sleep Quality but Does Not Change Body Composition in Healthy Elderly Women

Thiago Matheus da Silva Sousa,[1] Bruno Rodrigues,[2] Marco Carlos Uchida,[2] Olivia de Moraes Ruberti,[2] Paulo Adriano Schwingel,[3] Tânia Maria Gaspar Novais,[1] Paula de Lourdes Lauande Oliveira,[1] Fabiano de Jesus Furtado Almeida,[1,4] Janaína Oliveira Bentivi Pulcherio,[4] and Bruno Bavaresco Gambassi[1,2]

[1]*Physical Education Department, Ceuma University, São Luis, MA, Brazil*
[2]*Faculty of Physical Education, University of Campinas (UNICAMP), Campinas, SP, Brazil*
[3]*Human Performance Research Laboratory, University of Pernambuco, Petrolina, PE, Brazil*
[4]*Health Science Graduate Programs, Federal University of Maranhão, São Luis, MA, Brazil*

Correspondence should be addressed to Bruno Bavaresco Gambassi; professorbrunobavaresco@gmail.com

Academic Editor: Jean-Francois Grosset

The aim of this study was to investigate the effects of a novel combined training protocol on sleep quality and body composition of healthy elderly women. The study sample consisted of 8 sedentary elderly individuals with mean (±SD) of 67 (±8) years of age, 96.0 (±7.8) mg/dL fasting blood glucose, 94.4 (±36.1) mg/dL triglycerides, 179.1 (±22.4) mg/dL total cholesterol, 57.2 (±15.7) mg/dL high-density lipoprotein (HDL), 103.1 (±25.2) mg/dL low-density lipoprotein (LDL), 125.3 (±8.4) mmHg systolic blood pressure, and 72.6 (±10.1) mmHg diastolic blood pressure. The training protocol consisted of resistance training exercises (approximately 18-minute duration) combined with aerobic exercises (approximately 26-minute duration), performed interspersed in the same session, for 8 weeks (3 times a week), with a 24-hour interval rest between each session. Continuous variables were expressed as the mean (±standard deviation) and the paired sample t-test compares baseline with final measurement. The results showed a significant improvement ($p = 0.01$) in quality of sleep (4.9 ± 1.5 versus 3.8 ± 1.8 for total PSQI index) without body significant improvements in the fat-free mass (59.9 ± 4.0 versus 60.5 ± 4.4; $p = 0.20$) and fat mass (40.1 ± 4.0 versus 39.5 ± 4.4; $p = 0.20$) in healthy elderly women. In this sense, the novel combined training proposed may be an effective alternative or adjunct to present therapies aimed at improving the sleep quality in this population.

1. Introduction

Aging is a multifactorial process which depends on changes occurring at the cellular and molecular level and is associated with a morphofunctional decline affecting all physiological systems with a high degree of interindividual variability [1, 2].

Problems with sleep are common during aging; usually, increasing light sleep and shortening REM sleep can occur [3, 4]. These alterations may cause damage to coronary artery, increase in sympathetic tone, and negative changes in blood pressure [5, 6]. In addition, sleep problems are related to depression, obesity, arthritis, stroke, and lung diseases [6]. Additionally, as we age, there is also an increase in body fat, along with structural and functional changes in the muscular system [7–9]. Poor sleep quality and increased body fat increase the risk of developing cardiovascular and metabolic diseases [5, 6, 10].

On the other hand, the practice of physical exercises may improve sleep quality and body composition of the elderly [11–20]. The findings of Gambassi et al. [12], Ferris et al. [13], and Cai et al. [14] have shown that both resistance training and aerobic training were effective in improving sleep quality.

Additionally, some studies have found positive effects of resistance training on bone mineral density, muscle mass, and body fat of elderly women [15, 16, 21]. Moreover, other investigations have demonstrated positive effects of aerobic training on autonomic parameters and hemodynamic profile of older women [22–24]. In view of these results, we may speculate that combining the two modalities might expand the benefits of physical exercise for elderly women.

In this sense, the studies undertaken by Bonardi et al. [11], Rossi et al. [18], Burich et al. [19], and Guedes et al. [20] have all demonstrated that combined training improves sleep quality and promotes significant positive changes in body composition of older women.

In addition to the benefits of combined training practice in older women [11, 18–20], the American College of Sports Medicine (ACSM) [25] recommends the weekly practice of aerobic exercises (3 to 5 days per week) associated with resistance exercises (2 to 3 days per week). However, by having to fulfill several personal tasks, many people cannot practice physical exercises every day. Given this, we designed a dynamic combined training approach, which intersperses resistance and aerobic training, thus addressing the time limitation of the subjects and increasing adherence of the participants. This approach may also reduce monotony and mirror more faithfully the typical daily physical needs of the elderly, which are made up of a mixture of aerobic with resistance activities.

To the best of our knowledge, this is the first study investigating the effects of 8 weeks of combined exercise training (resistance training and aerobic exercises interspersed in the same session) on sleep quality and body composition in healthy elderly women.

We hypothesize that the 8-week practice of this novel alternative combined training protocol may improve the variables investigated.

2. Materials and Methods

2.1. Experimental Approach to the Problem. In the first visit to the laboratory, a meeting was held to explain the research proposal for the elderly. Furthermore, an informal but detailed lecture described and carefully laid out the exercises that would be performed by the elderly. For a week, the physical training protocol was performed only with the purpose of familiarizing the elderly with the combined training protocol proposed. After these adjustments, measurements of sleep quality and body composition were carried out. The same set of measurements were undertaken after 8 weeks of combined exercise training practice.

All participants, after being properly informed about the study proposal, the procedures they would be undergo, and their potential risks and benefits, signed a free informed consent form. This study was approved by the Research Ethics Committee of the University Ceuma (number 813,886), as recommended by the Resolution 466/12 of the National Health Council.

2.2. Subjects. The sample was selected using convenience sampling. Exclusion criteria were as follows: being physically active and having any impairment in the musculoskeletal system and/or chronic degenerative diseases. To ensure participants met the criteria, all subjects were asked to undergo the following tests: fasting blood glucose, triglycerides, total cholesterol, low-density lipoprotein (LDL), and high-density lipoprotein (HDL).

The study sample consisted of 8 sedentary elderly individuals with mean (±SD) of 67.0 (±8.0) years of age, 96.0 (±7.8) mg/dL fasting blood glucose, 94.4 (±36.1) mg/dL triglycerides, 179.1 (±22.4) mg/dL total cholesterol, 57.2 (±15.7) mg/dL HDL cholesterol, 103.1 (±25.2) mg/dL LDL cholesterol, 125.3 (±8.4) mmHg systolic blood pressure, and 72.6 (±10.1) mmHg diastolic blood pressure.

2.3. Procedures. Data collection was performed by physical education undergraduate students from the Ceuma University. They had been previously trained by researchers and professors from the Physical Education Department at Ceuma University, Sao Luis, Brazil.

2.4. Sleep Quality Assessment. The Pittsburgh Sleep Quality Index (PSQI) was used to assess sleep quality. This questionnaire encompasses components of subjective quality, habitual efficiency, latency, disorders, medication use, duration, and diurnal dysfunctions. Each component was evaluated on a scale of zero to three points and given the same value, with three points marking the negative end of the scale. The sum of the values constitutes the total PSQI index; scores between 0 and 4 would indicate good sleep quality, 5 and 10 poor sleep quality, and above 10 sleep disturbance [26].

2.5. Evaluating Body Composition. Total body mass in kilograms (kg) and height in centimeters (cm) were measured using an anthropometric scale PL-200 (Filizola S.A. Pesagem e Automacão, São Paulo, SP, Brazil), with an accuracy of 50 g and 0.1 cm, and properly calibrated (NBR ISO/IEC 17025:2005). Following these evaluations, body composition (fat mass and fat-free mass) was measured through a bioimpedance analyser (Maltron BF-906, Maltron International Ltd., Essex, UK). All participants were hydrated and refrained from using any diuretics for 7 days and eating solid food for 4 hours prior to the test. They were advised to urinate prior to evaluation, to wear light clothing, and to not carry any metal objects during body composition evaluation [27].

2.6. Combined Training Program. This novel proposal of combined exercise training consisted of resistance training (approximately 18 min) combined with aerobic exercise (approximately 26 min), performed interspersed in the same session, for 8 weeks (three times a week) with a 24-hour interval rest between each session. We used values between 11 and 13 of Borg scale [28] for measuring the intensity of physical training for walking.

The resistance training protocol [15] consisted of running leg press at 180°, seated row, leg curl, bench press, abductor machine, push-down, adductor machine, and biceps curl, alternated with a segment of 3 sets of 8 repetitions maximum

TABLE 1: Sleep quality and body composition before (in baseline) and after 8 weeks of a dynamic combined training program (n = 8).

Variables	Test moments		p values
	Before (n = 8) Mean ± SD	After (n = 8) Mean ± SD	
Sleep quality			
Total PSQI index	4.9 ± 1.5	3.8 ± 1.8*	0.01
Body composition			
Fat-free mass (%)	59.9 ± 4.0	60.5 ± 4.4	0.20
Fat mass (%)	40.1 ± 4.0	39.5 ± 4.4	0.20

SD: standard deviation of the mean; kg: kilograms; *significant difference between the pre- and posttest results.

performed with a rest interval of 1-min between sets. In this sense, the load enabled the attainment of a specified number of repetitions per set until reaching concentric fatigue. The exercises were performed by isotonic contraction lasting 3 seconds for the concentric phase and 3 seconds for the eccentric phase (6 seconds per repetition) [25].

We used the combined training protocol proposed by Gambassi et al. [29]. This program consists of stimulating the neuromuscular and cardiovascular systems in an intercalated fashion from beginning to end of a session. As the proposal of the present study is very dynamic, our group named the program *dynamic combined training method.*

Each session included the following (in this sequence): 10 minutes of walking; leg press at 180°; 2 minutes of walking; seated row; 2 minutes of walking; leg curl; 2 minutes of walking; bench press; 2 minutes of walking; abductor machine; 2 minutes of walking; push-down; 2 minutes of walking; adductor machine; 2 minutes of walking; biceps curl; 2 minutes of walking.

The elderly women were divided into 3 groups before performing this sequence. All of them remained under the close supervision of students and the researcher. This division allowed for better load control, rest interval, and the application of the Borg scale [28].

2.7. Statistical Analyses. The data were processed and analyzed using PRISM software (GraphPad Software, San Diego, CA, USA, Release 5.01). Initially, descriptive statistics were applied to the Kolmogorov–Smirnov test and to Bartlett's criteria. Continuous variables were expressed as the mean (±standard deviation) and the t-test paired sample compared baseline (pre-) with final (post)measurement. All analyses are two-tailed, confidence intervals (CI) are exact, and p values were calculated using a significance level of 5%. The magnitude of the differences in variables was calculated from the effect size [30].

3. Results and Discussion

Significant differences in the quality of sleep (p = 0.01; Δ = −1.1) were determined by comparing baseline and post-combined training results. In relation to this variable, large negative effect sizes were verified after 8 weeks of combined training [p = 0.01; d = −1,2 (95% CI −1,95 to −0,29)]. Changes were observed in fat-free mass (%) (p = 0.20; Δ = 0.6) and in body fat (%) (p = 0.20; Δ = −0.6). However, we did not find any significant differences between these variables (see Table 1 and Figure 1).

The findings of the present study partially confirm our hypothesis, since the dynamic combined training program (resistance training exercises combined with aerobic exercises interspersed in the same session) provided significant improvement in the sleep quality among healthy elderly women.

These findings emphasize the importance of physical training as a nonpharmacological strategy for improving sleep quality. In line with our results, Bonardi et al. [11] have demonstrated benefits of combined training (strength training plus aerobic exercise) on the quality of sleep in hypertensive elderly women. The combined training protocol adopted by these researchers was carried out for 10 weeks on alternate days for a total of 30 uninterrupted sessions. The protocol consisted of performing strength training with 50 to 60% of one repetition maximum (RM) intensity (one circuit with leg press at 45°, bench press, extensor bench, handle front, flexor bench-sitting, upright row, plantar flexion, seated row, and abdominals from 1st to 4th week, with a progression to 2 circuits between 5th and 10th week) plus aerobic exercises performed on treadmill for 20 minutes, from the 1st to the 4th week, with a progression to 30 minutes from the 5th to the 10th week.

Studies investigating the effects of combined training on sleep quality of the elderly remain scarce in the literature; however, some research has found that aerobic or resistance training improves sleep quality in the elderly and in postmenopausal women. Gambassi et al. [12] have compared elderly people practicing moderate-intensity resistance training for 12 weeks to sedentary elderly and found that the active population presented better sleep quality. Additionally, Ferris et al. [13] have shown that resistance training (circuit training method) performed for 3 months resulted in a significant improvement in sleep quality in the elderly.

As to aerobic training of moderate to high intensity, with a frequency of 3 times per week for 10 weeks, Cai et al. [14] have found and increase in melatonin and a significant improvement in sleep quality of postmenopausal women after 10 weeks of training. Each session of the exercise program of the study was comprised of warm-up with 10 to 15 minutes of stretching exercises for major muscles, step aerobics exercise in which the target HR was reached in the

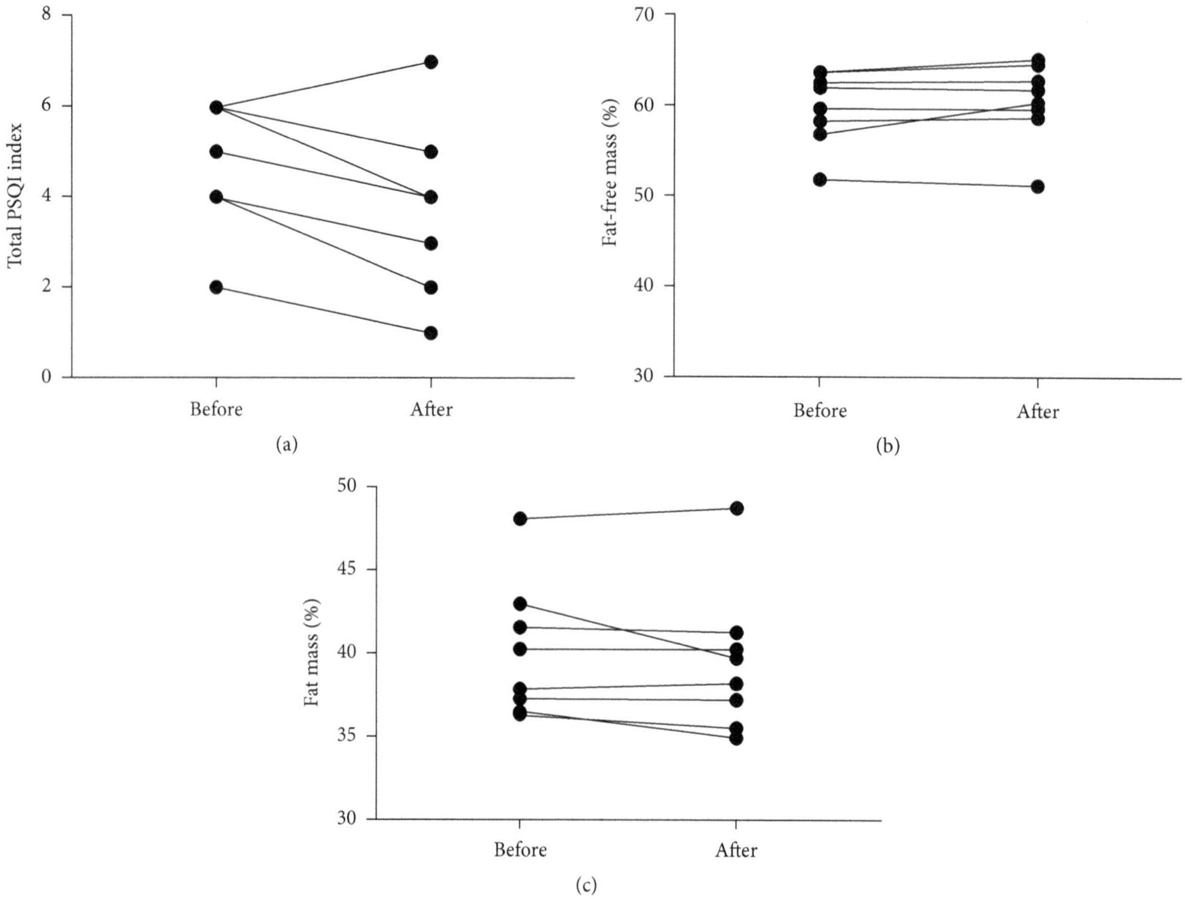

FIGURE 1: Changes in quality of sleep (a), fat-free mass (%) (b), and fat mass (%) (c) for each elderly woman before (in baseline) and after 8 weeks of a dynamic combined training program.

first 5 to 10 minutes and held for another 30 to 35 minutes, balance and cool-down for 10 to 15 minutes, and stretching and relaxation for 10 to 15 minutes. Additionally, Bonardi et al. [11] have also demonstrated positive effects on the sleep quality of elderly hypertensive patients after 10 weeks of aerobic training (exercises performed on the treadmill for 20 minutes from the 1st to the 4th week, with progression to 30 minutes from the 5th to the 10th week).

The findings of Bonardi et al. [11], Gambassi et al. [12], Ferris et al. [13], and Cai et al. [14] have shown that combined, resistance, or aerobic training was effective in improving sleep quality. Theories of energy conservation, thermoregulation, and body restoration are among the hypotheses to explain the mechanisms of sleep quality improvement through the practice of physical exercises [31]. However, more randomized controlled trials are needed to account for the mechanisms underlying exercise-induced improvements in sleep quality in the elderly.

As previously mentioned, in addition to the loss of strength during the aging process, negative changes affect body composition [7–9]. In the present study, we observed a reduction of fat percentage and increase in fat-free mass; however, no significant differences were found for these variables. In line with the results of the present study, Campos et al. [32] have not found any significant changes in body composition after the 12-week practice of 2 models of training (treadmill aerobic training plus strength training and strength training followed by aerobic treadmill training) performed by active elderly women. In both combined training protocols of their study [32], the traditional periodization was used (decreasing the volume and increasing the intensity over the weeks).

Unlike our study, the research carried out by Rossi et al. [18] has demonstrated significant benefits on body composition with increased fat-free mass and decreased fat mass in elderly women. These changes were observed after 16 weeks of combined training (27 min resistance training session plus 30 min aerobic training session performed in the same day). The intensity of the resistance training was adjusted every 4 weeks with increases in the RM zone. Concerning aerobic training, the intensity was adjusted after 4 weeks through the critical velocity.

Similarly, after performing the combined training, Burich et al. [19] have observed a significant reduction in body fat and in the waist-to-hip ratio in elderly. The combined training consisted of 20 minutes of cycling at 65% of heart rate reserve, followed by 20 minutes of strength training (3 sets of 15 RM in weeks 1 to 4; 3 sets of 12 RM in weeks 4 to 8; and 3 sets of 10 RM in weeks 8 to 12) three times a week for 12 weeks. Regarding the increase of muscular mass, the study corroborates the research undertaken by Rossi et al. [18]; Guedes et al. [20] have found an increase in the size of the vastus lateralis muscle after 8 weeks of combined training (2 sessions per week, consisting of 1 session of aerobic training and 1 session of resistance training lasting no more than 30 minutes a day, performed on different days).

The studies undertaken by Rossi et al. [18], Burich et al. [19], and Guedes et al. [20] have demonstrated that combined training promotes significant positive changes in the body composition of the elderly persons. However, we could not observe these changes in the present study, and our small sample might account for this discrepancy. A study conducted by Campos et al. [32] with a small number of participants (combined training with 5 participants) did not find any significant changes in body fat. Lack of dietary control may be another possible explanation for the results associated with body composition in our study.

The findings of the present study may inform strength and conditioning professionals on the possibility of achieving benefits on the quality of sleep of elderly women through a novel combined training approach.

The protocol used in this study (resistance and aerobic exercises interspersed in the same session) was not used in any of the other studies mentioned above. However, other training protocols have demonstrated positive effects on the variables investigated in our research [11, 18–20]. We should stress that the 24-session duration of our protocol presented benefits similar to studies using longer intervention time [11, 18–20]. Thus, the quality of sleep may be improved with our 8-week combined training protocol.

Our study has some limitations worth commuting upon. In this study, the absence of a control group, the lack of randomization, the small sample size, and the lack of diet control may be regarded as limitations. However, as a preliminary study, we raise issues for novel areas of research. In addition, we did not have the resources to assess aerobic capacity (VO2max) and perform exams at baseline after the combined training program. We found it difficult to have the elderly performing the 1 repetition maximum test in our previous research, since they manifested fear and the evaluation was underestimated. Thus, our groups have always adopted maximum repetitions protocols.

4. Conclusions

We conclude that the dynamic combined training program (resistance training and aerobic exercises interspersed in the same session) may provide benefits on the quality of sleep of elderly. However, our findings need further investigation, and adding randomized controlled trial would be required to lend support to our dynamic approach as an effective alternative or adjunct to present therapies aimed at improving sleep in this population

Conflicts of Interest

The authors report no conflicts of interest.

Authors' Contributions

All authors participated in the development of the research project, analysis and interpretation of the data, and preparation of the manuscript.

Acknowledgments

The authors are grateful to the volunteers who participated in this study. Bruno Rodrigues received grants from the Conselho Nacional de Desenvolvimento Científico e Tecnológico (BPQ-CNPq) and Fundaçao de Amparo à Pesquisa do Estado de São Paulo (FAPESP).

References

[1] E. N. de Moraes, F. L. de Moraes, and S. D. P. P. Lima, "Características biológicas e psicológicas do envelhecimento," *Revista Medicina Minas Gerais*, vol. 20, no. 1, pp. 67–73, 2010.

[2] H. J. Coelho Júnior, S. D. S. Aguiar, I. D. O. Gonçalves et al., "Sarcopenia is associated with high pulse pressure in older women," *Journal of Aging Research*, vol. 2015, Article ID 109824, 6 pages, 2015.

[3] J. R. Cooke and S. Ancoli-Israel, "Normal and abnormal sleep in the elderly," *Handbook of Clinical Neurology*, vol. 98, no. C, pp. 653–665, 2011.

[4] C. R. King, K. L. Knutson, P. J. Rathouz, S. Sidney, K. Liu, and D. S. Lauderdale, "Short sleep duration and incident coronary artery calcification," *Journal of the American Medical Association*, vol. 300, no. 24, pp. 2859–2866, 2008.

[5] M. Yuksel, A. Yildiz, M. Demir et al., "Effect of sleep quality on hemodynamic response to exercise and heart rate recovery in apparently healthy individuals," *Clinical and Investigative Medicine*, vol. 37, no. 6, pp. E352–E362, 2014.

[6] D. Foley, S. Ancoli-Israel, P. Britz, and J. Walsh, "Sleep disturbances and chronic disease in older adults: results of the 2003 national sleep foundation sleep in america survey," *Journal of Psychosomatic Research*, vol. 56, no. 5, pp. 497–502, 2004.

[7] J. A. Faulkner, L. M. Larkin, D. R. Claflin, and S. V. Brooks, "Age-related changes in the structure and function of skeletal muscles," *Clinical and Experimental Pharmacology and Physiology*, vol. 34, no. 11, pp. 1091–1096, 2007.

[8] T. Lang, T. Streeper, P. Cawthon, K. Baldwin, D. R. Taaffe, and T. B. Harris, "Sarcopenia: etiology, clinical consequences, intervention, and assessment," *Osteoporosis International*, vol. 21, no. 4, pp. 543–559, 2010.

[9] M. V. Narici and N. Maffulli, "Sarcopenia: characteristics, mechanisms and functional significance," *British Medical Bulletin*, vol. 95, no. 1, pp. 139–159, 2010.

[10] U. J. Jung and M. S. Choi, "Obesity and its metabolic complications: the role of adipokines and the relationship between obesity, inflammation, insulin resistance, dyslipidemia and nonalcoholic fatty liver disease," *International Journal of Molecular Sciences*, vol. 15, no. 4, pp. 6184–6223, 2014.

[11] J. M. T. Bonardi, L. G. Lima, G. O. Campos et al., "Effect of different types of exercise on sleep quality of elderly subjects," *Sleep Medicine*, vol. 25, pp. 122–129, 2016.

[12] B. B. Gambassi, F. J. F. Almeida, B. A. Sauaia et al., "Resistance training contributes to variability in heart rate and quality of the sleep in elderly women without comorbidities," *Journal of Exercise Physiology Online*, vol. 18, no. 6, pp. 112–123, 2015.

[13] L. T. Ferris, J. S. Williams, C. L. Shen, K. A. OKeefe, and K. B. Hale, "Resistance training improves sleep quality in older adultsa pilot study," *Journal of Sports Science and Medicine*, vol. 4, no. 3, pp. 354-60, 2005.

[14] Z.-Y. Cai, K. W.-C. Chen, and H.-J. Wen, "Effects of a group-based step aerobics training on sleep quality and melatonin levels in sleep-impaired postmenopausal women," *Journal of Strength and Conditioning Research*, vol. 28, no. 9, pp. 2597–2603, 2014.

[15] B. B. Gambassi, B. Rodrigues, D. J. Feriani et al., "Effects of resistance training of moderate intensity on heart rate variability, body composition, and muscle strength in healthy elderly women," *Sport Sciences for Health*, vol. 12, no. 3, pp. 389–395, 2016.

[16] S. W. Huang, J. W. Ku, L. F. Lin, C. D. Liao, L. C. Chou, and T. H. Liou, "Body composition influenced by progressive elastic band resistance exercise of sarcopenic obesity elderly women: a pilot randomized controlled trial," *European Journal of Physical and Rehabilitation Medicine*, 2017.

[17] S.-M. Park, Y.-S. Kwak, and J.-G. Ji, "The effects of combined exercise on health-related fitness, endotoxin, and immune function of postmenopausal women with abdominal obesity," *Journal of Immunology Research*, vol. 2015, Article ID 830567, 2015.

[18] F. E. Rossi, A. C. S. Fortaleza, L. M. Neves et al., "Combined training (aerobic plus strength) potentiates a reduction in body fat but demonstrates no difference on the lipid profile in post-menopausal women when compared with aerobic training with a similar training load," *Journal of Strength and Conditioning Research*, vol. 30, no. 1, pp. 226–234, 2016.

[19] R. Burich, S. Teljigović, E. Boyle, and G. Sjøgaard, "Aerobic training alone or combined with strength training affects fitness in elderly: randomized trial," *European Journal of Sport Science*, vol. 15, no. 8, pp. 773–783, 2015.

[20] J. M. Guedes, M. G. Bortoluzzi, L. P. Matte et al., "Effects of combined training on the strength, endurance and aerobic power in the elderly women," *Revista Brasileira de Medicina do Esporte*, vol. 22, no. 6, pp. 480–484, 2016.

[21] W. Kemmler, K. Engelke, D. Lauber, J. Weineck, J. Hensen, and W. A. Kalender, "Exercise effects on fitness and bone mineral density in early postmenopausal women: 1-Year EFOPS results," *Medicine and Science in Sports and Exercise*, vol. 34, no. 12, pp. 2115–2123, 2002.

[22] P. K. Stein, A. A. Ehsani, P. P. Domitrovich, R. E. Kleiger, and J. N. Rottman, "Effect of exercise training on heart rate variability in healthy older adults," *American Heart Journal*, vol. 138, no. 3 I, pp. 567–576, 1999.

[23] P. Carvalho, G. Barros, T. Melo, P. Santos, G. Oliveira, and I. DAmorim, "Efeito dos treinamentos aeróbio, resistido e concorrente na pressão arterial e morfologia de idosos normotensos e hipertensos," *Revista Brasileira de Atividade Física and Saúde*, vol. 3, no. 363, 2013.

[24] R. Perini, N. Fisher, A. Veicsteinas, and D. R. Pendergast, "Aerobic training and cardiovascular responses at rest and during exercise in older men and women," *Medicine and Science in Sports and Exercise*, vol. 34, no. 4, pp. 700–708, 2002.

[25] American College of Sports Medicine, *Diretrizes do ACSM para os Testes de Esforço e sua Prescrição*, Editora Guanabara Koogan, 2007.

[26] D. J. Buysse, C. F. Reynolds III, T. H. Monk, S. R. Berman, and D. J. Kupfer, "The Pittsburgh Sleep Quality Index: a new instrument for psychiatric practice and research," *Psychiatry Research*, vol. 28, no. 2, pp. 193–213, 1989.

[27] H. C. Lukaski, "Requirements for clinical use of bioelectrical impedance analysis (BIA)," *Annals of the New York Academy of Sciences*, vol. 873, pp. 72–76, 1999.

[28] G. Borg, *Borgs Perceived Exertion and Pain Scales*, Champaign: Human Kinetics, 1998.

[29] B. B. Gambassi, M. C. Uchida, T. M. S. Sousa, P. A. Schwingel, J. O. B. Pulcherio, and F. J. F. Almeida, "Effects of a new combined training approach on components of the functional autonomy of healthy elderly women," *Journal of Exercise Physiology Online*, vol. 20, no. 3, pp. 45–52, 2017.

[30] J. Cohen, *Statistical Power Analysis for the Behavioral Sciences*, Lawrence Erlbaum Associate, Routledge, Hillsdale, Mich, USA, 2nd edition, 1988.

[31] P. J. F. Martins, M. T. D. Mello, and S. Tufik, "Exercício e sono," *Revista Brasileira de Medicina do Esporte*, vol. 7, no. 1, pp. 28–36, 2001.

[32] A. L. P. Campos, L. D. S. Del Ponte, A. S. Cavalli, M. D. R. Afonso, J. F. G. Schild, and F. F. Reichert, "Efeitos do treinamento concorrente sobre aspectos da saúde de idosas," *Revista Brasileira de Cineantropometria e Desempenho Humano*, pp. 437–447, 2013.

22

Matrix Metalloproteinase-1 Gene Polymorphism Associated with Ultrasound-Assessed Carotid Thickness among Older Adults

Gilberto Santos Morais Junior,[1] Nathalia Oliveira Rodrigues,[1] Adriane Dallanora Henriques,[1] Audrey Cecília Tonet-Furioso,[1,2] Ciro José Brito,[3] Lucy Oliveira Gomes,[2] Clayton Franco Moraes,[1,2] and Otávio Toledo Nóbrega[1]

[1]*Universidade de Brasília, 70910-900 Brasília, DF, Brazil*
[2]*Universidade Católica de Brasília, 71966-700 Águas Claras, DF, Brazil*
[3]*Universidade Federal de Juiz de Fora, 36036-330 Juiz de Fora, MG, Brazil*

Correspondence should be addressed to Otávio Toledo Nóbrega; otnobrega@gmail.com

Academic Editor: Carmela R. Balistreri

Background and Aim. Due to the high incidence of vascular diseases, it is necessary to identify new circulating or structural markers for predicting risk for chronic diseases. Some studies suggest that MMP1 gene polymorphisms are associated with the enzyme expression levels in situ (e.g., in atherosclerotic plaques). *Objectives.* Thus, the study of this polymorphism may help understanding the pathophysiology of coronary disease. *Methods.* We performed cross-sectional clinical and laboratory evaluations (including measurement of intima-media thickness of carotid arteries) and genotyping of the MMP1 SNP rs495366 (A/G) in 366 elderly people. *Results.* No significant differences between genotypes were noted for biochemical, metabolic, inflammatory, or clinical variables except for a significant difference in intima-media thickness for the left carotid artery and a trend toward significance for the right counterpart. *Conclusion.* Carriers of the allele associated with lower MMP1 expression (allele A) presented greater carotid thickness. We suggest that the phenomenon can be explained by impaired remodeling of the arterial wall (poor degradation of collagen fibers in this scenario), yielding carotid wall thickening and a greater intrinsic risk for cerebrovascular events.

1. Introduction

The World Health Organization (WHO) reports that 60% of deaths worldwide are due to chronic diseases, mainly vascular-related disorders [1], and estimates that this value will reach 80% in developing countries by 2020 [2]. In Brazil, approximately one-third of the deaths of individuals over 60 years of age are caused by vascular events, a proportion similar to that in the Federal District [3]. Circulatory disorders associate with clinical and biological findings such as obesity, systemic arterial hypertension, type 2 diabetes mellitus, dyslipidemias, and genetic factors that, altogether, interact and act as risk factors to the onset and progression of vascular diseases and consequently with the mortality of affected patients. In this context, atherosclerosis stands out as an underlying cause, as it triggers the highest proportion of fatal or disabling events [4].

Atherosclerosis results from chronic inflammation of the arterial wall triggered in response to endogenously modified structures, particularly oxidized lipoproteins. It is widely recognized that stimulation by circulating mediators of innate and adaptive immune responses leads to further vascular wall damage, promoting disease progression [5] with evidence that the imbalance between pro- and anti-inflammatory factors plays a critical role in early vascular endothelial dysfunction [6].

Atherosclerosis is a progressive and irreversible process resulting from a series of specific cellular and molecular factors that affect large and medium elastic or muscular arteries [7]. The main concern is the possibility of causing thrombosis or severe arterial stenosis, leading to life-threatening adverse events, such as myocardial infarction, stroke, and ischemic injuries of the kidneys and intestines, as well as other manifestations. Avoiding morbidity and mortality from circulatory causes justifies the significant interest in the identification of asymptomatic patients at risk. In this context, the thickening of the intima-media layer of the common carotid artery is a subclinical biomarker that is easy to measure with reasonable predictive capacity for relevant vascular events [8]. There is a body of evidence in the literature that associates measurements of carotid intima-media thickness (cIMT) with cardiovascular risk [9–11]. On what concerns the cerebrovascular setting, Eigenbrodt et al. [12] and Baldassarre et al. [13] independently presented evidence for an association between carotid thickness and stroke events, suggesting that this measure can be a valuable prognostic biomarker.

The development of a vulnerable atherosclerotic plaque involves intense inflammation in the presence of lymphocytes, macrophages, and mast cells. In this milieu, matrix metalloproteinases (MMPs) are typically secreted by macrophages that progressively degrade the collagenous components of the fibrous capsule. MMPs are endopeptidases that contain zinc and/or calcium within their active sites and degrade extracellular matrix proteins, such as collagen fibers, thus compromising the integrity of the endothelial basement membrane and plaque stability with risk of rupture of advanced atheromas [4, 14].

Because cardiovascular diseases remain the leading cause of death worldwide, it is necessary to identify new circulating or structural markers for predicting risk for chronic diseases. Studies on the expression of matrix metalloproteinases are important for understanding the biological processes such as cell differentiation and function, related to pathological processes [15], such as coronary artery disease [16]. Some studies suggest that MMP1 gene polymorphisms are associated with enzyme expression levels, including in situ levels (e.g., in atherosclerotic plaques) [17]. For example, MMP1 gene expression may be influenced by a single-nucleotide polymorphism (SNP) in the promoter region of the gene located at the 11q22.3 position, which results in differential MMP1 expression according to the allelic variant [15, 17].

In this context, Chen et al. [18] used the high-throughput, genome-wide scanning procedure that identified an association between the rs495366 SNP of the MMP1 gene and the circulating, serum levels of MMP1. Thus, the study of this polymorphism may help elucidate the pathophysiology of vascular diseases. The general objective of the present study was to test the association between the rs495366 polymorphism of the MMP1 gene with vascular risk factors found in samples of an elderly population of the Brazilian Federal District.

2. Methods

2.1. Sample. A sample of noninstitutionalized patients aged 60 years or older without clinical symptoms of severe atherosclerosis were recruited between 2011 and 2013 in two general geriatrics outpatient clinics (Geriatric Unit of the Catholic University of Brasília (UCB) and Medical Center for the Elderly of the University of Brasília (UnB)) located in the Metropolitan Region of the Federal District, Brazil. The sample was used to assess the risk for vascular events through a cross-sectional evaluation. Patients recruited at UnB were sent to the Hospital of the Catholic University of Brasília (HUCB) to obtain a standardized baseline evaluation with a clinical protocol conducted by the same medical team.

Inclusion criteria enrolled patients spontaneously seeking primary or secondary care for vascular events at the aforementioned health sites. The exclusion criteria consisted of presenting (i) a clinical history of autoimmune disease or neoplasms of any type, current or past; (ii) report of a pulmonary condition compatible with severe symptomatic obstruction; (iii) severe chronic renal disease determined by creatinine clearance $<25\,\text{ml}\cdot\text{min}^{-1}$; and/or (iv) a clinical history of recurrent infections or chronic inflammation.

The project was approved by the Research Ethics Committee of the School of Medicine of UnB under Protocol number 061/2011. All participants signed an informed consent form.

2.2. Clinical and Biochemical Evaluations. The clinical examination consisted of a general evaluation of the patient with measurement of resting blood pressure (BP), cardiac and pulmonary auscultation, superficial and deep palpation of the abdomen, and inspection and digital palpation of the lower limbs according to routine semiological standards. A questionnaire was also administered to obtain information about the socioeconomic profile and medication used, recording the active principles consumed and their classification. Previous circulatory events, such as myocardial infarction or stroke, as well as lifestyle aspects, such as sedentary lifestyle and smoking, were also recorded.

The diagnosis of type 2 diabetes included self-reporting of the condition and fasting glycated hemoglobin (HbA1c) ≥ 6.5%, considering the consumption of hypoglycemic agents or insulin. Individuals were considered to be physically active if they reported 30 minutes or more of exercise for at least four days of the week, whereas smoking was defined as consumption of >100 cigarettes in a lifetime. For the metabolic analysis, the following measurements were obtained according to routine clinical biochemistry and are expressed in standard units: blood glucose, glycated hemoglobin (HbA1c), total cholesterol and fractions, triglycerides, high-sensitivity C-reactive protein, and thyroid-stimulating hormone (TSH). The anthropometric analyses evaluated the body mass index (BMI, in kg/m^2) and the waist circumference (cm) of each subject.

2.3. Measurement of Intima-Media Thickness. The carotid intima-media thickness (cIMT) was determined noninvasively in all participants using a high-resolution ultrasound (Philips, model IE 33) with a 3–9 MHz linear transducer. Measurements of cIMT were performed bilaterally on the distal wall of the common carotid artery bulb and on the origin of the internal carotid artery, using an automated edge-detection software that is capable of displaying the maximum value of 150 measurements of any 10 mm segment [19]. The maximum cIMT was measured manually as the mean of three independent measurements. All clinical procedures and imaging evaluations were performed at the UCB Hospital.

2.4. MMP1 Genotyping. Total genomic DNA was obtained using a commercial extraction kit (QIAamp DNA Mini Kit, Qiagen, Brazil). Genotyping reactions were performed using qPCR (real-time PCR) with TaqMan® Universal Master Mix reagent and an assay specific for SNP rs495366 from Thermo Fisher (Massachusetts, USA), with probes designed to detected the flanking regions and the polymorphic variation based on the TTGACCTAAATTTCTGCAAACTATA[R]TCTTATGG TTATGACTCTTTTTGT sequence. The denaturation/ extension times and number of cycles used followed the standard program on the equipment used, the QuantStudio 3 Real-Time PCR System (Thermo Fisher®, Massachusetts, USA).

2.5. Assessment of Inflammation. At the time of the biochemical evaluations, whole blood was collected. The serum obtained was frozen at −80°C and later thawed for evaluation of immunological mediators. Cytokine concentrations were assessed by traditional immunoenzymatic assays (ELISA) using specific kits manufactured by BD Biosciences (San Diego, CA, USA) used according to the manufacturer's protocols.

Briefly, each serum sample was processed in duplicate together with the standard sample of the mediator provided by the kit, and the readings were made in a BioTek® reader (Winooski, VT, USA). Standard curves for each cytokine were generated by linear regression, and the concentration in each serum sample was determined by interpolation from the corresponding curve.

2.6. Statistical Analysis. To test for differences between clinical, biochemical, and anthropometric measures in the sample according to MMP1 genotypes, our statistical analyses compared measures of central tendency by the Mann–Whitney test (continuous variables) or frequencies by the chi-square test. The normal distribution of all variables was assessed using the Kolmogorov–Smirnov test. For these analyses, $P \leq 0.05$ was adopted as the significance level. All analyses were performed with the Statistical Package for Social Sciences (SPSS) for Windows (version 17.0).

Table 1: Anthropometric, clinical, metabolic, and inflammatory variables of the sample according to the genotypic group.

Variables	rs495366 genotypes GG (n = 174)	A_ (n = 192)	P
Age (years)	79.5 ± 9.3	79.2 ± 8.3	0.745
Male (%)	32.2	28.1	0.398
BMI (kg·m^{-2})	26.9 ± 4.9	26.9 ± 5.1	0.841
WC (cm)	96.3 ± 12.4	94.7 ± 11.4	0.169
SBP (mm Hg)	138.8 ± 20.4	142.0 ± 21.2	0.150
DBP (mm Hg)	78.1 ± 11.0	77.2 ± 11.5	0.268
SAH (%)	76.4	76.0	0.929
Glucose level (mg·dl^{-1})	101.8 ± 22.6	105.4 ± 43.0	0.659
HbA1c (%)	6.0 ± 0.9	6.1 ± 1.3	0.365
DM2 (%)	25.3	21.4	0.374
Total cholesterol (mg·dl^{-1})	194.4 ± 40.0	203.2 ± 84.2	0.297
Triglycerides (mg·dl^{-1})	131.5 ± 58.8	135.3 ± 62.6	0.498
HDL-c (mg·dl^{-1})	51.7 ± 12.9	51.5 ± 13.2	0.988
LDL-c (mg·dl^{-1})	113.2 ± 34.1	115.9 ± 36.2	0.407
VLDL-c (mg·dl^{-1})	29.3 ± 13.4	30.0 ± 13.9	0.482
Creatinine clearance (ml·min^{-1})	60.3 ± 26.4	55.6 ± 24.1	0.120
CRP (mg·dl^{-1})	1.61 [2.25]	1.70 [3.10]	0.636
TSH (mIU·l^{-1})	2.16 [2.05]	2.15 [2.53]	0.976
TNF	0.00 [0.60]	0.00 [0.34]	0.684
IL12	0.00 [8.92]	0.00 [8.93]	0.551
IL10	0.84 [2.84]	1.24 [2.94]	0.599
Sedentary (%)	59.2	63.0	0.453
Smoker (%)	19.5	17.2	0.561
Right cIMT (mm)	1.28 ± 0.60	1.40 ± 0.66	0.087
Left cIMT (mm)	1.27 ± 0.60	1.44 ± 0.64	0.041

Data are expressed as average ± standard deviation for normally distributed continuous parameters, relative frequencies within genotype for categorical features, and median with the interquartile range in brackets for nonnormally distributed continuous variables. BMI = body mass index; WC = waist circumference; HbA1c = glycated hemoglobin A1c; DM2 = type 2 diabetes mellitus; VLDL-c = very low-density lipoprotein cholesterol; LDL-c = low-density lipoprotein cholesterol; HDL-c = high-density lipoprotein cholesterol; SBP = systolic blood pressure; DBP = diastolic blood pressure; SAH = systemic arterial hypertension; CRP = C-reactive protein; TSH = thyroid-stimulating hormone; cIMT = carotid intima-media thickness.

3. Results

A total of 366 people aged 60 years and over without clinical symptoms of severe atherosclerosis consecutively treated at the geriatrics units of the participating institutions were included in the study. SNP rs495366 genotyping revealed that homozygotes for the A allele constituted a minority (n = 30) and were added to the heterozygous group to form a single group (n = 174) of carriers of the A (A_) allele. The GG genotype group included 192 patients with similar mean age and sex ratio. The genotype proportions did not violate the Hardy–Weinberg equilibrium ($P > 0.05$).

Inferential statistics of the anthropometric, metabolic, and biochemical variables analyzed the individuals according to the genotype groups defined and are presented in Table 1. In purely descriptive terms, the sample was marked by a high prevalence of biochemical and metabolic disorders such as overweight, type 2 diabetes, dyslipidemia, and systemic arterial hypertension, as expected in elderly individuals from a developing country [20]. However, no variations in frequencies or mean values of these findings were found according to MMP1 genotypes.

Similar to the biochemical and metabolic variables, no significant differences between groups were noted for clinical variables except for a sufficient difference in intima-media thickness on the left carotid artery (P = 0.041) and a trend toward a significance difference on the right counterpart territory (P = 0.087). Regarding the behavioral variables that increase the risk for vascular events, such as sedentary lifestyle or smoking, no statistically or clinically significant differences were observed.

4. Discussion

The main finding of the present study was a significant difference in the intima-media thickness of the left carotid, which was 0.17 mm thicker in carriers of the rs495366 A allele compared with carriers of the GG genotype. The left common carotid artery may be considered more vulnerable to atherosclerosis compared with the right and may be more prone to the development of atherosclerotic plaques and consequently strokes [21, 22] due to greater blood flow in this region, potentiating health problems [23]. Based on the increase in intima wall thickness evidenced here, we can assume that carriers of the A allele of rs495366 SNP may be more prone to stroke, as Lorenz et al. [24] demonstrated that an increase in carotid thickness of 0.10 mm increases the risk for stroke by 17%.

Several genetic factors are considered determinants for the development of atherosclerotic disease. Approximately 400 genes may be involved in the regulation of various factors, such as endothelial function, coagulation, inflammation, and lipid metabolism [25]. Among these, we highlight the MMP1 (collagenase-1) polymorphism given that an imbalance in its activity is reported in the literature as a factor that contributes to plaque instability in atheromas [26].

Increased MMP1 expression in the early stages of an atherosclerotic process may be a compensatory response that involves tissue remodeling under physiological stress to delay the progression to thromboembolic events [26]. However, one cannot ignore the hypothesis that MMP1 plays a pathophysiological role via excessive accumulation as a result of smooth muscle cell accumulation in a necrotic core under a fibrous cap where it weakens high-stress regions [6], predisposing the plaque to rupture [4, 27]. Despite this hypothesis, MMP1 activation is essential for vascular wall remodeling to prevent excessive growth of the intima layer in response to lesions mainly by migration or reprogramming of vascular smooth muscle cells. In this sense, it is plausible that the observed association arises from an impaired ability to promote remodeling among carriers of the A allele, which is associated with reduced enzyme expression in the tissues of carriers of this allelic form [6]. Galon et al. [16] suggested that lower MMP1 expression leads to the accumulation of extracellular matrix proteins, contributing to the early formation of vascular lesions and structural changes that promote rupture of atheromatous plaques.

The protective role of enhanced MMP1 expression is supported by Lemaître et al. [28] and by Ye et al. [26], suggesting that increased MMP1 expression during atherogenesis results in smaller and less severe lesions with a lower collagen content, which is compatible with negative remodeling (degradation of the collagen matrix) that delays the progression of atherogenesis and results in more stable lesions.

Regarding the validity of our findings, assuming that both genotypic groups were approximately equal in size, the equation by Whitley and Ball [29] was used to calculate a posteriori the power of our study to detect a change in carotid thickness. Taking into account the left carotid measurements where the difference in mean values between genotypes was 0.17 mm and the general standard deviation of the variable was 0.62 mm, the standardized difference to be detected was 0.17/0.62 = 0.274 (0.3). Thus, the number of participants needed to detect a difference with a discriminatory power of 80% and a 5% statistical significance level was calculated as 176 subjects in each group. Our study was very close to the sample size needed to consider it representative, as it was only short two individuals in the group of G homozygotes.

It should be recognized that the onset of atherosclerotic plaques is multifactorial mostly due to unhealthy lifestyle habits, such as a diet rich in lipids and carbohydrates, a sedentary lifestyle, and smoking. Although it was not possible to investigate the dietary intake of the patients, our study contributes to the literature by demonstrating that the latter aspects were similar between groups and thus did not significantly influence the conclusions presented. Similarly, and consistent with several studies that analyzed the impact of different risk factors for stroke in several populations worldwide [30–34], the frequencies of classic risk factors for stroke (namely, hypertension, dyslipidemias, obesity, and diabetes) did not differ between genotype groups, possibly revealing an allelic effect that outweighs the classic determinants when homogeneous between groups. Even systemic inflammatory factors, which are associated with lateral inequality between carotid branches [35], do not seem to have an effect in our recent findings. And despite the lack of an actual assessment on MMP1 levels, the authors consider that such limitation was addressed and, to some extent, lessened by an investigation that relied precisely on a genetic variation with solid evidence for an effect on MMP1 levels. Therefore, our conditions considered the best possible proxy.

However, it is important to recognize that matrix degradation is determined not only by the tissue expression of metalloproteinases but also by the activation pattern of the enzymes in the extracellular space, the degree of inhibition promoted by endogenous inhibitors, and the presence and activity of enzymes that do not directly degrade the metalloprotease matrix. Thus, a better understanding of the elements involved and the dynamics of matrix degradation in the fibrous plaque in high-stress regions is needed to provide information on the progression of stable and unstable plaques in the circulatory tree [6].

5. Conclusion

In this study, subjects carrying the allele associated with lower MMP1 expression exhibited increased left carotid intima-media thickness, and this finding is presumed to increase the risk of stroke among elderly outpatients. When imbalanced, MMP1 activity in advanced atheroma may be one of the contributing factors of plaque instability. Thus, we assume that increased MMP1 expression in the early stages of atherogenesis may be a beneficial adaptive response.

Conflicts of Interest

The authors declare that no potential conflicts of interest exist.

Authors' Contributions

Gilberto Santos Morais Junior and Nathalia Oliveira Rodrigues assessed MMP1 genotypes; Audrey Cecília Tonet-Furioso and Adriane Dallanora Henriques executed genotyping quality control procedures; Lucy Oliveira Gomes and Clayton Franco Moraes executed the medical component of the study; Gilberto Santos Morais Junior and Ciro José Brito conducted anthropometric assessments on subjects; Clayton Franco Moraes and Otávio Toledo Nóbrega designed and coordinated the study as well as analyzed the results; Gilberto Santos Morais Junior, Nathalia Oliveira Rodrigues, and Otávio Toledo Nóbrega participated in the preparation of the original manuscript.

Acknowledgments

The research was supported with Grants nos. 445692/2014 and 442925/2014 from CNPq as well as with Grant nos. 193.000.967-2015 and 193.001.240 2016 from FAPDF, with a stipend to Gilberto Santos Morais Junior (CAPES) and a fellowship for productivity in research to Otávio Toledo Nóbrega (CNPq).

References

[1] World Health Organization, *Global Status Report on Noncommunicable Diseases 2014*, WHO, Geneva, Switzerland, 2014.

[2] Á. Avezum, L. N. Maia, and M. Nakazone, "Cenário das Doenças Cardiovasculares no Mundo Moderno," in *Manual de Cardiologia*, pp. 1–5, Atheneu, São Paulo, SP, Brazil, 2012.

[3] E. N. Gaui, G. M. M. Oliveira, and C. H. Klein, "Mortality by heart failure and ischemic heart disease in Brazil from 1996 to 2011," *Arquivos Brasileiros de Cardiologia*, vol. 102, no. 6, pp. 557–565, 2014.

[4] G. H. Tison, M. Guo, M. J. Blaha et al., "Multisite extracoronary calcification indicates increased risk of coronary heart disease and all-cause mortality: the Multi-Ethnic Study of Atherosclerosis," *Journal of Cardiovascular Computer Tomography*, vol. 9, no. 5, pp. 406–414, 2015.

[5] Z. Mallat, "Matrix metalloproteinase-8 and the regulation of blood pressure, vascular inflammation, and atherosclerotic lesion growth," *Circulation Research*, vol. 105, no. 9, pp. 921–929, 2009.

[6] A. C. Newby, "Dual role of matrix metalloproteinases (matrixins) in intimal thickening and atherosclerotic plaque rupture," *Physiological Reviews*, vol. 85, no. 1, pp. 1–31, 2005.

[7] M. Gottlieb, G. Bonardi, and E. Moriguchi, "Fisiopatologia e aspectos inflamatórios da aterosclerose," *Scientia Medica*, vol. 15, no. 3, pp. 203–207, 2005.

[8] R. Flore, F. R. Ponziani, G. Tinelli et al., "New modalities of ultrasound-based intima-media thickness, arterial stiffness and non-coronary vascular calcifications detection to assess cardiovascular risk," *European Review Medical and Pharmacological Sciences*, vol. 19, no. 8, pp. 1430–1441, 2015.

[9] E. S. Adamsson, G. Östling, M. Rosvall et al., "Carotid intima-media thickness is associated with incidence of hospitalized atrial fibrillation," *Atherosclerosis*, vol. 233, no. 2, pp. 673–678, 2014.

[10] Y. Zhang, E. Guallar, Y. Qiao et al., "Is carotid intima-media thickness as predictive as other noninvasive techniques for the detection of coronary artery disease?," *Arteriosclerosis, Thrombosis, and Vascular Biology*, vol. 34, no. 7, pp. 1341–1345, 2014.

[11] T. Z. Naqvi and M. S. Lee, "Carotid intima-media thickness and plaque in cardiovascular risk assessment," *JACC: Cardiovascular Imaging*, vol. 7, no. 10, pp. 1025–1038, 2014.

[12] M. L. Eigenbrodt, G. W. Evans, K. M. Rose et al., "Bilateral common carotid artery ultrasound for prediction of incident strokes using intima-media thickness and external diameter: an observational study," *Cardiovascular Ultrasound*, vol. 11, no. 22, p. 1, 2013.

[13] D. Baldassarre, A. Hamsten, F. Veglia et al., "Measurements of carotid intima-media thickness and of interadventitia common carotid diameter improve prediction of cardiovascular events: results of the IMPROVE (carotid intima media thickness [IMT] and IMT-progression as predictors of vascular events in a high risk European population) study," *Journal of the American College of Cardiology*, vol. 60, no. 16, pp. 1489–1499, 2012.

[14] S. H. Da Silva and R. N. Moresco, "Cardiac biomarkers for assessment of acute coronary syndrome," *Scientia Medica*, vol. 21, no. 3, pp. 132–142, 2011.

[15] Y. C. Cheng, W. H. L. Kao, B. D. Mitchell et al., "Genome-wide association scan identifies variants near matrix metalloproteinase (MMP) genes on chromosome 11q21-22 strongly associated with serum MMP-1 levels," *Circulation: Cardiovascular Genetics*, vol. 2, no. 4, pp. 329–337, 2009.

[16] M Z. Galon, G. C. Meireles, S. Kreimer et al., "Clinical and angiographic profile in coronary artery disease: hospital outcome with emphasis on the very elderly," *Arquivos Brasileiros de Cardiologia*, vol. 95, no. 4, pp. 422–429, 2010.

[17] H. L. Huang, S. Wu, L. A. Hsu et al., "Genetic variants associated with circulating MMP1 levels near matrix metalloproteinase genes on chromosome 11q21-22 in Taiwanese: interaction with obesity," *BMC Medical Genetics*, vol. 14, no. 14, p. 30, 2013.

[18] Y. Chen, N. B. Nixon, P. T. Dawes, and D. L. Mattey, "Influence of variations across the MMP-1 and -3 genes on the serum levels of MMP-1 and -3 and disease activity in rheumatoid arthritis," *Genes and Immunity*, vol. 13, no. 1, pp. 29–37, 2012.

[19] L. E. Chambless, M. M. Zhong, D. Arnett et al., ""Variability in B-mode ultrasound measurements in the Atherosclerosis Risk in Communities (ARIC) study," *Ultrasound in Medicine and Biology*, vol. 22, no. 5, pp. 545–554, 1996.

[20] O. T. Nóbrega, V. P. Faleiros, and J. L. Telles, "Gerontology in the developing Brazil: Achievements and challenges in public policies," *Geriatrics Gerontology International*, vol. 9, no. 2, pp. 135–139, 2009.

[21] X. Luo, Y. Yang, T. Cao, and Z. Li, "Differences in left and right carotid intima-media thickness and the associated risk factors," *Clinical Radiology*, vol. 66, no. 5, pp. 393–398, 2011.

[22] C. Yuan, C. W. K. Lai, L. W. C. Chan et al., "Cumulative effects of hypertension, dyslipidemia, and chronic kidney disease on carotid atherosclerosis in Chinese patients with type 2 diabetes mellitus," *Journal of Diabetes Research*, vol. 2014, Article ID 179686, 7 pages, 2014.

[23] K. F. Layton, D. F. Kallmes, H. J. Cloft, E. P. Lindell, and V. S. Cox, "Bovine aortic arch variant in humans: clarification of a common misnomer," *American Journal of Neuroradiology*, vol. 27, no. 7, pp. 1541-1542, 2006.

[24] M. W. Lorenz, H. S. Markus, M. L. Bots, M. Rosvall, and M. Sitzer, "Prediction of clinical cardiovascular events with carotid intima-media thickness: a systematic review and meta-analysis," *Circulation*, vol. 115, no. 4, pp. 459–467, 2007.

[25] P. A. Doevendans, W. Jukema, W. Spiering, J. C. Defesche, and J. J. P. Kastelein, "Molecular genetics and gene expression in atherosclerosis," *International Journal of Cardiology*, vol. 80, no. 2-3, pp. 161–172, 2001.

[26] S. Ye, C. R. Gale, and C. N. Martyn, "Variation in the matrix metalloproteinase-1 gene and risk of coronary heart disease," *European Heart Journal*, vol. 24, no. 18, pp. 1668–1671, 2003.

[27] E. Cavusoglu, J. D. Marmur, S. Hegde et al., "Relation of baseline plasma MMP-1 levels to long-term all-cause mortality in patients with known or suspected coronary artery disease referred for coronary angiography," *Atherosclerosis*, vol. 239, no. 1, pp. 268–275, 2015.
[28] V. Lemaître, T. K. O'Byrne, A. C. Borczuk et al., "ApoE knockout mice expressing human matrix metalloproteinase-1 in macrophages have less advanced atherosclerosis," *Journal of Clinical Investigation*, vol. 107, no. 10, pp. 1227–1234, 2001.
[29] E. Whitley and J. Ball, "Statistics review 4: sample size calculations," *Critical Care*, vol. 6, no. 4, pp. 335–341, 2002.
[30] M. L. F. Chaves, "Acidente vascular encefálico: conceituação e fatores de risco," *Revista Brasileira de Hipertensão*, vol. 7, no. 4, pp. 372–382, 2000.
[31] T. Gezmu, D. Schneider, K. Demissie, Y. Lin, and M. S. Gizzi, "Risk factors for acute stroke among South Asians compared to other racial/ethnic groups," *PLoS One*, vol. 9, no. 9, Article ID e108901, 2014.
[32] A. P. Mansur, M. F. M. de Souza, A. Timerman et al., "Tendência do Risco de Morte por Doenças Circulatórias, Cerebrovasculares e Isquêmicas do Coração em 11 Capitais do Brasil de 1980 a 1998," *Arquivos Brasileiros de Cardiologia*, vol. 87, no. 5, pp. 641–648, 2002.
[33] M. G. dos Santos, M. Pegoraro, F. Sandrini, and E. C. Macuco, "Risk factors for the development of atherosclerosis in childhood and adolescence," *Arquivos Brasileiros de Cardiologia*, vol. 90, no. 4, pp. 276–283, 2008.
[34] L. Copstein, J. G. Fernandes, and G. A. N. Bastos, "Prevalence and risk factors for stroke in a population of Southern Brazil," *Arquivos de Neuro-Psiquiatria*, vol. 71, no. 5, pp. 294–300, 2013.
[35] W. Machado-Silva, A. D. Henriques, G. D. Souza et al., "serum immune mediators independently associate with atherosclerosis in the left (but not right) carotid territory of older individuals," *Journal of Stroke and Cerebrovascular Diseases*, vol. 25, no. 12, pp. 2851–2858, 2016.

23

The Influence of Video Game Training with and without Subpatelar Bandage in Mobility and Gait Speed on Elderly Female Fallers

Isabela Feitosa de Carvalho,[1] **Gianluca Loyolla Montanari Leme**,[1] **and Marcos Eduardo Scheicher**[1,2]

[1]*Human Development and Technologies, UNESP, Rio Claro, SP, Brazil*
[2]*Physical Therapy, UNESP, Marília, SP, Brazil*

Correspondence should be addressed to Isabela Feitosa de Carvalho; isabelafeitosa.fisio@gmail.com

Academic Editor: Jean-Francois Grosset

Objectives. The aim of the study was to investigate the effect of balance training with Nintendo Wii technology, with and without the use of additional sensory information (subpatellar bandage), in the functional mobility and gait speed of elderly female fallers. *Methods.* Twenty elderly women were divided into two groups: group I: trained with the use of the Nintendo Wii; group II: trained using the Nintendo Wii and the addition of sensory information (subpatellar bandage). The functional mobility was assessed with the *Timed up and Go* test (TUG) and gait speed with the 10 m test. The tests were carried out with and without the use of the subpatellar bandage. The training was carried out within sessions of 30 minutes, twice a week, using three different games (*Penguin Slide*, *Table Tilt*, and *Tightrope*). *Results.* There was an increase in the gait speed and a decrease in the TUG time in both groups, independently of the sensory condition used ($p < 0.05$). In the short term, the subpatellar bandage improved the TUG time ($p < 0.05$) and the gait speed ($p < 0.01$). *Conclusion.* The training for postural balance with virtual reality was effective for improving functional mobility and gait speed of elderly female fallers. The subpatellar bandage did not maximize the effect of training.

1. Introduction

The use of video games for the training of postural balance is increasing in research related to the elderly population, due to the favorable results on the improvement of posture control, as well as a decrease in the risk of falls [1–3].

Studies in elderly established that many aspects of motor control are affected by aging, causing slower movement and less coordinated [4]. The negative effect of age on balance stability is attributed primarily to sensorimotor dysfunctions [5, 6], muscle weakness [7], and structural changes in brain grey and white matter [8, 9].

For balance maintenance, the postural control system uses mainly information from three sensory systems (visual, vestibular, and somatosensory), which provide information about the relative positions of the body segments and the magnitude of the forces acting on this body, which are not constant [10–12]. Because of this, it is reasonable to suggest that the body orientation is obtained by a relationship between sensory information and motor action. In this case, sensory information influences the performance of the motor actions related to the postural control and, simultaneously, the accomplishment of these motor actions influences the obtaining of sensory information [12].

In this sense, some studies have investigated the effect of somatosensory information on postural control [13–16]. These studies indicate that sensory information can be added with a contact on a touch bar or with a subpatellar bandage, causing a reduction in body oscillation. In these studies, the beneficial effects of the use of additional sensory information

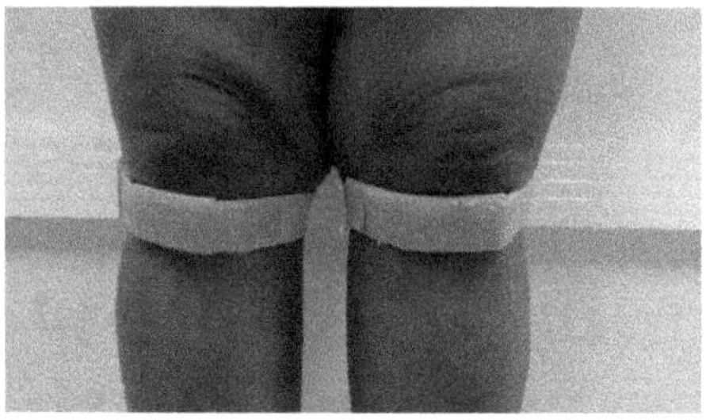

Figure 1: Subpatellar bandage.

were observed in healthy individuals and in individuals with an anterior cruciate ligament injury. In other studies, similar results have been found in the elderly fallers [17–19] using a subpatellar bandage as additional sensory information.

In a recent research paper, Botelhos and Bonfim [20] showed that the effects of a sensorimotor training can be improved with the use of the additional sensory information in healthy individuals.

However, although these studies demonstrate a positive effect of the use of additional sensory information on postural control, there is no evidence that this increasement in sensory input can contribute in a dynamic intervention process, such as in postural balance training with video games in elderly fallers.

Therefore, the objective of this study was to investigate the effect of balance training with Nintendo Wii® technology, with and without the use of additional sensory information (subpatellar bandage), in the functional mobility and gait speed of elderly female fallers.

2. Methodology

Twenty elderly women who live in Marilia, Sao Paulo, 60 years old or over, classified as sedentary according to the Brazilian Society of Sports Medicine and the Brazilian Society of Geriatrics and Gerontology [21], with a history of one or more falls in the last 12 months were recruited for the study [22]. All patients were recruited in geriatrics clinics, community centers, primary care assistance, basic health units, and so on.

Only the women who had the ability of independent ambulation without the use of walking aid devices were selected. Their cognitive abilities were evaluated with the Mini-Mental State Examination (MMSE) and the elderly who obtained scores considered normal for their respective years of study were included in the study [23]. The women who presented sequelae of neuromusculoskeletal diseases, arthritis, uncorrected vision problems, and postural hypertension and reported the continuous use of sedatives, antidepressants, and hypnotics were not included in the study.

All participants answered questionnaires regarding their personal data, history of falling (place, number, and sequelae), marital status, and number of medications.

The participants were separated into two groups:

(1) Training without additional sensory information (untaped condition, control group)

(2) Training with additional sensory information (taped condition): subpatellar bandage condition with a pad, a width of 2 cm, Salvape® brand, maintaining contact with the skin bilaterally, in an orthostatic position (Figure 1).

3. Assessment Section

3.1. Functional Mobility. The mobility was evaluated with the TUG test, before and after training. The test measures the time (in seconds) necessary for a person to rise from a chair with armrests, walk 3 meters at a comfortable walking speed, turn, return to the chair, and sit down [24].

The test was performed twice in the untaped and taped condition, first for familiarization and then for time recording [24]. The TUG test is highly recommended as a means of assessing the risk of falling for the elderly because it identifies the deficit of balance and gait speed. Therefore, lower scores indicate better functional mobility, better posture, and an increased gait speed [25].

3.2. Gait Speed. In order to evaluate the gait speed, a simple 10-meter walking test was carried out. The usual gait speed is a simple measure, and there is no need for expensive and sophisticated equipment, but simply the use of a timer and some walking space. In order to eliminate any anomalies, the participants had to begin walking 1.2 meters before the timing and finish 1.2 meters after [26]. A single examiner using a digital stopwatch with a 1/100 of a second reading (Cronobio SW-2018®, Pastbio, SP, Brazil) recorded the walking time of all volunteers.

The test was carried out three times in order to eliminate any variables; the shortest durations were used in the data and were analyzed. The participants were told to continue walking to the next point, in their regular speed as soon as they were ready [26, 27].

4. Balance Training with Virtual Reality

The postural balance training was carried out within sessions of 30 minutes, twice a week. The exercises were done with commercialized games of *Wii Fit by Nintendo®* in sync with the *Wii Balance Board®*. This platform is wireless and connects to the *Nintendo Wii* console via Bluetooth. It has a rectangular design and includes sensory pressure that detects the center of pressure and movement of the user [28, 29].

Three different games were used for postural balance training: *Penguin Slide*, where the participants had to catch fish while balanced on a piece of ice by shifting their weight from side to side; *Table Tilt*, where the participants had to shift body weight in multiple directions to get balls into a series of holes; and *Tightrope*, where the participants had to cross a tightrope by marching in place and do verticals jumps by bending and extending their knees to avoid dynamic obstacles. The personal profile of the participant was entered into the system so that his or her progress could be tracked and difficulty levels could be adjusted to each person's training program according to his/her progress [28]. All the evaluations were carried out by the same evaluator.

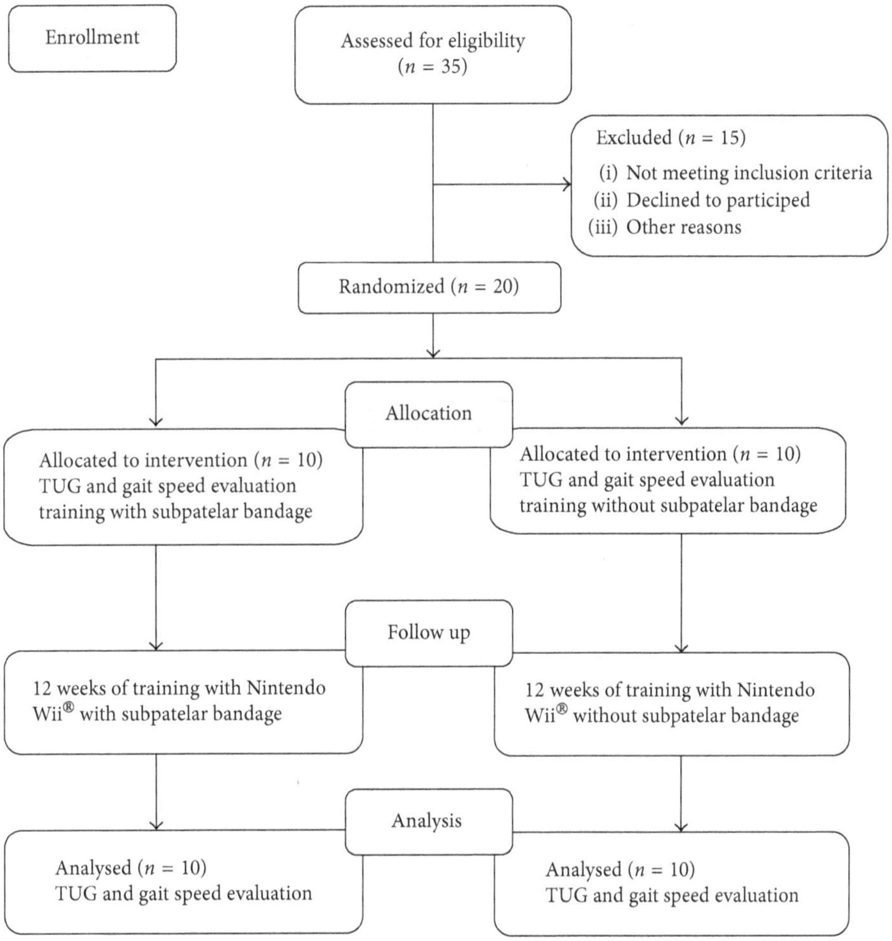

FIGURE 2: Methodology flowchart.

Each game had a duration of 10 minutes [30]. The participants observed the body movements on a multimedia projector, providing greater visual feedback.

The intervention went on for 12 weeks, with two sessions per week on different days. The methodology flowchart can be seen in Figure 2. At the beginning and the end of each session, the blood pressure, heart rate, and breathing were checked.

Written informed consent was obtained from all participants before enrollment. The study was approved by the Research Ethics Committee of the Faculty of Philosophy and Sciences–UNESP (process no. 0982/2014) and published in the Brazilian Registry for Clinical Trials (RBR-54jrwd).

5. Data Analysis

The normality of the distribution of data was evaluated by the *Shapiro–Wilk* test. A repeated measures ANOVA with Bonferroni posttest (within-subjects) was used to compare the data. All analysis were made using GraphPad Instat software, with $p < 0.05$.

6. Results

The Shapiro–Wilk test showed that the data had a normal distribution. Table 1 demonstrates the participants' characterizations in terms of age, test scores (MMSE), and their number of falls. Of the sample evaluated, 50% of the women reported that their falls had been frequent the year before. All the participants used medication, and 70% of them used more than one type of medication per day. Figure 3 represents the measurements of the TUG test before and after training, with additional sensory information, along with the subpatellar bandage. Both groups presented a decrease in results in the TUG test independently of the sensory condition. The statistical tests revealed a significant difference between evaluations with and without additional sensory information ($p < 0.05$) but did not show significance with the use of the subpatellar bandage during video game training.

The gait speed data evaluations before and after training with and without the use of the subpatellar bandage are represented in Figure 4. Both groups had an increase in gait speed after training, independently of the sensory condition of the group. The participants also represented an increase in the gait speed during the evaluations after training with the use of additional sensory information.

7. Discussion

Research on the benefits brought to the elderly by video game technologies, especially in terms of postural balance

Table 1: Sample characterization.

	Group taped (n = 10) Mean (SD)	Group untaped (n = 10) Mean (SD)
Age (years)	70.1 (6.33)	69.5 (8.07)
MMSE	24.9 (2.99)	26.2 (2.74)
Number of falls	2.0 (0.66)	1.2 (0.70)

MMSE: Mini-Mental State Examination; SD: standard deviation.

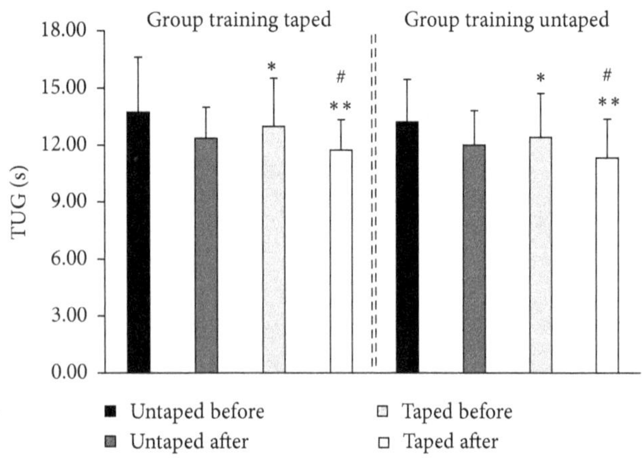

Figure 3: Comparison of TUG test between taped and untaped groups before and after training. $^*p < 0.05$ in comparison to untaped before; $^{**}p < 0.01$ in relation to untaped before; $^{\#}p < 0.05$ in comparison to taped before.

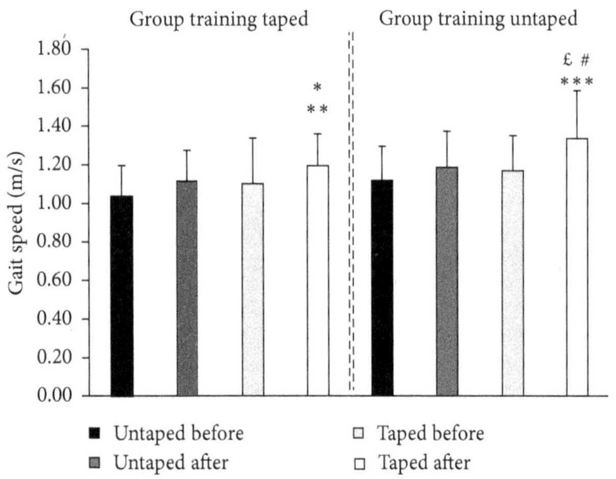

Figure 4: Comparison of gait speed between taped and untaped groups before and after training. Group training taped: $^*p < 0.001$ in relation to untaped before; $^{**}p < 0.05$ in relation to taped before; group training untaped: $^{***}p < 0.001$ in relation to untaped before; $^{\#}p < 0.01$ in relation to untaped after; $^{£}p < 0.001$ in relation to taped before.

and risk of falling, has increased in recent years [28, 29]. Also, it has been shown that the addition of sensory information decreases postural imbalance in young and elderly people [13–19]. There is no evidence that this increasement in sensory input can contribute in a dynamic intervention process, such as in postural balance training with video games, for example. Therefore, the objective of this study was to investigate the effect of balance training with Nintendo Wii technology, with and without the use of additional sensory information (subpatellar bandage), in the functional mobility and gait speed of elderly female fallers.

The results obtained revealed an increase in the gait speed and a decrease in the TUG time in both groups, independently of the sensory condition used. In addition, the effects of the additional sensory information were demonstrated after training in both groups.

The use of the video game technologies in elderly populations presents beneficial results regarding the decrease in risks of falls, fragilities, dependence, and deaths, associated with the aspect of motivation and entertainment, considering it an effective strategy to improve the physical health of the elderly [28, 31].

A study by Fu et al. [32], showed that training with the Nintendo Wii promoted an improvement in reaction timing, quadriceps strength, and body oscillation. These findings were found in the comparison with conventional physiotherapy and virtual reality as a means of potential therapy.

The games give feedback in real time for the participants, which is necessary for learning new abilities, especially for rehabilitation. The visual feedback in real time improves training, when compared to the conventional training, assisting the individual with body movement corrections and alignment [33].

There was a reduction in TUG time after training in both groups. This result shows the efficiency of training proposed in the functional mobility of the elderly who fall frequently. These results corroborate with those of Walker et al. [34], which demonstrated an improvement in the TUG test after training with visual feedback.

Gait speed also improved with the training in both groups. There are few studies associating walking gait speed and the use of video games technologies, but the present study suggests the beneficial effect of this training modality to improve the mean gait speed, especially in the elderly. The gait speed is a kinematical parameter; its assessment is simple, cheap, and reliable and may be interesting to assess the mobility of subjects, being possible to avoid complications such as falling, hospital visits, and possibly death. The research by Hardy et al. [35] and Hollman et al. [36], suggests that the reduction of 0.1 m/s in gait speed could increase the risk of the elderly falling by 7% and that the improvement of mean speed could decrease by 17.7% the risk of deaths.

Although the research demonstrated the efficiency of training with Nintendo Wii, the hypothesis that the additional sensory information could maximize this effect was rejected despite a trend of improvement of the parameters.

In contrast, the evaluations demonstrated that the subpatellar bandage presents a good effect in short term.

Only one study evaluated the effects of a sensorimotor training with the use of the additional sensory information showing good results [20]. In our study, this hypothesis has not been verified. One reason for this may be that the training in our study was different from the Botelhos study. Although it cannot be generalized, the results suggest that the use of subpatellar bandage improves balance and mobility and can be used to reduce the risk of falls among the elderly, in a short time. In addition, other studies should be done with a larger number of participants to show whether subpatellar bandage may potentiate the effects of treatments. The video game technologies represent a good acceptance for the geriatric population due to a playful component and the audio-visual feedback given in each game. The facility of using the tool in addition to its mobility improvements could turn video game technologies' training into an important ally to the conventional physiotherapy methods [37–39].

8. Conclusion

The training for postural balance with Nintendo Wii balance board, with and without the inclusion of additional sensory information was effective for the improvement of the functional mobility and gait speed of elderly fallers. The subpatellar bandage had a short-term effect, but it was not possible to show its potential to amplify the training effect; however, there was a trend for improvement.

Conflicts of Interest

The authors declare that they have no conflicts of interest.

References

[1] G. Duque, D. Boersma, G. Loza-Diaz et al., "Effects of balance training using a virtual-reality system in older fallers," *Clinical Interventions in Aging*, vol. 8, pp. 257–263, 2013.

[2] C. H. Lai, C. W. Peng, Y. L. Chen, C. P. Huang, Y. L. Hsiao, and S. C. Chen, "Effects of interactive video-game based system exercise on the balance of the elderly," *Gait & Posture*, vol. 37, no. 4, pp. 511–515, 2013.

[3] D. K. A. Singh, B. S. Rajaratnam, V. Palaniswamy, H. Pearson, V. P. Raman, and P. S. Bong, "Participating in a virtual reality balance exercise program can reduce risk and fear of falls," *Maturitas*, vol. 73, no. 3, pp. 239–243, 2012.

[4] P. Linortner, M. Jehna, H. Johansen-Berg et al., "Aging associated changes in the motor control of ankle movements in the brain," *Neurobiology of Aging*, vol. 35, no. 10, pp. 2222–2229, 2014.

[5] M. P. Boisgontier, I. Olivier, O. Chenu, and V. Nougier, "Presbypropria: the effects of physiological ageing on proprioceptive control," *Age*, vol. 34, no. 5, pp. 1179–1194, 2012.

[6] N. Bugnariu and J. Fung, "Aging and selective sensorimotor strategies in the regulation of upright balance," *Journal of NeuroEngineering and Rehabilitation*, vol. 4, no. 1, p. 19, 2007.

[7] C. I. Morse, J. M. Thom, M. G. Davis, K. R. Fox, K. M. Birch, and M. V. Narici, "Reduced plantarflexor specific torque in the elderly is associated with a lower activation capacity," *European Journal of Applied Physiology*, vol. 92, no. 1-2, pp. 219–226, 2004.

[8] M. P. Boisgontier, B. Cheval, S. Chalavi et al., "Individual differences in brainstem and basal ganglia structure predict postural control and balance loss in young and older adults," *Neurobiology of Aging*, vol. 50, pp. 47–59, 2017.

[9] A. Van Impe, J. P. Coxon, D. J. Goble, M. Doumas, and S. P. Swinnen, "White matter fractional anisotropy predicts balance performance in older adults," *Neurobiology of Aging*, vol. 33, no. 9, pp. 1900–1912, 2012.

[10] M. Duarte and S. M. S. F. Freitas, "Revision of posturography based on force plate for balance evaluation," *Revista Brasileira de Fisioterapia*, vol. 14, no. 3, pp. 183–192, 2010.

[11] F. Horak and J. Macpherson, "Postural orientation and equilibrium: interaction and coordination," in *Handbook of Physiology*, L. Rowell and J. Shepard, Eds., pp. 255–292, Oxford University Press, New York, NY, USA, 1996.

[12] J. A. Barela, "Estratégias de controle em movimentos complexos: ciclo percepção-ação no controle postural," *Revista de Educação Física*, vol. 14, no. 3, pp. 79–88, 2000, https://www.revistas.usp.br/rpef/article/viewFile/139616/134916.

[13] J. J. Jeka and J. R. Lackner, "The role of haptic cues from rough and slippery surfaces in human postural control," *Experimental Brain Research*, vol. 103, no. 2, pp. 267–276, 1995.

[14] J. J. Jeka, "Light touch contact as a balance aid," *Physical Therapy*, vol. 77, no. 5, pp. 476–487, 1997.

[15] J. J. Jeka and J. R. Lackner, "Fingertip contact influences human postural control," *Experimental Brain Research*, vol. 100, no. 3, pp. 495–502, 1994.

[16] T. R. Bonfim, D. B. Grossi, C. A. J. Paccola, and J. A. Barela, "Additional sensory information reduces body sway of individuals with anterior cruciate ligament injury," *Neuroscience Letters*, vol. 441, no. 3, pp. 257–260, 2008.

[17] I. F. de Carvalho, T. B. Bortolotto, L. C. S. Fonseca, and M. E. Scheicher, "Uso da bandagem infrapatelar no desempenho físico e mobilidade funcional de idosas com história de quedas," *Revista Brasileira de Geriatria e Gerontologia*, vol. 18, no. 1, pp. 119–127, 2015.

[18] G. L. M. Leme, I. F. de Carvalho, and M. E. Scheicher, "Improvement of postural balance in elderly women with the use of additional sensory information," *Fisioterapia e Pesquisa*, vol. 24, no. 1, pp. 68–73, 2017.

[19] M. E. Scheicher, L. C. S. Fonseca, T. B. Bortolloto, and I. F. de Carvalho, "A patellar bandage improves mobility but not static balance in elderly female fallers," *Journal of Bodywork and Movement Therapies*, 2017. In press.

[20] D. C. Botelhos and T. R. Bonfim, "Influência da informação sensorial adicional no treinamento sensório-motor," *Fisioterapia e Pesquisa*, vol. 19, no. 3, pp. 268–274, 2012.

[21] A. C. L. da Nóbrega, E. V. de Freitas, M. A. B. de Oliveira et al., "Posicionamento Oficial da Sociedade Brasileira de Medicina do Esporte e da Sociedade Brasileira de Geriatria e Gerontologia : Atividade Física e Saúde no Idoso," *Revista Brasileira de Medicina do Esporte*, vol. 5, no. 6, pp. 207–211, 1999.

[22] F. V. Siqueira, L. A. Facchini, D. S. da Silveira et al., "Prevalence of falls in elderly in Brazil: a countrywide analysis," *Cadernos de Saúde Pública*, vol. 27, no. 9, pp. 1819–1826, 2011.

[23] S. M. D. Brucki, R. Nitrin, P. Caramelli, P. H. F. Bertolucci, and I. H. Okamoto, "Sugestões para o uso do mini-exame do estado mental no Brasil," *Arquivos de Neuro-Psiquiatria*, vol. 61, no. 3, pp. 777–781, 2003.

[24] D. Podsiadlo and S. Richadson, "The timed "Up and Go" test: a test of basic functional mobility for frail elderly persons," *Journal of the American Geriatrics Society*, vol. 39, no. 2, pp. 142–148, 1991.

[25] D. Schoene, S. M. S. Wu, A. S. Mikolaizak et al., "Discriminative ability and predictive validity of the timed up and go test in identifying older people who fall: systematic review and meta-analysis," *Journal of the American Geriatrics Society*, vol. 61, no. 2, pp. 202–208, 2013.
[26] R. D. Novaes, A. S. Miranda, and V. Z. Dourado, "Usual gait speed assessment in middle-aged and elderly Brazilian subjects," *Revista Brasileira de Fisioterapia*, vol. 15, no. 2, pp. 117–122, 2011.
[27] S. S. E. Abreu and C. P. Caldas, "Gait speed, balance and age: a correlational study among elderly women with and without participation in a therapeutic exercise program," *Brazilian Journal of Physical Therapy*, vol. 12, no. 4, pp. 324–330, 2008.
[28] M. Yamada, T. Aoyama, M. Nakamura et al., "The reliability and preliminary validity of game-based fall risk assessment in community-dwelling older adults," *Geriatric Nursing*, vol. 32, no. 3, pp. 188–194, 2011.
[29] M. G. Prata and M. E. Scheicher, "Effects of strength and balance training on the mobility, fear of falling and grip strength of elderly female fallers," *Journal of Bodywork and Movement Therapies*, vol. 19, no. 4, pp. 646–650, 2015.
[30] H. Bateni, "Changes in balance in older adults based on use of physical therapy vs the Wii Fit gaming system: a preliminary study," *Physiotherapy*, vol. 98, no. 3, pp. 211–216, 2012.
[31] B. C. Kwok, K. Mamun, M. Chandran, and C. H. Wong, "Evaluation of the Frails' fall efficacy by comparing treatments (EFFECT) on reducing fall and fear of fall in moderately frail older adults: study protocol for a randomised control trial," *Trials*, vol. 12, no. 1, pp. 155–162, 2011.
[32] A. S. Fu, K. L. Gao, A. K. Tung, W. W. Tsang, and M. M. Kwan, "Effectiveness of exergaming training in reducing risk and incidence of falls in frail older adults with a history of falls," *Archives of Physical Medicine and Rehabilitation*, vol. 96, no. 12, pp. 2096–2102, 2015.
[33] K. Laver, B. Lange, S. George, J. Deutsch, G. Saposnik, and M. Crotty, "Virtual reality for stroke rehabilitation," *Cochrane Database of Systematic Reviews*, vol. 20, 2011.
[34] C. Walker, B. J. Brouwer, and E. G. Culham, "Use of visual feedback in retraining balance following acute stroke," *Physical Therapy*, vol. 80, no. 9, pp. 886–895, 2000.
[35] S. E. Hardy, S. Perera, Y. F. Roumani, J. M. Chandler, and S. A. Studenski, "Improvement in usual gait speed predicts better survival in older adults," *Journal of the American Geriatrics Society*, vol. 55, no. 11, pp. 1727–1734, 2007.
[36] J. Hollman, B. Beckman, R. Brandt, E. Merriwether, R. Williams, and J. Nordrum, "Minimum detectable change in gait velocity during acute rehabilitation following hip fracture," *Journal of Geriatric Physical Therapy*, vol. 31, no. 2, pp. 53–56, 2008.
[37] W. Young, S. Ferguson, S. Brault, and C. Craig, "Assessing and training standing balance in older adults: a novel approach using the "Nintendo Wii" Balance Board," *Gait & Posture*, vol. 33, no. 2, pp. 303–305, 2011.
[38] R. A. Clark, A. L. Bryant, Y. Pua, P. McCrory, K. Bennell, and M. Hunt, "Validity and reliability of the Nintendo Wii Balance Board for assessment of standing balance," *Gait & Posture*, vol. 31, no. 3, pp. 307–310, 2010.
[39] C. Basak, W. R. Boot, M. W. Voss, and A. F. Kramer, "Can training in a real-time strategy video game attenuate cognitive decline in older adults?," *Psychology and Aging*, vol. 23, no. 4, pp. 765–777, 2008.

24

Can Driving-Simulator Training Enhance Visual Attention, Cognition, and Physical Functioning in Older Adults?

Mathias Haeger [1] **Otmar Bock** [1] **Daniel Memmert,** [2] **and Stefanie Hüttermann** [2]

[1] *Institute of Physiology and Anatomy, German Sport University Cologne, Am Sportpark Müngersdorf 6, 50933 Cologne, Germany*
[2] *Institute of Training and Computer Science in Sport, German Sport University Cologne, Am Sportpark Müngersdorf 6, 50933 Cologne, Germany*

Correspondence should be addressed to Mathias Haeger; m.haeger@dshs-koeln.de

Academic Editor: Jean-Francois Grosset

Virtual reality offers a good possibility for the implementation of real-life tasks in a laboratory-based training or testing scenario. Thus, a computerized training in a driving simulator offers an ecological valid training approach. Visual attention had an influence on driving performance, so we used the reverse approach to test the influence of a driving training on visual attention and executive functions. Thirty-seven healthy older participants (mean age: 71.46 ± 4.09; gender: 17 men and 20 women) took part in our controlled experimental study. We examined transfer effects from a four-week driving training (three times per week) on visual attention, executive function, and motor skill. Effects were analyzed using an analysis of variance with repeated measurements. Therefore, main factors were group and time to show training-related benefits of our intervention. Results revealed improvements for the intervention group in divided visual attention; however, there were benefits neither in the other cognitive domains nor in the additional motor task. Thus, there are no broad training-induced transfer effects from such an ecologically valid training regime. This lack of findings could be addressed to insufficient training intensities or a participant-induced bias following the cancelled randomization process.

1. Introduction

Many studies strongly suggest that attention declines with advancing age. This has been documented via several components of visual attention, such as selective attention [1, 2], sustained attention [1], distributed attention [3, 4], and divided attention [2]. There is also a decline of executive functions in old age, which is indicated by reduced inhibitory control, declined working memory, or slower cognitive flexibility [5–7]. The age-related deficits of executive functions [7–10] and visual attention can be ameliorated by practice [11, 12]. Thus, the purpose of our study is to evaluate a training approach for these cognitive functions.

Cognitive functions can be trained by classic cognitive training [13], computerized brain training programs [12], and video games [7, 14–18] (for a corresponding review, see [19]). A further review in healthy older adults showed that computerized training could improve working memory, cognitive speed of processing, or visuospatial abilities, but not executive functions or attention [20]. The authors conducted domain-specific analyses for cognitive functions but neglected differences regarding the kind of computerized training. Thus, different types of programs might have different effects since action video games, for example, are probably effective based on fast reactions and management of multiple tasks at the same time [21].

It has been suggested that cognitive training based on video/computer games is more attractive than cognitive training based on standard laboratory tasks, as it is diverse and motivating rather than stereotyped and dull [22–24]. However, training benefits seem to be smaller rather than larger if compared to laboratory-type training [19, 22, 25]. One possible explanation is that trained activities were not familiar and realistic; that is, they lacked ecological validity [26, 27]: the cognitive benefits of training regimes are thought to increase when trained activities are similar to situations of everyday life [28]. Thus, an ecologically valid training reflects everyday actions and could be helpful, especially for older adults, to pass demanding situations (i.e., driving on dangerous crossroads). In such situations, people also have to manage multiple tasks at the same time, and studies including multitasking training have already showed cognitive benefits [14].

One possible approach for a diverse, motivating, and ecologically valid cognitive training regime is driving in a car simulator. It requires selective, sustained, distributed, and divided attention as well as executive abilities, that is, cognitive skills which are known to decay in older age (see above). Furthermore, there is some evidence that visual attention [29, 30] and working memory [31] are connected with real-life driving performance. Although two earlier studies found little benefits of driving-simulator training for older participants' attention, training quantity was limited to 10 × 40 minutes in one [23] and 2 × 120 minutes in the other study [32]. Additionally, results from Casutt and colleagues [23] only showed effects in an overall cognitive score with the greatest impact on simple and complex choice reaction times. It remains questionable whether components of visual attention were improved. Furthermore, task realism and benefits for visual attention were reduced by using only one central screen to display the driving scenarios. We believe that more substantial benefits of driving-simulator training are conceivable since they already have been observed in reciprocal approaches, in which cognitive training targeting speed of processing [11, 32, 33] or attention and dual-tasking training [34] improved driving performance. In our approach, we want to reevaluate the cognitive benefits of driving-simulator training using more and longer sessions as well as a larger visual display. We reasoned that a larger display may provide a more immersive experience and thus facilitate top-down modulation of visual attention (i.e., upcoming moving obstacles near the lane), which was recently connected with the prefrontal cortex (PFC) [2, 35]. Furthermore, there is growing evidence that the PFC moreover regulates the focus of attention, selects information, and controls executive functions [36]. So, we decided to expand the scope of outcome variables and include executive functions. Besides the theoretical connection, executive functions are known to be associated with driving performance [37] but have not been evaluated yet in the context of driving-simulator training.

A further aspect that has also not been evaluated before is functional mobility as a far transfer from driving-simulation training. We took that into consideration because driving involves limb movements and requires complex visual processing—two abilities associated with mobility and risk of falls in older adults [38–40]—and also because there is an association between cognition (i.e., executive function and dual tasking) and gait parameters (i.e., walking speed) [41]. So, we decided to assess functional mobility by the Timed Up-and-Go (TUG) test, an established marker of reduced mobility [42]. From our point of view, it is an interesting insight concerning a relationship between a computerized training (i.e., including cognitive and coordinative aspects) and a functional parameter, which was slightly examined before [43].

Summing up, we reevaluated driving-simulation training in older adults [23, 32] to extend existing knowledge about effects on visual attention, executive functions, and mobility. Since other computerized training regimes showed benefits on different cognitive functions [19, 20, 44], we hypothesized that our ecologically valid training (1) would improve different parameters of visual attention (distributed, divided, selective, and sustained attention); (2) would improve core executive functions (working memory and task switching); and (3) would show a positive far transfer from cognitive training on functional abilities, as it is suggested in literature [43].

2. Method

2.1. Sample. Required sample size was calculated by G-Power® 3.1 as follows: earlier attention studies yielded effect sizes ranging from $f = 0.105$ to $f = 0.47$ [14–16, 23, 32], so we expect an effect size of $f = 0.25$. For the interaction term of a 2 (group) × 2 (time) analysis of variance with $f = 0.25$, alpha = 0.05, and beta = 0.80, correlation among repetitive measures = 0.40, G-Power yielded a required total sample size of 40 participants. Participants were recruited by distributing flyers on the university campus and, in the city, sending them out through mailing lists, uploading them on the Internet, and adding them to newspapers.

We initially planned a randomized controlled trial, using a computerized block-randomized (two per block, balanced for groups) allocation; however, we had to abort this process after a few participants because a lot of interested people refused their participation (i.e., they only were interested in one: intervention or control group). Additionally, recruitment was slow and the dropout rate was high because of the high time demand of this study. So, we asked all respondents personally who met our inclusion criteria to take part in the intervention group, and if they refused because of the high time demand, we asked them to participate in the control group. There was no additional investigator blinding. Finally, we had a controlled experimental design without randomization (Figure 1).

Inclusion criteria were 65 to 80 years of age, no neurological disease, MMSE >23, normal or corrected-to-normal vision, and car driving experience of no more than 20 hours per month within the last six months. Exclusion criteria were a low MMSE score (<24), previous or actual neurological diseases (i.e., stroke, multiple sclerosis), and daily driving routine. These criteria were formulated to bring in older, not cognitive-impaired drivers with minor driving routine. It was met by 47 respondents, of whom four dropped out later on because of time limitations and six because of simulator sickness. In effect, 16 men and women were retained in the intervention and 21 in the control group.

2.2. Training. We used a commercially available driving simulator (Carnetsoft BV, Groningen, NL) which consists of a computer, three rendering monitors, a steering wheel, pedals, and a gear shift (Figure 2). The monitors have a 48″ diagonal and a 100 HZ frame rate and were positioned on laboratory tables at eye level in front of a black shroud which

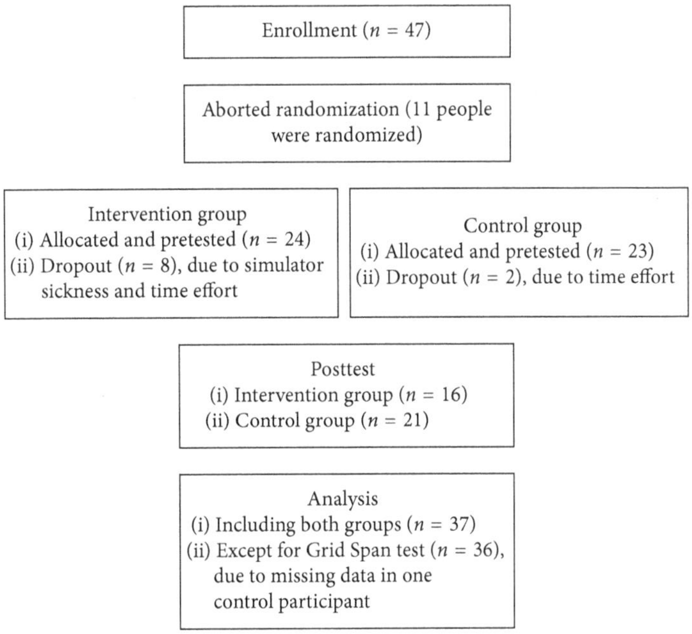

Figure 1: Study flowchart describing participants' allocation in both groups. Enrollment started in November 2015, and the study was finished in September 2016.

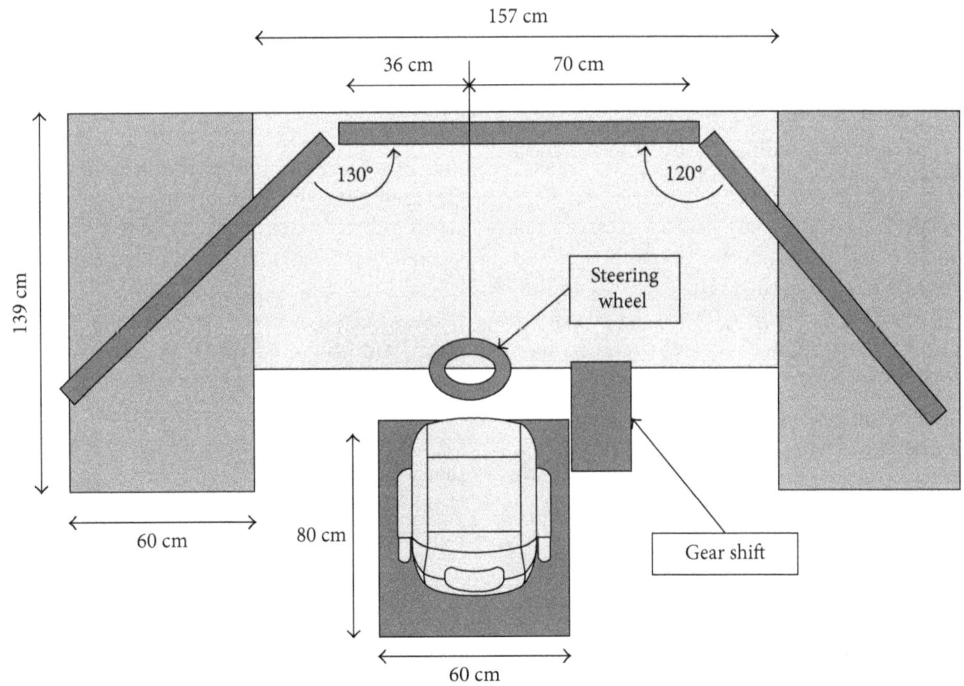

Figure 2: Top view of the driving simulator including tables, monitors, seat, gear shift, and steering wheel. Pedals are under the table (not shown).

blocked vision of the laboratory room. Pedals and the driver's seat were adjusted individually for comfort. Steering wheel, seat, pedals, and gear shift were placed mid between the center and the left edge of the middle screen to imitate the drivers' position in a real car.

The Carnetsoft® software includes a curriculum with multiple driving scenarios from which the following were used for training: learn to drive, using a gear shift, emergency breaking in different road settings, driving ecologically, noticing road signs during the drive, and danger of driving after consuming alcohol. Scenarios consist of rural areas, towns, highways, or combinations of them and include leading or oncoming vehicles. During the drive, a female voice gave driving directions. In addition, participants received short informal feedback from the instructor after each session (i.e., driving errors). Therefore, we recorded some driving parameters (i.e., velocity and lane-adherence) as well as errors (i.e., missing a stop sign) and reported those afterwards. Additionally, we yielded information for safer driving (i.e., scanning the upcoming lane for potential danger). Training took four weeks with three training sessions of about 50–60 minutes per week. It began with simple scenarios whose difficulty level increased gradually in three main steps. So, the first session was for familiarization of our participants with the car dynamics of the driving simulator (i.e., using pedals and gear shift). The following five sessions had more complex requirements: participants had to enter motorways, overtake slow driving cars, or drive over a longer period. During those scenarios we increased traffic (i.e., approaching cars and slower cars ahead), driving durations, and complexity of scenarios (i.e., from a rural area to a city including pedestrians). Finally, the last six sessions consisted of a randomized order of more challenging tasks: participants should drive while paying attention to traffic signs (i.e., we presented additional signs on the left and right display), long highway driving sessions including a lot of traffic as well as traffic jams, and brake-reaction tasks. During these scenarios, we additionally recorded reaction times (i.e., brake reaction or seeing traffic signs) to inform participants about their results in each session (see above: feedback). A single training session took place during the week between 9 a.m. and 4 p.m., depending on availability of our participants.

2.3. Outcome Measures. The following test battery was administered before and after training in the intervention group and four weeks apart in the control group:

(i) The Precue task [45, 46] is a measure of distributed/spatial attention. Participants respond after a correct, false, or neutral cue to visual stimuli presented on the right or left side of a central fixation point. Performance is quantified as a mean reaction time for correct, false, and neutral cues.

(ii) The D2-Attention task [47] is a measure of selective and sustained attention. In a computerized version of this test, participants watch a sequence of items from the list {d„ d, d d' d" d,' p„ p, p p' p" p,'} and have to select all instances of a letter "d" followed by two dashes (d„ d" d,') over a time period of six minutes. Performance is quantified as the number of correct answers minus the number of errors.

(iii) The Attention Window task [4, 48] is a measure of multistream divided attention [2]. Participants watch a sequence of two simultaneously presented patterns, each consisting of four objects, dark or light grey triangles and circles. Following the presentation of each pair, they are asked to indicate the number of light grey triangles in both patterns, without being pressed for time. Successive pattern pairs vary quasi-randomly in the number of light grey triangles and in the distance from a central fixation point. Performance is quantified as percentage of correct responses to both patterns in a pair on each axis (diagonal, horizontal, and vertical).

(iv) The Grid Span task [49–51] is a measure of spatial working memory which is related to executive control. Participants watch a sequence of crosses in a 4×4 grid and are asked to replicate the sequence immediately thereafter. Sequence length increases from trial to trial, and performance is quantified as length of last correctly replicated sequence.

(v) The Switching task [52] is a measure of executive flexibility. Participants watch a sequence of small and large fruits and vegetables and have to indicate either the size (task A) or their nature (fruit versus vegetable; task B). In single blocks, only one task is asked for; in switching blocks, the task sequence AABBAABB and so on is asked for. Performance is quantified as mean reaction time in each task.

(vi) The PAQ-50+ [53] is a retrospective physical activity assessment, covering the preceding four weeks.

(vii) The Timed Up-and-Go task [42, 54] is a functional test of gait and balance. Participants stand up from a chair upon command, walk three meters, turn, and walk back to sit down again, all with their habitual velocity. Performance is quantified as mean completion time across three test repetitions.

(viii) The Mini-Mental State Examination (MMSE) [55] was administered as a screening tool on pretests only.

2.4. Procedure. The study was preapproved by the Ethics Committee of the German Sport University Cologne, and all participants signed an informed consent before testing started. Each participant was tested individually. During an initial interview, participants were informed about the test battery. Control persons were told that a follow-up evaluation will check whether performing the test battery had lasting effects, and training persons were told about the driving intervention and its possible effects. In sum, testing took approximately one and a half hours. Each session took place during the week between 9 a.m. and 5 p.m., and we tried to maintain the individual testing times from pre- to posttesting.

First, MMSE and PAQ-50+ were completed in the form of an interview. Next, computerized versions of Precue, D2-Attention, Grid Span, Switching, and Attention Window tasks were administered in a randomized order, which was the same during pre- and posttest. Finally, the TUG was conducted three times using a manually operated clock and a chair without armrest.

We preregistered our study in the Open Science Framework (OSF) but unfortunately had to change two methodological aspects later on. Due to slow participant recruitment and limited availability of laboratory space, we had to give up randomized group assignment and cancel the retention test twelve weeks after training.

2.5. Statistics. Data from the D2-Attention task, each axis of the Attention Window task, the Grid Span task, and TUG

Table 1: Mean values (and standard deviation) of demographic characteristics, MMSE, and PAQ-50+ scores in the intervention and control group.

		Intervention	Control	Statistics
Age (years)		70.25 (±3.77)	72.38 (±4.17)	$t_{(35)} = -1.61,\ p > 0.05$
Gender (men/women)		8/8	9/12	—
Education (1/2)		8/8	9/12	$c^2_{(1,N=37)} = 0.19,\ p > 0.05$
Driving time (hours per month)		10.63 (±7.21)	9.88 (±8.39)	$t_{(35)} = 0.02,\ p > 0.05$
MMSE (score)		28.63 (±1.09)	28.62 (±1.20)	$t_{(35)} = 0.28,\ p > 0.05$
PAQ-50+ (MET/week)	Pre	126.37 (±67.60)	125.35 (±66.84)	T: $F_{(1,35)} = 2.66,\ p > 0.05,\ \eta^2 = 0.071$
	Post	102.50 (±39.06)	119.40 (±65.76)	G*T: $F_{(1,35)} = 0.96,\ p > 0.05,\ \eta^2 = 0.027$

Statistics included t-tests, chi-square test (for education: 1 = A level, 2 = O level), and ANOVA (G = group effects, T = time effects) to analyze group differences.

were submitted to a 2 (group: intervention and control) × 2 (time: pre and post) analysis of variance (ANOVA) with repeated measures on the latter factor. For the Switching task, we used a 2 (group) × 2 (time) × 3 (trial: single, non-switching, and switching) ANOVA with repeated measures on the latter two factors. For the Precue task, we conducted a 2 (group) × 2 (time) × 3 (cue: correct, neutral, and false) ANOVA with repeated measures on the latter two factors. Furthermore, we conducted the Mauchly test for sphericity for the Switching task and the Precue task and used a Greenhouse–Geisser correction in case of a sphericity violation. Regarding this number of tests, we conducted a Bonferroni–Holm correction for multiple testing to adjust p values. Training benefits should emerge as significant group × time interactions in these analyses. Interaction effects (i.e., group × time) represent our primary outcome; main effects of these tests are secondary outcome.

As further secondary outcome, we analyzed participants' characteristics using an independent t-test, a two-dimensional (group and education) chi-square test, and a 2 (group) × 2 (time) ANOVA to reveal differences between our groups.

3. Results

Table 1 shows the demographic characteristics of all participants ($n = 37$) included in data analysis. None of the scores differed significantly between groups at the pretest. Furthermore, there were no group- or time-dependent effects in subjective physical activity ($F_{(1,35)} = 0.96$, MSE = 1516.202, $p > 0.05$).

As expected, the Precue task yielded with Greenhouse–Geisser correction ($\chi^2_{(2)} = 7.01$, $p = 0.03$, $\varepsilon = 0.843$) a significant main effect for cue ($F_{(1.69,59.01)} = 19.75$, MSE = 786.476, $p < 0.01$). There were no other significant differences, notably not for group × time × cue ($F_{(1.70,59.62)} = 0.79$, MSE = 523.931, $p > 0.05$). The D2-Attention task yielded a significant main effect for time ($F_{(1,35)} = 13.25$, MSE = 418.892, $p < 0.01$), but no other significant effects, in particular not for group × time ($F_{(1,35)} = 0.00$, MSE = 418.892, $p > 0.05$). For the Attention Window task, we found a significant group × time interaction for the horizontal axis ($F_{(1,35)} = 4.46$, MSE = 0.003, $p = 0.04$, $\eta^2 = 0.113$); however, this effect did not remain after Bonferroni–Holm correction. There was also neither a significant effect for the other two axes (diagonal: $F_{(1,35)} = 0.14$, MSE = 0.008, $p > 0.05$, $\eta^2 = 0.004$; vertical: $F_{(1,35)} = 0.01$, MSE = 0.007, $p > 0.05$, $\eta^2 = 0.000$) nor any other effects. Figure 3 illustrates that, in the Attention Window task, accuracy on the horizontal axis increased from pre to post in the intervention group but decreased in the control group; this tendency was absent on the other two axes.

There were no significant effects on the Grid Span task, notably no significant group × time interaction ($F_{(1,34)} = 1.86$, MSE = 0.627, $p > 0.05$). The Switching task yielded with Greenhouse–Geisser correction ($\chi^2_{(2)} = 17.03$, $p < 0.01$, $\varepsilon = 0.717$) significant effects for trial ($F_{(1.44,50.22)} = 37.39$, MSE = 12091.056, $p < 0.01$) and trial × time ($F_{(1.61,56.33)} = 3.71$, MSE = 5061.153, $p = 0.04$); but again after Bonferroni–Holm correction the trial × time interaction did not remain significant ($p > 0.01$). Finally, the Timed Up-and-Go task yielded no significance, notably not for group × time (TUG: $F_{(1,35)} = 3.72$, MSE = 0.291, $p > 0.05$). Table 2 summarizes all outcome scores. Further statistical outcomes are presented in an additional table as Supplementary Material (Table S1).

4. Discussion

We evaluated a four-week training program in a driving simulator with a wide field of view, administering three sessions of about one hour duration per week. Outcome measures comprised visual attention, executive functions, and physical abilities. Because of recruitment problems and a 28% dropout rate in the intervention group due to simulator sickness, only 16 participants completed in the intervention group and 21 completed in the control group. We found significant benefits of training for divided visual attention along the horizontal axis; however, statistical significance disappeared after correction for multiple testing. Furthermore, we did not find any significant effects neither for other cognitive measures nor for functional mobility. The lack of more substantial training benefits cannot be attributed to group differences regarding demographic, cognitive, or physical baseline scores (Tables 1 and 2).

First, we will discuss our results in relation to other driving-simulator studies. Casutt and colleagues [15] described a significant training benefit on overall cognitive performance, but regarding visual attention, those authors presented only descriptive statistics with small effects ($d = 0.13$–0.31) for selective attention, field of vision, and divided attention. Roenker and colleagues [32] described no

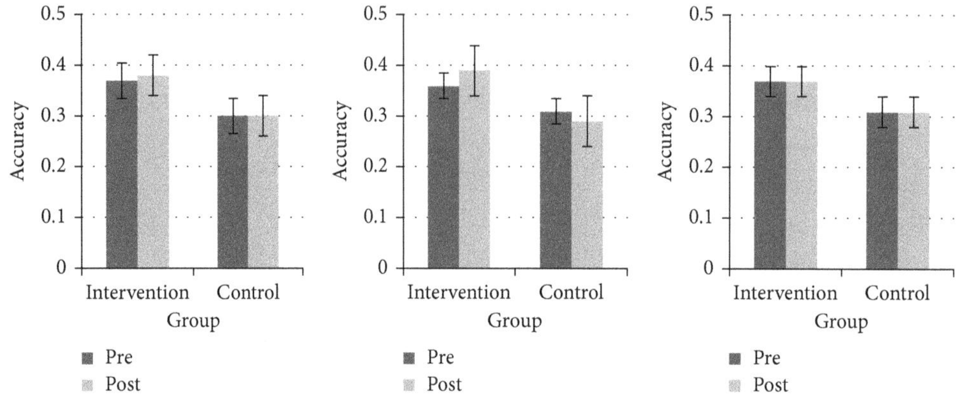

Figure 3: Response accuracy in the Attention Window test, plotted separately for the three axes and for the intervention group and the control group. Boxes indicate across-participant means and error bars the pertinent standard errors. (a) Diagonal. (b) Horizontal. (c) Vertical.

Table 2: Mean values and standard deviation of pre- and posttest scores in the intervention and control group as well as statistical results (T = time, C = cue, G = group, Tr = trial).

Test		Intervention	Control	Statistics
Precue "false" (ms)	Pre	371.63 (±64.96)	393.75 (±71.48)	T: $F_{(1,35)} = 0.15$, $p > 0.05$, $\eta^2 = 0.004$
	Post	374.38 (±76.03)	391.77 (±77.68)	T*G: $F_{(1,35)} = 0.05$, $p > 0.05$, $\eta^2 = 0.001$
Precue "neutral" (ms)	Pre	362.88 (±61.16)	377.48 (±60.41)	C: $F_{(1.69,59.01)} = 19.75$, $p < 0.00$, $\eta^2 = 0.361$
	Post	355.16 (±50.90)	372.71 (±66.04)	C*G: $F_{(1.69,59.01)} = 1.68$, $p > 0.05$, $\eta^2 = 0.046$
Precue "correct" (ms)	Pre	358.92 (±68.31)	357.26 (±41.64)	T*C: $F_{(1.70,59.62)} = 0.46$, $p > 0.05$, $\eta^2 = 0.013$
	Post	348.70 (±53.34)	359.86 (±63.12)	G*T*C: $F_{(1.70,59.62)} = 0.79$, $p > 0.05$, $\eta^2 = 0.022$
D2 (score)	Pre	141.13 (±37.81)	134.29 (±36.76)	T: $F_{(1,35)} = 13.25$, $p < 0.01$, $\eta^2 = 0.275$
	Post	158.75 (±36.67)	151.62 (±31.74)	G*T: $F_{(1,35)} = 0.00$, $p > 0.05$, $\eta^2 = 0.000$
Grid Span (score)	Pre	5.63 (±0.72)	4.75 (±0.91)	T: $F_{(1,34)} = 0.09$, $p > 0.05$, $\eta^2 = 0.003$
	Post	5.31 (±1.14)	4.95 (±1.00)	G*T: $F_{(1,34)} = 1.86$, $p > 0.05$, $\eta^2 = 0.052$
Switching "single" (ms)	Pre	839.75 (±120.60)	808.43 (±84.38)	T: $F_{(1,35)} = 0.82$, $p > 0.05$, $\eta^2 = 0.023$
	Post	790.35 (±105.56)	758.51 (±122.16)	T*G: $F_{(1,35)} = 0.24$, $p > 0.05$, $\eta^2 = 0.007$
Switching "nonswitch" (ms)	Pre	884.69 (±157.93)	840.80 (±102.71)	Tr: $F_{(1.44,50.22)} = 37.39$, $p < 0.00$, $\eta^2 = 0.517$
	Post	855.24 (±123.44)	836.59 (±156.47)	Tr*G: $F_{(1.44,50.22)} = 0.02$, $p > 0.05$, $\eta^2 = 0.000$
Switching "switch" (ms)	Pre	951.24 (±146.64)	905.39 (±153.74)	T*Tr: $F_{(1.61,56.33)} = 3.71$, $p = 0.04$, $\eta^2 = 0.096$
	Post	940.00 (±144.86)	932.36 (±174.00)	G*T* Tr: $F_{(1.61,56.33)} = 0.43$, $p > 0.05$, $\eta^2 = 0.012$
TUG (s)	Pre	8.70 (±1.40)	8.52 (±1.67)	T: $F_{(1,35)} = 0.57$, $p > 0.05$, $\eta^2 = 0.016$
	Post	8.37 (±1.41)	8.67 (±1.75)	G*T: $F_{(1,35)} = 3.72$, $p > 0.05$, $\eta^2 = 0.096$

Data from the attention window test are presented in Figure 2.

training benefits on the Useful Field of View (UFOV®), a test of various aspects of visual attention and perception. The present study is therefore in line with earlier work since training had no substantial benefits for most cognitive functions. In a first analytical step, we found benefits for the horizontal component of divided visual attention, which did not remain after a further statistical correction. However, we calculated an effect size for that component (overall effect size for divided attention, $\eta^2 = 0.039$; conversion according to [56, 57]) as $d = 0.403$, which is slightly more than the value reported by Casutt et al. [23]. We attribute this stronger effect in our study to the dramatically wider field of view of our simulator (see Introduction).

Our results can also be compared to those on video-game training. Action video games, characterized by moving objects, fast responses, and multiple tasks [21, 58], led to improvements in selective [16] and sustained attention [14], but this was not necessarily the case for other types of video games: a review of computerized cognitive training in older adults confirmed training benefits for visuospatial abilities but not for attention [20]. However, the authors of this review did not differentiate, for example, between computerized cognitive training (e.g., [12]) and video games (e.g., [15]). Especially, in the case of visual attention, a more detailed differentiation would be needed since action video games appeared to be more effective than "slower" video games [21]. So, for action video games, a recent review showed moderate benefits for older adults in attention and visuospatial abilities [44]. We assume that, in our study, improvements of attention were limited since fast responses and multitasking occurred less frequently than in action video games.

Regarding our results, we have to reject our first hypothesis that there is a broad impact on older people's visual attention from our driving-simulator training. This is partly in line with previous driving-simulator studies and "slower" video games.

Unlike earlier driving-simulator studies, earlier video game research also evaluated the effects of training on executive functions. Improvements of working memory [14] and task switching [59] were reported, but a generalized effect on executive functioning is still under discussion [19, 20]. However, a recent review described moderate effects on executive functions from action video games [44]. Thus, in executive functions, the same differentiation like in visual attention might be necessary. We found no effects of driving-simulator training in executive functions, and our data are therefore in agreement with the more pessimistic views. In view of these results, we also had to reject our second hypothesis that driving-simulator training would induce transfer effects on executive functions. The use of engaging and ecologically valid training regimes seems not enough to ensure improved executive functions. Possibly, training has to specifically address those functions, as was the case in the studies by Anguera et al. [14] and Montani et al. [59], since the transfer of training benefits to unpracticed tasks may be limited [60].

Another point of criticism pertains to the software used: the simulated driving tasks were possibly not difficult enough to challenge participants' executive and attentional abilities. At last, we had only six sessions including complex situations that might be not enough for experienced drivers. There should be more visual stimulation to facilitate top-down modulation, which forms an important part in visual attention and executive functions [2, 36]. Further studies should also record participants' training sessions to analyze the training progress. Thus, it would be possible to regulate the training process individually.

In view of functional mobility, we observed no training benefits for participants' as assessed by the TUG test. We again conclude that our ecologically valid training regimes are no guarantee for a strong transfer of training benefits to untrained abilities. So, taking into account that there were also no cognitive training benefits, we rejected our third hypothesis of a positive far transfer from cognitive training on functional abilities.

There are also a few more methodological aspects that should be discussed. First, our recruited older participants were healthy, physically active, and still able to drive a car. Regarding this, benefits might only occur in more inactive people [61], and further studies should also control whether participants additionally use their car during the intervention. Secondly, we used an inactive control group and aborted our randomization process. Therefore, possible differences in motivation, expert knowledge (i.e., in computerized training), or individual arrangements of physical activities (i.e., an inactive control group has more leisure time) could affect our measurements. Further studies should take these points into account.

5. Limitations

We preregistered our study protocol in the Open Science Framework (OSF) but have to indicate some methodological changes. First, we encountered substantial recruitment problems because of the time and effort involved in participating. As a consequence, we had to cancel the planned randomization and instead assigned the first 24 participants to the intervention group. Second, six participants from the intervention group dropped out because of simulator sickness. Third, only a few participants were willing to undergo follow-up testing, and we therefore had to cancel that part of our study. Possibly, research with older participants became so popular in recent years that the willingness of older persons to contribute to yet another study has been overstrained. As a consequence of these methodological issues, there could also be a bias based on group-related differences: possibly, our intervention group was more familiar with a computerized training, more motivated, or there occurred group differences in other driving-related traits. Regarding the last point, we also missed to analyze personality traits (e.g., motivation, self-efficacy, and driving behavior) which could further explain differences between our groups. We also should have chosen fewer (in view of multiplicity of analyses) and perhaps other cognitive (i.e., a driving-related dual task) or functional tests (i.e., leg/hand coordination task). At last, we did not save results from individual training sessions for a further analysis (i.e., to detect learning curves); in this regard, it would also be beneficial to evaluate motivation during the training process since our tasks were too easy and motivation possibly dropped as time passes.

6. Conclusion

We found no evidence that our diverse and realistic driving-simulator training would improve attention, executive functions, and functional mobility. The only marked training benefit was the one on the horizontal component of divided attention, probably because this component was specifically trained in our horizontally wide display; however, it did not remain after statistical corrections. Perhaps, this lack of findings in our study could be based on a range of methodological aspects. For example, a more complex training including fast reactions and an individual training progress might be more stimulating for visual attention and executive functions. So, in view of further diverse and ecologically valid interventions, the training process and other methodological aspects should be reflected.

Consent

All participants signed an informed consent before their testing started.

Conflicts of Interest

The authors declare that they have no conflicts of interest with respect to the authorship or publication of this article.

Acknowledgments

Thanks are due to Katharina Reingen and Franziska Gliese for their assistance in testing and training.

References

[1] L. P. McAvinue, T. Habekost, K. A. Johnson et al., "Sustained attention, attentional selectivity, and attentional capacity across the lifespan," *Attention, Perception, and Psychophysics*, vol. 74, no. 8, pp. 1570–1582, 2012.

[2] T. P. Zanto and A. Gazzaley, "Attention and ageing," in *The Oxford Handbook of Attention*, A. C. Nobre and S. Kastner, Eds., pp. 927–971, Oxford University Press, Oxford, UK, 2014.

[3] K. Ball, C. Owsley, and B. Beard, "Clinical visual perimetry underestimates peripheral field problems in older adults," *Clinical Vision Sciences*, vol. 5, no. 2, pp. 113–125, 1990.

[4] S. Hüttermann, O. Bock, and D. Memmert, "The breadth of attention in old age," *Ageing Research*, vol. 4, no. 1, p. e10, 2012.

[5] J. Kray, K. Z. H. Li, and U. Lindenberger, "Age-related changes in task-switching components: the role of task uncertainty," *Brain and Cognition*, vol. 49, no. 3, pp. 363–381, 2002.

[6] T. Strobach, *Executive Functions Modulated by Context, Training, and Age*, Humboldt-Universität zu Berlin, Berlin, Germany, 2014.

[7] A. Diamond, "Executive functions," *Annual Review of Psychology*, vol. 64, no. 1, pp. 135–168, 2013.

[8] T. Strobach, T. Salminen, J. Karbach, and T. Schubert, "Practice-related optimization and transfer of executive functions: a general review and a specific realization of their mechanisms in dual tasks," *Psychological Research*, vol. 78, no. 6, pp. 836–851, 2014.

[9] S. Enriquez-Geppert, R. J. Huster, and C. S. Herrmann, "Boosting brain functions: improving executive functions with behavioral training, neurostimulation, and neurofeedback," *International Journal of Psychophysiology*, vol. 88, no. 1, pp. 1–16, 2013.

[10] B. Wollesen and C. Voelcker-Rehage, "Training effects on motor–cognitive dual-task performance in older adults," *European Review of Aging and Physical Activity*, vol. 11, no. 1, pp. 5–24, 2014.

[11] J. D. Edwards, E. G. Valdés, C. Peronto et al., "The efficacy of insight cognitive training to improve useful field of view performance: a brief report," *Journals of Gerontology Series B: Psychological Sciences and Social Sciences*, vol. 70, no. 3, pp. 417–422, 2013.

[12] C. Peretz, A. D. Korczyn, E. Shatil, V. Aharonson, S. Birnboim, and N. Giladi, "Computer-based, personalized cognitive training versus classical computer games: a randomized double-blind prospective trial of cognitive stimulation," *Neuroepidemiology*, vol. 36, no. 2, pp. 91–99, 2011.

[13] L. Bherer, A. F. Kramer, M. S. Peterson, S. Colcombe, K. Erickson, and E. Becic, "Training effects on dual-task performance: are there age-related differences in plasticity of attentional control?," *Psychology and Aging*, vol. 20, no. 4, pp. 695–709, 2005.

[14] J. A. Anguera, J. Boccanfuso, J. L. Rintoul et al., "Video game training enhances cognitive control in older adults," *Nature*, vol. 501, no. 7465, pp. 97–101, 2013.

[15] C. Basak, W. R. Boot, M. W. Voss, and A. F. Kramer, "Can training in a real-time strategy videogame attenuate cognitive decline in older adults?," *Psychology and Aging*, vol. 23, no. 4, pp. 765–777, 2008.

[16] P. Belchior, M. Marsiske, S. M. Sisco et al., "Video game training to improve selective visual attention in older adults," *Computers in Human Behavior*, vol. 29, no. 4, pp. 1318–1324, 2013.

[17] C. S. Green and D. Bavelier, "Action video game modifies visual selective attention," *Nature*, vol. 423, no. 6939, pp. 534–537, 2003.

[18] C. S. Green and D. Bavelier, "Action video game experience alters the spatial resolution of vision," *Psychological Science*, vol. 18, no. 1, pp. 88–94, 2007.

[19] A. M. Kueider, J. M. Parisi, A. L. Gross, and G. W. Rebok, "Computerized cognitive training with older adults: a systematic review," *PLoS One*, vol. 7, no. 7, article e40588, 2012.

[20] A. Lampit, H. Hallock, M. Valenzuela et al., "Computerized cognitive training in cognitively healthy older adults: a systematic review and meta-analysis of effect modifiers," *PLoS Medicine*, vol. 11, no. 11, p. e1001756, 2014.

[21] B. Hubert-Wallander, C. S. Green, and D. Bavelier, "Stretching the limits of visual attention: the case of action video games," *Wiley Interdisciplinary Reviews: Cognitive Science*, vol. 2, no. 2, pp. 222–230, 2010.

[22] J. C. Binder, J. Zöllig, A. Eschen et al., "Multi-domain training in healthy old age: hotel plastisse as an iPad-based serious game to systematically compare multi-domain and single-domain training," *Frontiers in Aging Neuroscience*, vol. 7, p. 137, 2015.

[23] G. Casutt, N. Theill, M. Martin, M. Keller, and L. Jäncke, "The drive-wise project: driving simulator training increases real driving performance in healthy older drivers," *Frontiers in Aging Neuroscience*, vol. 6, pp. 1–14, 2014.

[24] M. N. Lees, J. D. Cosman, J. D. Lee, and N. Fricke, "Translating cognitive neuroscience to the driver's operational environment: a neuroergonomic approach," *American Journal of Psychology*, vol. 123, no. 4, pp. 391–411, 2010.

[25] K. Murphy and A. Spencer, "Playing video games does not make for better visual attention skills," *Journal of Articles in Support of the Null Hypothesis*, vol. 6, no. 1, pp. 1–20, 2009.

[26] N. Chaytor and M. Schmitter-Edgecombe, "The ecological validity of neuropsychological tests: a review of the literature on everyday cognitive skills," *Neuropsychology Review*, vol. 13, no. 4, pp. 181–197, 2003.

[27] C. Deniaud, V. Honnet, B. Jeanne, and D. Mestre, "The concept of "presence" as a measure of ecological validity in driving simulators," *Journal of Interaction Science*, vol. 3, no. 1, p. 1, 2015.

[28] D. Moreau and A. R. A. Conway, "The case for an ecological approach to cognitive training," *Trends in Cognitive Sciences*, vol. 18, no. 7, pp. 334–336, 2014.

[29] O. J. Clay, V. G. Wadley, J. D. Edwards, D. L. Roth, D. L. Roenker, and K. K. Ball, "Cumulative meta-analysis of the relationship between useful field of view and driving performance in older adults: current and future implications," *Optometry and Vision Science*, vol. 82, no. 8, pp. 724–731, 2005.

[30] H. Sakai, Y. Uchiyama, M. Takahara et al., "Is the useful field of view a good predictor of at-fault crash risk in elderly Japanese drivers?," *Geriatrics and Gerontology International*, vol. 15, no. 5, pp. 659–665, 2015.

[31] S. M. Cox, D. J. Cox, M. J. Kofler et al., "Driving simulator performance in novice drivers with autism spectrum disorder: the role of executive functions and basic motor skills," *Journal of Autism and Developmental Disorders*, vol. 46, no. 4, pp. 1379–1391, 2015.

[32] D. L. Roenker, G. M. Cissell, K. K. Ball, V. G. Wadley, and J. D. Edwards, "Speed-of-processing and driving simulator training result in improved driving performance," *Human*

Factors: The Journal of the Human Factors and Ergonomics Society, vol. 45, no. 2, pp. 218–233, 2003.

[33] J. D. Edwards, C. Myers, L. A. Ross et al., "The longitudinal impact of cognitive speed of processing training on driving mobility," *The Gerontologist*, vol. 49, no. 4, pp. 485–494, 2009.

[34] N. D. Cassavaugh and A. F. Kramer, "Transfer of computer-based training to simulated driving in older adults," *Applied Ergonomics*, vol. 40, no. 5, pp. 943–952, 2009.

[35] A. Gazzaley and A. C. Nobre, "Top-down modulation: bridging selective attention and working memory," *Trends in Cognitive Sciences*, vol. 16, no. 2, pp. 129–135, 2012.

[36] A. H. Lara and J. D. Wallis, "The role of prefrontal cortex in working memory: a mini review," *Frontiers in Systems Neuroscience*, vol. 9, no. 173, pp. 1–7, 2015.

[37] J. Adrian, V. Postal, M. Moessinger, N. Rascle, and A. Charles, "Personality traits and executive functions related to on-road driving performance among older drivers," *Accident Analysis and Prevention*, vol. 43, no. 5, pp. 1652–1659, 2011.

[38] E. E. Freeman, B. Muñoz, G. Rubin, and S. K. West, "Visual field loss increases the risk of falls in older adults: the Salisbury eye evaluation," *Investigative Opthalmology and Visual Science*, vol. 48, no. 10, pp. 4445–4450, 2007.

[39] C. Owsley and G. J. McGwin, "Association between visual attention and mobility in older adults," *Journal of the American Geriatrics Society*, vol. 52, no. 11, pp. 1901–1906, 2004.

[40] J. R. Reed-Jones, S. Dorgo, M. K. Hitchings, and J. O. Bader, "Vision and agility training in community dwelling older adults: incorporating visual training into programs for fall prevention," *Gait and Posture*, vol. 35, no. 4, pp. 585–589, 2012.

[41] G. Yogev-Seligmann, J. M. Hausdorff, and N. Giladi, "The role of executive function and attention in gait," *Movement Disorders*, vol. 23, no. 3, pp. 329–342, 2008.

[42] R. W. Bohannon, "Reference values for the timed up and go test: a descriptive meta-analysis," *Journal of Geriatric Physical Therapy*, vol. 29, no. 2, pp. 64–68, 2006.

[43] M. E. Kelly, D. Loughrey, B. A. Lawlor, I. H. Robertson, C. Walsh, and S. Brennan, "The impact of cognitive training and mental stimulation on cognitive and everyday functioning of healthy older adults: a systematic review and meta-analysis," *Ageing Research Reviews*, vol. 15, pp. 28–43, 2014.

[44] P. Wang, H.-H. Liu, X.-T. Zhu, T. Meng, H.-J. Li, and X.-N. Zuo, "Action video game training for healthy adults: a meta-analytic study," *Frontiers in Psychology*, vol. 7, no. 907, pp. 1–13, 2016.

[45] M. A. Posner, "Orienting of attention," *Quarterly Journal of Experimental Psychology*, vol. 32, no. 1, pp. 3–25, 1980.

[46] J. T. Coull, "Neural Correlates of attention and arousal: insight from electrophysiology, functional neuroimaging and Psychopharmacology," *Progress in Neurobiology*, vol. 55, no. 4, pp. 343–361, 1998.

[47] R. Brickenkamp, *Test d2 Aufmerksamkeits-Belastungs-Test Manual 9. überarb*, Hogrefe, Göttingen, Germany, 2002.

[48] S. Hüttermann, D. Memmert, D. J. Simons, and O. Bock, "Fixation strategy influences the ability to focus attention on two spatially separate objects," *PLoS One*, vol. 8, no. 6, article e65673, 2013.

[49] S. Hale, N. S. Rose, J. Myerson et al., "The structure of working memory abilities across the adult life span," *Psychology and Aging*, vol. 26, no. 1, pp. 92–110, 2011.

[50] A. Miyake, N. P. Friedman, M. J. Emerson, A. H. Witzki, and A. Howerter, "The unity and diversity of executive functions and their contributions to complex "Frontal Lobe" tasks: a latent variable analysis," *Cognitive Psychology*, vol. 41, no. 1, pp. 49–100, 2000.

[51] A. Baddeley, "Working memory: theories, models, and controversies," *Annual Review of Psychology*, vol. 63, no. 1, pp. 1–29, 2012.

[52] J. Karbach and J. Kray, "How useful is executive control training? Age differences in near and far transfer of task-switching training," *Developmental Science*, vol. 12, no. 6, pp. 978–990, 2009.

[53] C. Huy and S. Schneider, "Instrument für die erfassung der physischen aktivität bei personen im mittleren und höheren erwachsenenalter: entwicklung, prüfung und anwendung des "German-PAQ-50+"," *Zeitschrift für Gerontologie und Geriatrie*, vol. 41, no. 3, pp. 208–216, 2008.

[54] B. R. Greene, A. O'Donovan, R. Romero-Ortuno, L. Cogan, C. N. Scanaill, and R. A. Kenny, "Quantitative falls risk assessment using the timed up and go test," *IEEE Transactions on Biomedical Engineering*, vol. 57, no. 12, pp. 2918–2926, 2010.

[55] M. F. Folstein, S. E. Folstein, and P. R. McHugh, "Mini-mental state; a practical method for grading the cognitive state of patients for the clinician," *International Journal of Geriatric Psychiatry*, vol. 12, no. 3, pp. 189–198, 1975.

[56] J. Cohen, *Statistical Power Analysis for the Behavioral Sciences*, p. 567, New York, NY, USA, Lawrence Erlbaum Associates, 1988.

[57] R. Rosenthal, "Parametric measures of effect size," in *The Handbook of Research Synthesis*, H. Cooper and L. V. Hedges, Eds., pp. 231–244, Russell Sage Foundation, New York, NY, USA, 1994.

[58] C. S. Green and D. Bavelier, "Learning, attentional control, and action video games," *Current Biology*, vol. 22, no. 6, pp. R197–R206, 2012.

[59] V. Montani, M. D. F. De Grazia, and M. Zorzi, "A new adaptive videogame for training attention and executive functions: design principles and initial validation," *Frontiers in Psychology*, vol. 5, pp. 1–12, 2014.

[60] J. Karbach and P. Verhaeghen, "Making working memory work: a meta-analysis of executive-control and working memory training in older adults," *Psychological Science*, vol. 25, no. 11, pp. 2027–2037, 2014.

[61] D. E. R. Warburton, C. W. Nicol, and S. S. D. Bredin, "Health benefits of physical activity: the evidence," *Canadian Medical Association Journal*, vol. 174, no. 6, pp. 801–809, 2006.

25

Implementation of an Evidence-Based Exercise Program for Older Adults in South Florida

Richard C. Palmer,[1] Anamica Batra,[1] Chelsie Anderson,[1] Timothy Page,[1] Edgar Vieira,[2] and Laura Seff[1]

[1] *Robert Stempel College of Public Health and Social Work, 11200 SW 8th Street, Miami, FL 33199, USA*
[2] *College of Nursing and Health Sciences, 11200 SW 8th Street, Miami, FL 33199, USA*

Correspondence should be addressed to Richard C. Palmer; richard.palmer@fiu.edu

Academic Editor: Elke Bromberg

Introduction. This study aimed to examine how well an evidence-based physical activity program could be translated for wide scale dissemination and adoption to increase physical activity among community-dwelling older adults. *Methods.* Between October 2009 and December 2012, reach, fidelity, dosage, ease of implementation, and barriers to translation of EnhanceFitness (EF) were assessed. To assess effectiveness, a pretest-posttest design was used to measure increases in functional fitness (chair stands, arm curls, and the up-and-go test). *Results.* Fourteen community-based agencies offered 126 EF classes in 83 different locations and reached 4,490 older adults. Most participants were female (72%). Thirty-eight percent of participants did not complete the initial 16-week EF program. The 25% who received the recommended dose experienced an increase in upper and lower body strength and mobility. Further, participants reported high satisfaction with the program. *Conclusion.* EF was successfully implemented in a variety of settings throughout South Florida and reached a large number of older adults. However, challenges were encountered in ensuring that those who participated received a program dose that would lead to beneficial gains in functional fitness.

1. Introduction

Regular physical activity can promote physical and psychological wellbeing and reduce risk of disability and vulnerability to chronic diseases in older adults [1–5]. Nevertheless, adults over 50 years of age are the least physically active segment of the US adult population [6–8]. Evidence-based exercise programs designed for older adults show promise as a way to increase opportunities for safe and effective physical activity [9]. However, little is known about how well these programs, which were tested and evaluated using controlled trials, are translated for wider use in community settings [10]. It is important to know if research-based programs will maintain their effectiveness when they are implemented in community settings [11]. Further, accurate interpretation of outcomes depends on knowing which aspects of the intervention were delivered and how faithful the delivery was to original program design [12].

The Healthy Aging Regional Collaborative (HARC) was established by the Health Foundation of South Florida (HFSF) to increase the adoption of evidence-based programs that promote and preserve the health of older adults in South Florida. Among the programs selected was EnhanceFitness (EF), which is an evidence-based group exercise program for older adults of all fitness levels [13, 14]. EF aims to help participants improve overall functional fitness and personal wellbeing. Intervention studies have documented the efficacy of EF and have shown that EF improves performance on fitness assessments, perceived physical functioning, social functioning, mental health, and decreases bodily pain [15–18]. Limited evidence exists demonstrating that EF can be translated to community-based settings and still achieve improvements in fitness and wellbeing [19]. Therefore, we investigated the ability of HARC to implement and sustain the EF program in South Florida over a three-year period. We examine if HARC was able to retain program fidelity, recommended dosage and exposure to the program, and comparable gains in functional fitness.

2. Methods

2.1. Setting. The Healthy Aging Regional Collaborative was created to increase local community capacity to offer accessible health promotion programs to older adults in South Florida. HARC was established by the HFSF and was designed to (1) disseminate evidence-based health promotion programs to address inactivity and chronic health conditions in older adults in South Florida; (2) establish a local group of trained professionals and lay leaders with the capacity to provide a range of evidence-based health promotion programs to older adults on an ongoing basis; and (3) provide a foundation for planning, coordination, technical assistance, and peer learning for present and future collaborative members. Community-based agencies that were interested in participating in HARC had to apply to HFSF and received funding to offer evidence-based programs, including EF. Funding covered licensing for use of the selected evidence-based program, instructor training, program implementation materials and equipment, and support for the administrative costs of implementation, including procurement of sites, instructors and participants, data collection, and data entry. Funded agencies were responsible for delivering EF. Agencies identified suitable sites to offer EF classes (i.e., churches, senior housing, senior centers, community centers, and parks) as well as recruited program participants.

2.2. EnhanceFitness Overview and Implementation. A one-hour EF class includes a 5-minute warm-up, a 20-minute low impact aerobic workout, a 5-minute cooldown, a 20-minute strength training workout, and 10 minutes of stretching and is offered three times per week. Instructors who were certified by a nationally recognized fitness organization (i.e., YMCA, ACE, or ACSM) and who received training in EF procedures at a two-day training conducted by EF program developers and EF master trainers led classes. All instructors were required to teach EF as outlined in EF training materials provided by the program developer. Individuals over the age of 50 who were interested in participating in EF were enrolled by agencies as long as they were cognitively and physically able to participate in the EF program.

2.3. Data Collection and Management. Multiple sources of data were collected to evaluate how well HARC agencies were able to implement EF. Descriptive/demographic data form, a health history, a fitness check (FC), and program satisfaction survey were collected. Participant data were collected at enrollment, with a second FC and the evaluation scheduled to be completed 16 weeks after enrollment as prescribed by the EF program. Program managers and instructors collected all participant data. All staff who administered the forms and collected data were trained regarding the meaning and importance of the items and shown the correct way to administer the three functional tests included on the FC during EF training sessions. Program managers submitted class registrations, new and ongoing participant data, and participant attendance records to HARC's evaluation team. An annual survey of program managers was also conducted online. Program fidelity was monitored by trained observers who observed randomly selected classes and then completed a fidelity observation checklist aimed at identifying implementation issues.

Prior to receiving any data from agencies, HARC's evaluation team received approval from the Institutional Review Board at Florida International University to conduct the evaluation of HARC.

2.4. Measures. The number of agencies, sites, classes, and participants were tracked as measures of EF implementation. Demographic characteristics of participants were self-identified on a form that included questions regarding gender, age, race and ethnicity, highest level of education, annual personal income, living situation (alone or with others), marital status, and primary spoken language. Participant satisfaction was measured using the satisfaction survey developed and provided by EF.

Effectiveness of the EF program was assessed based on changes in measures of functional fitness (30-second arm curl to assess upper extremity strength, the 30-second chair stand to measure lower extremity strength, and the timed eight-foot up-and-go circuit to measure balance and mobility), self-reported general health, and self-reported frequency (days per week) of exercise of at least 30-minute duration.

Additional measures included (1) the BRFSS general health measure, with a response scale from 1 = poor to 5 = excellent [20]; (2) self-reported number of days of exercise of at least 30-minute duration in a week, including EF sessions; and (3) a single item on the second FC to measure the self-reported degree of improvement in physical abilities (walking, bending, strength, moving around, and doing the activities you want to do) as a result of EF program participation, reported on a 10-point scale where 1 is no improvement and 10 is great improvement. Attendance records provided data regarding dose, average number of sessions attended by participants, and average duration of participant enrollment.

The annual survey of HARC program coordinators served as a process evaluation tool and identified implementation issues that agencies in HARC experienced. Questions specific to implementing EF were included each year and only agencies who offered the EF program completed these items. Items assessed ease of implementing the EF program, challenges with implementation, assessed participant recruitment activities, and also assessed long-term adoption and sustainability.

Observations of 30% of randomly selected classes assessed fidelity to the program design. Observers were staff members of the evaluation team and were trained on program specifications through a detailed review of the instructor manual. As part of the training, observers would accompany an experienced observer and interrater reliability would be assessed. Observers used a structured checklist that was based on the instructor manual and was developed by the evaluation team, EF master trainers, and HARC member agencies.

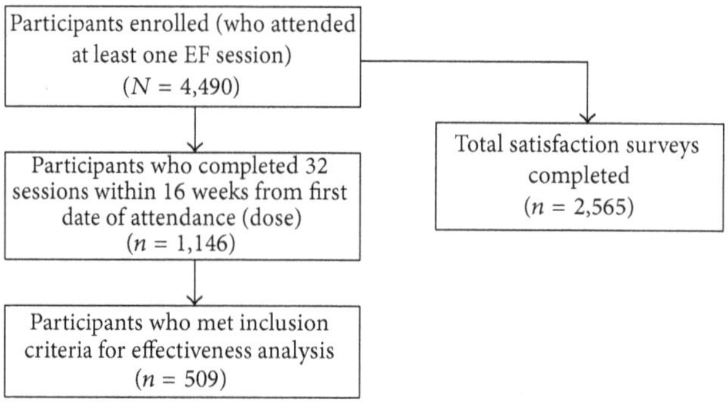

Figure 1: Number of participants by inclusion criteria.

The checklist specified observable elements related to the class environment, instructor, duration, and site. Each element was marked as observed or not observed. Discrepancies from the prescribed exercise routine were noted in a comment section.

2.5. Data Analysis. Of the 4,490 enrolled participants, 1,146 received the dose of the intervention proposed by Belza and colleagues [13] (Figure 1). Exclusion criteria for the current study include (1) no data for the pretest, the posttest, or both; (2) a first FC that did not fall within 30 days before and seven days after the first attendance date (to assure that baseline data reflected actual abilities prior to any benefits received from attending EF sessions); (3) a second FC completed before the recommended dose was attained; and (4) more than six months between the first and second fitness checks. With these exclusions, the sample used to calculate participant outcomes included 509 participants (Figure 1).

Data were extracted from the online database and imported into SPSS 22.0 for analysis. Data was first assessed for normality and outliers. Data on participant satisfaction, self-reported improvement in physical abilities, participant characteristics, participant attendance metrics, and program manager survey and fidelity observation data were analyzed using descriptive statistics. To test specific hypotheses about program effectiveness, the general linear model (GLM) was chosen to assess within-subject changes in outcome measures (arm curls, chair stands, and 8-foot up-and-go) at baseline and 6 weeks and controlled for potential differences in performance site [21].

3. Results

A total of 4,490 older adults enrolled and attended at least one EF session between October 1, 2009, and December 31, 2012. The majority of enrolled participants were women. Participant ages ranged from 29 to 107, with a mean age of 74.8 years (SD ± 9.9). The racial/ethnic composition of participants was diverse, with non-Hispanic whites and Hispanics making up the two largest groups (Table 1). The number of agencies, classes, sites, and participants, tracked in each of the first three years of the HARC as measures of EF implementation, are shown in Table 2, by year. Total number of participants reached increased every year. The largest number of new participants was reached in Year 1. After an expected reduction of new participants in Year 2, the number of new participants increased in Year 3, but not to the Year 1 level. At the end of the three-year period, nine agencies were funded and active, offering 70 ongoing EF classes at 56 sites (Table 2).

3.1. Fidelity. Sixty-nine EF classes were observed for fidelity by the evaluation team between, accounting for nearly 33% of all EF classes offered during the time period. Almost half of the observed classes, 47.8%, had no significant fidelity concerns in the measured dimensions. The most frequently cited concerns related to instructors not using key phrases developed to ensure participant safety, including checking if participants could see and hear the instructor (30%), and reminding participants not to do exercises their physician advised against (30%), not to do any exercises that were painful (16%), and to exercise at a pace that was comfortable (14%). Additionally, 41% of observed sessions lasted less than 60 minutes (Figure 2).

3.2. Dose. Of 4,490 participants enrolled in the HARC EF program between October 1, 2009, and December 31, 2012, who attended at least one session, an average of 26% received the minimum recommended dose [13] (Table 2). The ratio of completers to new participants enrolled declined in each of the three years. Other measures, potentially relevant in terms of dose, were examined. Three percent of enrolled participants attended only one session and 38% stopped attending within the initial 16 weeks. The average time between enrollment and last date of attendance was 1.1 years. The average number of sessions attended per participant was 59.

3.3. Ease of Implementation and Barriers. In the Year 1 program manager survey, six of seven program managers responsible for implementing EF reported that implementation was difficult or very difficult on a five-point scale from very easy to very difficult. In the Year 2 and Year 3 surveys, more than half of the program managers indicated that implementation was moderate, that is, half-way between very easy and very difficult on the measurement scale, showing

TABLE 1: Characteristics of EnhanceFitness participants.

	$N = 4{,}490^a$
Gender	
Female	3,216
Male	862
Age	
<60 years	176
60–69 years	948
70–79 years	1,462
80–89 years	936
90 years and over	276
County of residence	
Broward	1,588
Miami-Dade	1,920
Monroe	645
Race-ethnicity	
Hispanic/Latino	677
Haitian/other non-Hispanic Caribbeans	144
White, non-Hispanic	794
Black, non-Haitian	188
Other	44
Marital status	
Married/partnered	1,625
Single/not partnered	2,343
Annual income	
<$15,000	1,089
$15,000–$24,999	450
$25,000–$49,999	404
$50,000–$75,000	185
>$75,000	151
Education	
Less than high school	613
High school graduate	919
Some college	1,031
College graduate or higher	1,404
Other variables	
Frail/disabled	470
Has Medicare	2,641
Has Medicaid	807

[a]Reported values may not add up to total participant N due to missing data.

that ease of implementation improved over time. Implementation barriers most frequently cited over the three years remained relatively constant and included funding, inadequate staff, inadequate client interest, cultural norms of the community, and difficulty in recruiting class instructors. The most frequent barriers identified for recruiting participants included difficulty maintaining consistent participation and the seasonal residence of some participants in the South Florida area. The most frequent barriers to instructor recruitment included availability for the three weekly one-hour sessions, finding individuals who were committed to the EF program, and lack of transportation.

3.4. Effectiveness. Analysis revealed that participants who completed the recommended dose and received a posttest after participating in the program for four months significantly improved their scores on the three physical ability measures, self-reported general health, and frequency of daily exercise of at least 30-minute duration after participating in EF program (Table 3).

3.5. Participant Satisfaction. When asked on the second FC about improvements in physical abilities as a result of their EF participation, 71.5% of participants indicated improvement. Among the 2,565 EF participants who completed a program evaluation, 89% were satisfied or highly satisfied with the program. Additionally, 97% responded that they would take the class again and 92% would recommend the class to a friend.

4. Discussion

The HARC initiative described here is the largest scale translation of EF to a broad cross section of community agencies and settings within the same geographical area to date in the United States. Data reported here suggest that HARC was able to successfully implement EF throughout South Florida and reach a large number of older adults over the three-year period. These findings indicate that this effort to form a collaborative, sharing resources, training, and knowledge, was an effective approach for translating an evidence-based program to a wide array of community settings and sites.

Unlike controlled trials of EF, data reported here are based on the real world implementation of EF in a variety of community settings throughout South Florida. It was important to investigate if the community-based EF implementation produced participant changes similar to those reported in controlled EF efficacy studies. Our findings are consistent with prior controlled studies of EF and other fitness programs [13, 15, 16]. Participants in this study demonstrated statistically significant improvements in upper body strength, lower body strength, functional mobility, self-reported health status, and frequency of daily exercise of at least 30-minute duration over the follow-up period.

As with any adoption of a health promotion program, the potential for changes and deviations in the curriculum is a concern. Adaptation is a normal process, yet it can cause a program to be less effective if changes are made that undermine the program's effectiveness. In our evaluation, we assessed fidelity to determine how accurately EF agencies and instructors implemented the program. Surprisingly, very few concerns were identified for the core elements of the program. The majority of observed concerns involved safety warnings that instructors are supposed to use throughout the class.

Our evaluation did identify several areas that warrant comment and further investigation. A participant recruitment challenge relating to male participants existed. Only about 15% of participants were male, while the percentage of males in the total population in the three targeted Florida counties is much higher, at nearly 44% [22]. This rate of male participation is similar to findings of other programs

TABLE 2: HARC EnhanceFitness process measures.

Measure	Year 1 N	Year 2 N	Year 3 N	All years N
Participants	1,528	1,961	2,127	4,490
Percent completers	29.4%	24.3%	21.8%	25.5%
Agencies offering EF classes	8	9	9	14
EF classes offered	59	73	79	126
Classes observed for fidelity	18	25	26	69
Sites where EF classes were offered	51	60	63	83

EF: EnhanceFitness.

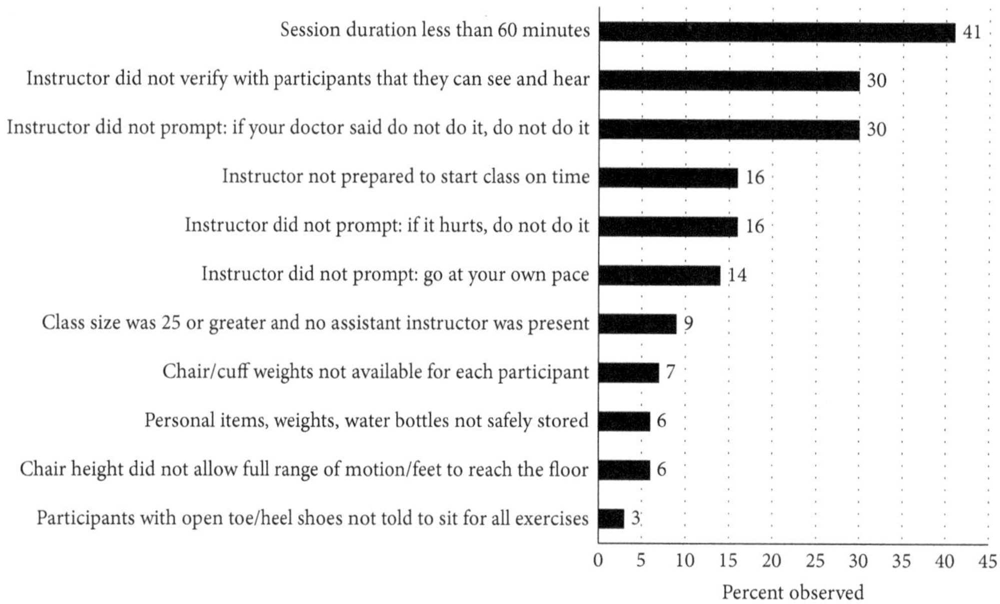

FIGURE 2: Frequency of fidelity concerns identified.

that serve older adults, although there is limited knowledge regarding why older men do not participate in health promotion programs [23, 24]. There is a need for research that explores how to overcome male resistance to such participation. Additionally, of the process issues identified, perhaps the most significant were frequency of attendance and attrition. There appears to be a problem with participants achieving the recommended dosage (32) sessions within a 16-week period that has been associated with functional fitness and mobility benefits [13]. Almost 41% of all EF participants in this region stopped attending within the initial 16-week period. Moreover, for those who did continue through the initial 16 weeks and beyond, only 26% attended at least 32 sessions in the first 16 weeks. In both cases, participants did not receive the dose that has been suggested as being optimal to obtain all the benefits associated with exercise and strength training. For EF to be effective, participants must participate regularly to achieve maximum benefits. Subsequently, more research is warranted to better understand the elements that affect attendance patterns of older adults at ongoing exercise programs and to explore strategies that effectively address these attendance barriers.

Although findings show that EF can be effectively implemented by a collaborative in South Florida and that participants can achieve benefits consistent with clinical trials if they participate regularly, this evaluation has certain limitations. As this was a community-based implementation and not a controlled research study, a randomized design could not be used. Participants self-selected into the program, so they may not be representative of the larger older adult population in South Florida. Bias could also be an issue if functional test results reflect the impact of health-promoting activities that participants engaged in other than EF. A large number of participants did not have documented follow-up measures, which reduced data available for analysis of fitness test results. Finally, functional test data are potentially subject to measurement bias because different instructors collected data on outcome measures. However, the rigorous training on data collection tools prior to being certified to teach an EF class, use of the same tool, and ongoing fidelity monitoring of instructors reduces the chances of measurement bias.

Even with these limitations, this study had strengths. The program was implemented by multiple agencies, and the diverse racial/ethnic mix of the South Florida participants is

TABLE 3: EnhanceFitness effectiveness measures.

Fitness test	N^a	Baseline mean (SD)	Follow-up mean (SD)	Change	P value
Number of chair stands in 30 seconds	491	11.78 (4.09)	15.41 (5.36)	3.63	<.001
Number of arm curls in 30 seconds	499	15.92 (5.85)	20.76 (7.34)	4.84	<.001
Number of seconds to complete up-and-go	487	8.62 (4.69)	7.40 (4.28)	−1.22	<.001

SD: standard deviation; N/A: not applicable.
[a]Reported values do not add up to total participant ($N = 509$) due to missing data.

likely different than demographic profiles found in previously described evaluations. Many measures of implementation used indicated successful introduction of the programs and ongoing fidelity to program design. A longer-term retrospective study of sustained fidelity and the program's impact on participant physical fitness, health status, frequency of exercise, and healthcare costs is needed to confirm that outcomes reported here endure over longer time periods.

5. Conclusions

Health promotion efforts targeting older adults are essential for improvement in quality of life, functional ability, and healthcare cost savings. HARC's innovative approach to rapid EF implementation on a wide scale shows that EF can be introduced in many different settings and delivered successfully. Moreover, there is reason to believe that community-based EF programs have the potential to offer access to an evidence-based physical activity with proven health benefits to a large percentage of older adults in the community. However, efforts are needed to ensure that community-based agencies that offer EF reinforce the importance of continued attendance to ensure the most benefit to program participants and that implementers continue to assess implementation fidelity of the program to the original design tested in controlled trials.

Competing Interests

The authors declare that there are no competing interests regarding the publication of this manuscript.

Acknowledgments

This study was supported by the Health Foundation of South Florida as part of the Healthy Aging Initiative. The authors would like to thank the member agencies of the Healthy Aging Regional Collaborative for their support and assistance with program implementation and data collection.

References

[1] US Department of Health and Human Services, *2008 Physical Activity Guidelines for Americans Summary*, 2008, https://health.gov/paguidelines/guidelines/summary.aspx.

[2] M. E. Cress, D. M. Buchner, T. Prohaska et al., "Physical activity programs and behavior counseling in older adult populations," *Medicine & Science in Sports & Exercise*, vol. 36, no. 11, pp. 1997–2003, 2004.

[3] R. S. Mazzero, P. Cavanagh, J. Evans et al., "American College of Sports Medicine. Position stand: exercise and physical activity for older adults," *Medicine & Science in Sports & Exercise*, vol. 30, no. 6, pp. 992–1008, 1998.

[4] W. J. Rejeski and S. L. Mihalko, "Physical activity and quality of life in older adults," *Journals of Gerontology Series A: Biological Sciences and Medical Sciences*, vol. 56, no. 2, pp. 23–35, 2001.

[5] F. Sun, I. J. Norman, and A. E. While, "Physical activity in older people: a systematic review," *BMC Public Health*, vol. 13, article 449, 2013.

[6] J. Kruger, S. A. Carlson, and D. Bucher, "How active are older Americans?" *Preventing Chronic Disease*, vol. 4, pp. 1–12, 2007.

[7] Centers for Disease Control and Prevention, *Behavioral Risk Factor Surveillance System Survey Data*, U.S. Department of Health and Human Services, Centers for Disease Control and Prevention, Atlanta, Ga, USA, 2006.

[8] C. A. Schoenborn and K. M. Heyman, "Health characteristics of adults aged 55 years and over: United States, 2004–2007," National Health Statistics Reports 16, National Center for Health Statistics, Hyattsville, Md, USA, 2009, http://www.cdc.gov/nchs/data/nhsr/nhsr016.pdf.

[9] A. C. King, W. J. Rejeski, and D. M. Buchner, "Physical activity interventions targeting older adults. A critical review and recommendations," *American Journal of Preventive Medicine*, vol. 15, no. 4, pp. 316–333, 1998.

[10] R. E. Glasgow, E. Lichtenstein, and A. C. Marcus, "Why don't we see more translation of health promotion research to practice? Rethinking the efficacy-to-effectiveness transition," *American Journal of Public Health*, vol. 93, no. 8, pp. 1261–1267, 2003.

[11] L. Dusenbury, R. Brannigan, W. B. Hansen, J. Walsh, and M. Falco, "Quality of implementation: developing measures crucial to understanding the diffusion of preventive interventions," *Health Education Research*, vol. 20, no. 3, pp. 308–313, 2005.

[12] J. A. Durlak and E. P. DuPre, "Implementation matters: a review of research on the influence of implementation on program outcomes and the factors affecting implementation," *American Journal of Community Psychology*, vol. 41, no. 3-4, pp. 327–350, 2008.

[13] B. Belza, S. Snyder, M. Thompson, and J. LoGerfo, "From research to practice: EnhanceFitness, an innovative community-based senior exercise program," *Topics in Geriatric Rehabilitation*, vol. 26, no. 4, pp. 299–309, 2010.

[14] Senior Services, Enhance Fitness, 2013, http://www.projectenhance.org/EnhanceFitness.aspx.

[15] T. L. Moore-Harrison, M. A. Johnson, M. E. Quinn, and M. E. Cress, "An evidence-based exercise program implemented in congregate-meal sites," *Journal of Physical Activity and Health*, vol. 6, no. 2, pp. 247–251, 2009.

[16] S. Snyder and B. Belza, "Eliminating disparities in communities of color through the Lifetime Fitness Program," 2005, http://www.cdc.gov/pcd/issues/2005/apr/04_0142j.htm.

[17] B. Belza, A. Shumway-Cook, E. A. Phelan, B. Williams, S. J. Snyder, and J. P. LoGerfo, "The effects of a community-based exercise program on function and health in older adults: the EnhanceFitness program," *Journal of Applied Gerontology*, vol. 25, no. 4, pp. 291–306, 2006.

[18] J. I. Wallace, D. M. Buchner, L. Grouthaus et al., "Implementation and effectiveness of a community-based health promotion program for older adults," *Journals of Gerontology Series A: Biological Sciences and Medical Sciences*, vol. 53, pp. M301–M306, 1998.

[19] M. Tomioka, N. Sugihara, and K. L. Braun, "Replicating the enhancefitness physical activity program in Hawai'i's multicultural population, 2007–2010," *Preventing Chronic Disease*, vol. 9, no. 3, Article ID 110155, 2012.

[20] Centers for Disease Control and Prevention, *Behavioral Risk Factor Surveillance System Survey Questionnaire*, U.S. Department of Health and Human Services, Centers for Disease Control and Prevention, Atlanta, Ga, USA, 2008.

[21] P. McCullagh and J. Nelder, *Generalized Linear Models*, Chapman and Hall/CRC, London, UK, 2nd edition, 1989.

[22] U.S Census Bureau, 2010 Census Data, http://www.census.gov/2010census/data/.

[23] W. H. Courtenay, "Constructions of masculinity and their influence on men's well-being: a theory of gender and health," *Social Science and Medicine*, vol. 50, no. 10, pp. 1385–1401, 2000.

[24] M. E. Addis and J. R. Mahalik, "Men, masculinity, and the contexts of help seeking," *American Psychologist*, vol. 58, no. 1, pp. 5–14, 2003.

26

Health Status and Social Networks as Predictors of Resilience in Older Adults Residing in Rural and Remote Environments

Christine McKibbin, Aaron Lee, Bernard A. Steinman, Catherine Carrico, Katelynn Bourassa, and Andrea Slosser

University of Wyoming, 1000 E. University Avenue, Laramie, WY 82071, USA

Correspondence should be addressed to Christine McKibbin; cmckibbi@uwyo.edu

Academic Editor: Enrica Menditto

Purpose. Health status and social networks are associated with resilience among older adults. Each of these factors may be important to the ability of adults to remain in rural and remote communities as they age. We examined the association of health status and social networks and resilience among older adults dwelling in a rural and remote county in the Western United States. *Methods.* We selected a random sample of 198 registered voters aged 65 years or older from a frontier Wyoming county. Hierarchical linear regression was used to examine the association of health status as well as social networks and resilience. We also examined health status as a moderator of the relationship between social networks and resilience. *Results.* Family networks ($p = 0.024$) and mental health status ($p < 0.001$) significantly predicted resilience. Mental health status moderated the relationship of family ($p = 0.004$) and friend ($p = 0.021$) networks with resilience. Smaller family and friend networks were associated with greater resilience when mental health status was low, but not when it was high. *Conclusion.* Efforts to increase mental health status may improve resilience among older adults in rural environments, particularly for those with smaller family and friends networks.

1. Introduction

Older rural adults comprise a large and increasing percentage of the population in the United States. As of 2014, more than 16% of the population aged 65 years and older were categorized as living in rural settings by the US Census Bureau [1]. The proportion of older adults in rural areas has grown rapidly due in part to aging in place, retirement transitions, and outmigration of younger families [2]. Frontier areas are the most remote and sparsely populated areas among these rural settings. While it is well known that most older adults would prefer to age in their homes and communities [3], older residents in the most remote areas may be far from healthcare and social services, social venues, and other necessities to promote engagement and independent living. Additionally, transportation is frequently lacking and traveling to larger towns and cities where necessities including healthcare are located can be difficult [4].

Shifting demographic trends in rural and remote communities will bring societal changes and challenges. Primary among them will be identifying effective resources to foster health, wellbeing, and independence of older people as they face many of the stressors that often accompany aging in rural environments. For example, with increasing age, risk escalates for adverse outcomes associated with physical and mental health [5], disability [6], declining social network size [7], and economic security [8]. These stressors may be compounded by living in low-density population regions and can impact the quality of life of older adults, especially when the resources they may have available to help them adapt to change may be suboptimal.

The concept of resilience has gained traction as a means to explain how some individuals are able to bounce back from adverse events and stressors and adapt to their changing life circumstances, while others continue to struggle or decline in the face of similar events. On an individual level, resilience is thought to be a personality attribute that helps to neutralize negative effects of high stress [9]. According to Wagnild [10] resilience comprises dimensions of equanimity, a sense of purpose, perseverance, and acceptance of one's life, and a belief in one's self and capabilities. As a general resource possessed by many older adults, resilience can serve to buffer the negative impacts of stress, promote adaptation to late life changes, and contribute to maintenance of independent functioning and wellbeing [11].

As a research construct, resilience has received increasing attention in recent years. For instance, resilience has been examined in relation to specific age-related stressors, including pain [12, 13], mental health outcomes [14], aging with HIV/AIDS [15], bereavement following loss of a spouse [16], and having low income [10]. These studies suggest that resilience may play an important role in promoting healthy response to age-related change.

Much of the previous research on resilience has focused on urban and suburban samples [17] and few studies have examined resilience of community-dwelling older adults in rural and remote settings. One exception is research by Wells [18], which examined resilience levels of older adults residing in rural New York as well as predictors of resilience levels. Wells found that resilience levels were high in participants of this study. Importantly, resilience was not associated with sociodemographic factors and was only weakly associated with social networks. Significant relationships were also reported between physical and mental health status and resilience. While this was one of the first studies examining resilience among rural adults, the study was conducted in one rural community in New York. It is not clear to what degree these results will generalize to other rural communities or to older adults living in not only rural but also remote areas. Moreover, several studies show relationships between social networks and health among older adults [19–21]. Additionally, the work of Li and Zhang showed that relationships between social networks and health among older adults may be bidirectional such that those who have poorer health rely on more restricted social networks [20]. To date, few studies have been conducted to examine whether health status may moderate the relationship between social networks and other constructs like resilience among older adults, especially those residing in rural or remote areas.

The purpose of this study was to extend this small but important body of research. As part of this study, we examined the relationships between resilience and both social networks and health status, in a sample of older adults living in a rural environment. This study differs from the previous work, in that we sampled a population that is relatively more remote than the sample analyzed by Wells [18, 22] and substantially more remote than many other areas in the United States. The Western US state of Wyoming is unique with regard to its topography and the distribution of its population. Cities and towns are widely dispersed across the state's 97,093 square miles and long distances between points of interest are common. Additionally, the population of the state is very small relative to other states. According to estimates produced by data from the American Community Survey (ACS), there were just fewer than 600,000 Wyoming residents in 2014, equating to only about 5.8 persons per square mile (compared to 87.4 persons per square mile, nationally) [1]. Thus, many older Wyoming residents live in an expansive frontier environment that creates unique challenges for them with respect to accessing resources and necessities. Additionally, residents in general may live long distances away from their families, friends, and neighbors, potentially reducing the support and resources available when stressors such as acute and chronic illnesses arise. Given these circumstances, it is reasonable to expect that health outcomes and individual characteristics such as resilience may differ in this type of environment, even compared to other areas that are also categorized as rural. We expected that, like the work of Wells [18], social networks and health status would predict resilience. To build upon existing research, we examined moderation effects of physical and mental health status on the relationship of social networks and resilience in rural, community-dwelling older adults. We hypothesized that both physical and mental health status would moderate the relationship between social networks and resilience.

2. Methods

2.1. Study Sample. The University of Wyoming's Institutional Review Board approved all study methods. We used random sampling methods to obtain a sample of older adults residing in a frontier Wyoming county. First, we used the United States Department of Agriculture (USDA) Economic Research Service's 2013 Rural-Urban Continuum Codes [23] to determine the rurality of all counties in the state. This scale ranges from 0 to 9, with nine being the most rural based on the degree of urbanization and proximity to metro areas. We chose Fremont County, which scores a 7 on the scale, as the basis for our sample (compared to a rating of 6 for the county analyzed in the study by Wells [18]). Fremont County is relatively more rural than the rest of Wyoming, with only 4.4 persons per square mile. A prospective pool of study participants over the age of 65 residing in Fremont County ($N = 3{,}368$) was identified using the 2009 voting registration electoral roll. From this population, a sample of 600 individuals (18%) was randomly selected to receive a mailed survey packet.

Mailings included four components: (1) a cover letter that described the project, (2) a consent form that explained the recipient's rights as a research participant, (3) a raffle entry slip that gave participants an opportunity to win a $50 gift card as incentive to participate, and (4) the survey instrument (described below). Postcards reminding prospective participations of our request were mailed two weeks after the initial mailing. Of the 600 packets that were sent, 80 (13%) were returned as undeliverable. Of the 520 successfully delivered surveys, 225 were returned with useable data, resulting in a return rate of about 43%. A total of 27 incomplete surveys with only partial demographic data completed were removed prior to analysis, yielding a sample of 198 respondents.

2.2. Measures. The survey comprised questionnaires assessing the following four components: (1) sociodemographics, (2) degree of resilience, (3) self-reported physical and mental health status, and (4) size and quality of social networks.

2.2.1. Sociodemographic Questionnaire. The sociodemographic questionnaire included items that assessed the age, gender, race/ethnicity, educational attainment, marital status, and employment status of participants.

2.2.2. Connor-Davidson Resilience Scale. We measured each participant's degree of resilience using the Connor-Davidson Resilience Scale (CD-RISC; [24]). The CD-RISC is a 25-item questionnaire that asks participants to rate their level of agreement over the last month with statements such as "*I am able to adapt when changes occur*" and "*I tend to bounce back after illness, injury, or other hardships.*" Each statement was rated on a 0 (not true at all) to 5 (*true nearly all the time*) scale. Item responses were summed to generate a total score, with higher scores indicating greater resilience. The CD-RISC has demonstrated convergent validity and good internal reliability ($\alpha = 0.89$) in previous work [24] as well as in the current study ($\alpha = 0.92$).

2.2.3. Short-Form Revised Health Survey. We assessed the physical and mental health status of participants using all twelve items of the Short-Form revised Health Survey (SF-12v2). Items in this instrument ask participants to rate their general health and to describe how physical and mental health issues limit or interfere with their daily activities and social activities. Weighted-items scores were used to calculate a Physical Component Summary score and a Mental Component Summary score. The SF-12v2 provides norms-based scores for the Physical Component Summary and the Mental Component Summary scores that are standardized (population mean = 50; standard deviation = 10) with higher scores reflecting greater functioning in each domain [25].

2.2.4. Lubben Social Network Scale-6. We used the abbreviated Lubben Social Network Scale-6 to assess the social networks and supports of participants [26]. The Lubben Social Network Scale-6 is comprised of two 3-item subscales, which assess the size and quality of family and friend social networks. Several items are designed to assess the number of regular social contacts. For example, respondents are asked, "*How many relatives do you see or hear from at least once a month?*" Responses to these items are made on a five-point scale ranging from 0 (*none*) to 5 (*nine or more*). Other items ask about frequency of contact with family and friends (e.g., "*How often do you hear from the relative with whom you have the most contact?*"). Responses to these items range from 0 (*less than monthly*) to 5 (*daily*). Finally, the quality and availability of social relationships are addressed using items such as "*How often is one of your relatives available for you to talk to when you have an important decision to make?*" Responses to these items range from 0 (*never*) to 5 (*always*). Higher scores on the Lubben Social Network Scale reflect more substantial social networks. Subscale scores less than or equal to 6 are suggestive of marginal family and friendship ties, and total scores less than or equal to 12 are indicative of social isolation. Both subscales have demonstrated convergent validity with measures of emotional support and social engagement [26]. The family and friend subscales have demonstrated good internal reliability in previous work (i.e., $\alpha = 0.89$ and 0.82, resp.) [26] as well as in the current study ($\alpha = 0.80$ and 0.81, resp.).

2.3. Statistical Analysis. All analyses were conducted using Statistical Package for the Social Sciences (SPSS) Version 22.0 [27]. Descriptive statistics (i.e., percentages, means, and standard deviations) were calculated to characterize the sample. Bivariate analyses were used to assess the zero-order correlations among SF-12vs component scores (i.e., Physical Component Summary and Mental Component Summary score), Lubben Social Network Scale subscale scores (family and friends), and resilience scores. A two-step hierarchical linear regression was used to simultaneously examine Physical Component Summary scores, Mental Component Summary scores, family network scores, and friend network scores as predictors of resilience while controlling for relevant sociodemographic variables. We entered age, gender, educational attainment (i.e., ≤ high school = 0; > high school = 1), marital status (i.e., single, divorced, or widowed = 0; married or long-term relationship = 1), and employment status (i.e., not employed = 0; employed = 1) in the first step of the model. In the second step of the model, we entered SF-12v2 Physical Component Summary and Mental Component Summary scores, as well as the family network and friend network scores. Tolerances were assessed for possible multicollinearity.

We used the PROCESS macro for SPSS to examine whether SF-12v2 Physical Component Summary scores and Mental Component Summary scores moderated the relationships between the social network subscales and resilience scores [28]. All predictors and covariates were mean centered. Heteroskedasticity consistent standard error estimators were used to guard against violations of homogeneity of variance [29]. Simple slopes were evaluated at one standard deviation above and below the mean of the moderator variable. The Johnson-Neyman approach was used to determine the boundary value of the moderator above and below which simple slopes were significantly different from zero [28, 30].

Bias-corrected and accelerated bootstrapping with 5,000 replications was used to estimate 95% confidence intervals ($CI_{95\%}$) for all correlation and unstandardized regression coefficients. Alpha was set to $p < 0.05$, and all tests were two-tailed.

3. Results

Table 1 depicts the result of descriptive analyses. The majority of survey respondents were female, non-Hispanic White, married, and retired. Age of participants ranged from 64 to 95 years and the average age was about 74 years. The mean resilience score was near 80 and comparable to the average resilience (i.e., CD-RISC) scores for the US general population (M = 80.4) [24]. Average social network scores for family and friends were each over 8 and greater than the suggested cut-point of 6 used for identifying marginal family and friendship networks among older adults [26]. Using a cut-score of 6 or lower, approximately 17% of the sample had marginal family networks and 24% of the sample had marginal friend networks. Physical Component Summary scores and Mental Component Summary scores of study participants were each slightly higher on average than the established population means for adults aged 65 years and

TABLE 1: Descriptive statistics for covariates, independent variables, and dependent variable (N = 198).

	M (SD)	n (%)
Sociodemographic		
Age	73.68 (6.90)	
Gender (female)		104 (52.5)
Race (white)		186 (93.9)
Non-Hispanic		198 (100)
Education (> high school)		149 (75.3)
Not employed		151 (76.3)
Married or having a long-term relationship		121 (61.1)
SF-12 health status		
MCS	53.49 (7.56)	
PCS	46.36 (10.50)	
Lubben Social Network Scale-6		
Friends	8.93 (2.85)	
Family	8.30 (3.18)	
CD-RISC	81.56 (12.23)	

Note. MCS: Mental Component Summary score; PCS: Physical Component Summary score; family: family network size; friend: friend network size; CD-RISC: resilience.

TABLE 2: Correlations among all independent variables and dependent variable (N = 198).

	PCS	Family	Friend	CD-RISC
MCS	0.11	$0.21^{\dagger}$	$0.22^{\dagger}$	$0.48^{\ddagger}$
PCS		0.08	0.14	0.16^{*}
Family			$0.56^{\ddagger}$	$0.33^{\ddagger}$
Friend				$0.28^{\ddagger}$

$^{*}p < 0.05$; $^{\dagger}p < 0.01$; $^{\ddagger}p < 0.001$.
Note. MCS: Mental Component Summary score; PCS: Physical Component Summary score; family: family network size; friend: friend network size; CD-RISC: resilience.

older (Physical Component Summary score, M = 43.73, and Mental Component Summary score, M = 53.15) [25]. Table 2 shows correlations among all key predictor and outcome variables. Notably, significant positive correlations were found between resilience and Physical Component Summary scores (p = 0.025), Mental Component Summary scores (p < 0.001), family networks (p < 0.001), and friend networks (p < 0.001).

Table 3 shows unstandardized regression coefficients, standard errors, and ΔR^2 values for the two-step hierarchical linear regression analysis. In step one of the analysis, the covariates (i.e., age, gender, educational attainment, marital status, and employment status) did not explain a significant amount of variance in resilience scores, and none of the variables independently predicted resilience scores. In the second step, the Physical Component Summary score, Mental Component Summary score, family network, and friend network scores accounted for a significant increase

TABLE 3: Regression results of resilience status on covariates and independent variables (N = 198).

	B	SE	ΔR^2	p
Step1			<0.01	0.994
Age	−0.01	0.15		0.974
Gender	0.51	1.81		0.786
Relationship status	0.67	1.95		0.726
Employed	−0.31	2.00		0.876
Education	0.77	2.15		0.715
Step2			0.29	<0.001
SF-12 MCS	0.67	0.11		<0.001
SF-12 PCS	0.10	0.08		0.165
LSNS-6 friend	0.23	0.29		0.424
LSNS-6 family	0.88	0.39		0.024
Full-model			0.30	<0.001

Note. MCS: Mental Component Summary score; PCS: Physical Component Summary score; LSNS-6 friend: friend network size; LSNS-6 family: family network size; CD-RISC: resilience.

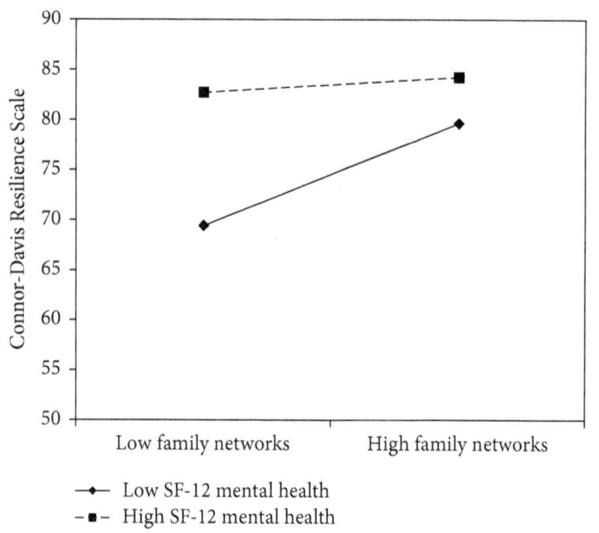

FIGURE 1: The simple slopes of Lubben Social Network Scale-6 family networks on Connor-Davis Resilience Scale scores at high and low levels of SF-12 Mental Health Component Summary scores.

in explained variance in resilience scores. Whereas, the Physical Component Summary scores and friend networks were not significant predictors of resilience, both the Mental Component Summary score and family network scores significantly predicted resilience scores while controlling for sociodemographic variables.

As shown in Figure 1, the bootstrapped test of moderation yielded a significant interaction of family network by Mental Component Summary scores on resilience scores (B = −0.10, SE = 0.03, $CI_{95\%}$ [−0.17, −0.03], and p = 0.004), when controlling for age, gender, educational attainment, marital status, and employment status. Specifically, family network scores significantly predicted resilience scores at low (i.e., −1 SD) values of Mental Component Summary

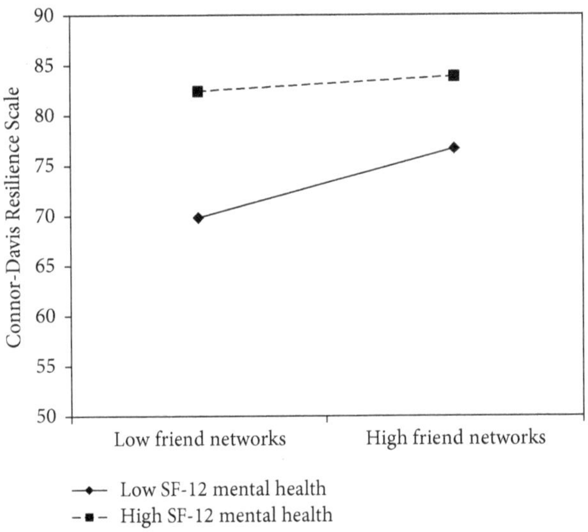

FIGURE 2: The simple slopes of Lubben Social Network Scale-6 friend networks on Connor-Davis Resilience Scale scores at high and low levels of SF-12 Mental Health Component Summary scores.

scores (B = 1.80, SE = 0.39, $CI_{95\%}$ [1.03, 2.57], and p < 0.001). However, no significant relationship between family networks and resilience was observed at high (i.e., +1 SD) values of Mental Component Summary scores (B = 0.27, SE = 0.42, $CI_{95\%}$ [−0.56, 1.10], and p = 0.529). Family networks significantly predicted resilience below, but not above, the Mental Component Summary score of 56.98. The majority of the sample (n = 117, 59.1%) scored below this boundary value.

Figure 2 shows the significant interaction of friend networks by Mental Component Summary scores on resilience scores (B = −0.06, SE = 0.02, $CI_{95\%}$ [−0.10, −0.01], and p = 0.021), when controlling for sociodemographic covariates. Analysis of simple slopes showed a significant positive association between friend networks and resilience at low (−1 SD) levels of Mental Component Summary scores (B = 1.07, SE = 0.32, $CI_{95\%}$ [0.45, 1.71], and p = 0.001). There was no significant association between friend networks and resilience at high (+1 SD) levels of Mental Component Summary scores (B = 0.23, SE = 0.28, $CI_{95\%}$ [−0.33, 0.78], and p = 0.425). Friend networks were significantly associated with resilience below, but not above, the Mental Component Summary score of 49.45, below which most participants scored (n = 115, 58.1%).

Contrary to our expectations, moderation analyses did not show any additional significant interactions between the Physical Component Summary scores and family (B = −0.02, SE = 0.04, $CI_{95\%}$ [−0.09, 0.05], and p = 0.619) or friend (B = −0.05, SE = 0.04, $CI_{95\%}$ [−0.13, 0.02], and p = 0.163) networks when controlling for age, gender, educational attainment, marital status, and employment status.

4. Discussion

Developing a better understanding of resilience in rural older adults and its interrelationships with social networks and health status can help determine who may struggle to adapt successfully to stressful age-related changes and, ultimately, who will experience poorer outcomes. Literature shows that older adults living in rural and remote areas possess varying degrees of resilience, as do individuals living in urban and suburban areas [20]. For some older adults, a rural environment with strong social networks can provide valuable caring environments for people as they age. For others, rural environments may be isolating.

Results of our study showed that resilience levels of older adults living in a rural and remote county in Wyoming are generally high. Our results also suggest that both family social networks and mental health status are important predictors of resilience among these individuals. According to Fiori et al. [31], many types of social networks may contribute to relationship satisfaction in older adults and ultimately to better or worse health outcomes. For example, unmarried older adults often report lower physical and psychological wellbeing than married couples, and widowed women with friend-focused social networks report higher wellbeing than unmarried individuals. Older adults vary in the types and quantities of support needed from their social networks at different times. Utilizing networks in ways that serve the specific needs of older individuals is a likely contributor to the goal of successful aging via physical and psychological benefits, which also have potential to foster resilience [31]. With respect to social networks, results from this study suggest that family members are particularly important social resources that are associated with resilience among rural and remote older residents. In regions of the country where populations are widely dispersed, formal support resources are less likely to be directly on hand to provide assistance when it is needed. Thus, compared to more densely populated areas, family members of older adults living in remote areas may be required to step in more frequently when crises occur. It is possible that resilience can be fostered among residents in rural and remote communities by policies and programs that provide support for family members who may provide care for older residents.

Our results suggest that rural and remote, older persons with better functioning in the mental health domain also have higher degrees of resilience. This finding corresponds with the research of Fiori et al. [31], who reported similar outcomes. There are a few possible explanations for the association. First, resilience itself functions as an adaptive resource for coping with stressful situations. It may be that flexibility and adaptability serve as a buffer to stressors. Because our data were gathered at a single point in time, it did not take into account the order in which mental health-related issues arose relative to resilience status. Therefore, it is possible that our results reflect mental wellness that resulted from having high resilience, rather than the other way around. Second, older adults whose perceived mental health scores reflect higher levels of functioning may have traits that are more likely to promote and support the development of resilience. For example, older individuals who are able to maintain a positive outlook in the face of aging-related stressors can direct more of their cognitive resources toward productive problem-solving strategies and fewer resources toward monitoring and maintaining their mental health. Regardless of the explanation, our results suggest that encouraging mental health services and supporting access to them by older people in rural and remote areas can have a positive impact on resilience status and coping mechanisms.

Results of this study also expand the previous work of Wells [18] by suggesting that family social network may be an important moderator of the relationship between mental health functioning and resilience. A moderating relationship is one in which a variable—in this case family social networks—increases or decreases the magnitude of the relationship between two different variables [32]. Our findings suggest that strong family social networks can buffer the impact of poor mental health functioning with respect to its influence on resilience. In other words, when older rural and remote individuals experience mental health problems, strong family networks and the support they provide can help to make up the difference and restore resilience to levels near to those without mental health issues.

Dumitrache and colleagues [33] suggested that types of stressors and cultural contexts could impact the effects of social support in promoting resilience. Among older adults, factors associated with rural or remote living might strengthen, modify, or diminish relationships between social support, physical health status, and resilience. For example, Moore and colleagues [34] examined the interrelationships of perceived stress, social support, and self-reported successful aging and found that the influence of perceived stress on the relationship between physical functioning and self-reported successful aging was stronger among those with high levels of social support. Among rural and remote older adults in our study, physical health status did not predict resilience as it did in the study by Wells [18] and, thus, did not moderate the relationship between social support and resilience. It could be that the influence of the rural, Western context of participants in this study had a different influence compared to the rural Eastern context in which Wells' participants were recruited. One variable that may differ between the two samples is perceived stress. While neither this study nor the study by Wells [18] included a measure of perceived stress, this construct may have influenced relationships among the variables in both studies. Additional work that incorporates other potentially influential variables such as perceived stress and coping strategies might lead to greater understanding of the relationships between these variables.

This study is important to consider within the context of several limitations. First, like Wells [18, 22], we used mailed surveys to collect our data. Employing self-reported responses acquired through a mailed survey may not have captured the actual average level of resilience in rural and remote community-dwelling older adults. Selection bias may have limited participation by individuals with lower levels of resilience. The response rate in this study was 43%. While this rate was good, those with better health status, social networks, or resilience may have been more likely to respond. Additionally, although surveys were printed in 14-point font, participants with low visual acuity, chronic conditions, or low literacy may have been less able and less likely to respond to the survey. If this were the case, then our results might not generalize to those populations. This study did not gather information on all nonresponders. Therefore, it is not possible to discern how health status, social networks, or resilience may have differed among responding and nonresponding groups. Third, while this study addressed size and quality of social networks, other related constructs such as social connectedness, isolation, and loneliness were not measured. Other social network-related constructs should be addressed in future research. Fourth, as noted above, our study design was cross-sectional and, therefore, it is not possible to know with certainty the order of effects that we reported (i.e., whether mental health status precedes resilience, or the other way around). Future research that utilizes longitudinal data to assess how associations between social networks, health dimensions, and resilience levels covary over time would improve understanding of causal associations between these constructs. Lastly, our study only included older adults residing in rural and remote areas. Therefore, comparison of resilience and relationships of social networks and health status to resilience between rural and urban samples was not possible. Work by Wells [22] showed that resilience levels of older adults did not statistically differ depending on whether participants lived in rural, urban, or suburban areas. Thus, it is possible that there are no differences among older adults in these settings and that these results could generalize to older adults regardless of the size of their communities. However, it is also possible that older adults in rural versus urban settings utilize healthcare and mental health resources differently and/or that family and friend networks play unique roles in the lives of rural older adults compared to their more urban counterparts. Therefore, future work should include samples of rural, urban, and suburban residents to understand better the interplay of these constructs in each subgroup.

In addition to its statistical contribution, this study has clinical implications that are worthy of mention. The Institute of Medicine Report "Retooling for an Aging America: Building a Better Workforce" [35] echoes the recognized need for a workforce that is trained to meet the growing healthcare demands of an aging population. This report calls for an expansion of the roles of many members of the healthcare workforce including informal caregivers and direct care workers to improve care access [35]. While much attention has been given to mental health screening in primary care, other members of the workforce should also be prepared to identify mental health symptoms common among older adults. Moreover, all members of the healthcare workforce should have access to tools to assess social isolation among older adults and refer those individuals who are isolated or at risk for social isolation to community resources in order to prevent isolation or increasing isolation.

The inclusion of social supports in mental health interventions may also serve in mental health access and improve outcomes among older individuals facing mental health challenges. While collaborative care models have shown success for improving mental health outcomes, modifications of these models to include peer specialists to assist with transportation and delivery of basic interventions have shown success in improving access to care within small practices, such as those found in rural areas [36]. The delivery of socialization interventions by way of telehealth is another strategy to improve access to mental health services as well as health outcomes. For example, recent work by Choi and colleagues showed that tele-problem-solving therapy delivered through a Skype video call was an efficacious treatment for low-income homebound older adults [37]. Similarly, Jimison and colleagues [38] designed an intervention to increase social contact time of older adults in the home by enrolling them and a remote family member in a Skype-based health-coaching project. This program included weekly activities to meet target socialization goals as part of an individualized plan. Whereas positive impacts of telehealth interventions implemented to increase contact with social networks are feasible, additional challenges persist, such as lack of adequate technological infrastructure in rural areas to support cutting edge advancements that older adults in more urban regions may take for granted. Thus additional studies are needed to examine the specific needs and resources of older rural residents and their communities and the efficacy of technology for building strong social networks and improving mental health and resilience outcomes among rural and remote older adults.

Competing Interests

The authors declare that they have no competing interests.

References

[1] US Census Bureau, *State & County QuickFacts*, United States Census Bureau, Suitland, Md, USA, 2014.

[2] N. Glasgow, "Rural/urban patterns of aging and caregiving in the United States," *Journal of Family Issues*, vol. 21, no. 5, pp. 611–631, 2000.

[3] A. Kochera, A. Straight, and T. Guterbock, *A Report to the Nation on Livable Communities: Creating Environments for Successful Aging*, AARP, Washington, DC, USA, 2005.

[4] S. T. Syed, B. S. Gerber, and L. K. Sharp, "Traveling towards disease: transportation barriers to health care access," *Journal of Community Health*, vol. 38, no. 5, pp. 976–993, 2013.

[5] P. de Souto Barreto, "Participation bias in postal surveys among older adults: the role played by self-reported health, physical functional decline and frailty," *Archives of Gerontology and Geriatrics*, vol. 55, no. 3, pp. 592–598, 2012.

[6] M. E. Miller, W. J. Rejeski, B. A. Reboussin, T. R. Ten Have, and W. H. Ettinger, "Physical activity, functional limitations, and disability in older adults," *Journal of the American Geriatrics Society*, vol. 48, no. 10, pp. 1264–1272, 2000.

[7] C. Wrzus, M. Hänel, J. Wagner, and F. J. Neyer, "Social network changes and life events across the life span: a meta-analysis," *Psychological Bulletin*, vol. 139, no. 1, pp. 53–80, 2013.

[8] J. M. Poterba, "Retirement security in an aging population," *The American Economic Review*, vol. 104, no. 5, pp. 1–30, 2014.

[9] Q. Q. Tiet, D. Huizinga, and H. F. Byrnes, "Predictors of resilience among inner-city youths," *Journal of Child and Family Studies*, vol. 19, no. 3, pp. 360–378, 2010.

[10] G. Wagnild, "Resilience and successful aging: comparison among low and high income older adults," *Journal of Gerontological Nursing*, vol. 29, no. 12, pp. 42–49, 2003.

[11] J. W. Rowe and R. L. Kahn, "Successful aging and disease prevention," *Advances in Renal Replacement Therapy*, vol. 7, no. 1, pp. 70–77, 2000.

[12] O. Friborg, O. Hjemdal, J. H. Rosenvinge, M. Martinussen, P. M. Aslaksen, and M. A. Flaten, "Resilience as a moderator of pain and stress," *Journal of Psychosomatic Research*, vol. 61, no. 2, pp. 213–219, 2006.

[13] P. Karoly and L. S. Ruehlman, "Psychological 'resilience' and its correlates in chronic pain: findings from a national community sample," *Pain*, vol. 123, no. 1-2, pp. 90–97, 2006.

[14] G. Netuveli, R. D. Wiggins, S. M. Montgomery, Z. Hildon, and D. Blane, "Mental health and resilience at older ages: bouncing back after adversity in the British Household Panel Survey," *Journal of Epidemiology and Community Health*, vol. 62, no. 11, pp. 987–991, 2008.

[15] C. A. Emlet, S. Tozay, and V. H. Raveis, "'I'm not going to die from the AIDS': resilience in aging with HIV disease," *The Gerontologist*, vol. 51, no. 1, pp. 101–111, 2011.

[16] K. M. Bennett, "How to achieve resilience as an older widower: turning points or gradual change?" *Ageing and Society*, vol. 30, no. 3, pp. 369–382, 2010.

[17] S. E. Hardy, J. Concato, and T. M. Gill, "Resilience of community-dwelling older persons," *Journal of the American Geriatrics Society*, vol. 52, no. 2, pp. 257–262, 2004.

[18] M. Wells, "Resilience in rural community-dwelling older adults," *Journal of Rural Health*, vol. 25, no. 4, pp. 415–419, 2009.

[19] T. D. Windsor, P. Rioseco, K. L. Fiori, R. G. Curtis, and H. Booth, "Structural and functional social network attributes moderate the association of self-rated health with mental health in midlife and older adults," *International Psychogeriatrics*, vol. 28, no. 1, pp. 49–61, 2016.

[20] T. Li and Y. Zhang, "Social network types and the health of older adults: exploring reciprocal associations," *Social Science & Medicine*, vol. 130, pp. 59–68, 2015.

[21] S. B. Rafnsson, A. Shankar, and A. Steptoe, "Longitudinal influences of social network characteristics on subjective well-being of older adults: findings from the ELSA study," *Journal of Aging and Health*, vol. 27, no. 5, pp. 919–934, 2015.

[22] M. Wells, "Resilience in older adults living in rural, suburban, and urban areas," *Journal of Rural Nursing & Health Care*, vol. 10, no. 2, pp. 45–54, 2010.

[23] Economic Research Service USDA: Rural-Urban Continuum Codes, 2013.

[24] K. M. Connor and J. R. T. Davidson, "Development of a new resilience scale: the Connor-Davidson resilience scale (CD-RISC)," *Depression and Anxiety*, vol. 18, no. 2, pp. 76–82, 2003.

[25] J. Ware, M. Kosinski, D. M. Turner-Bowker, and B. Gandek, *User's Manual for the SF-12v2 Health Survey*, Quality Metric Incoroporated, Lincoln, RI, USA, 2007.

[26] J. Lubben, E. Blozik, G. Gillmann et al., "Performance of an abbreviated version of the Lubben Social Network Scale among three European community-dwelling older adult populations," *The Gerontologist*, vol. 46, no. 4, pp. 503–513, 2006.

[27] IBM Corp, *IBM SPSS Statistics for Windows*, Version 22.0., IBM Corp, Armonk, NY, USA, 2013.

[28] A. F. Hayes, *PROCESS: A Versatile Computational Tool for Observed Variable Mediation, Moderation, and Conditional Process Modeling*, 2012.

[29] A. F. Hayes and L. Cai, "Using heteroskedasticity-consistent standard error estimators in OLS regression: an introduction and software implementation," *Behavior Research Methods*, vol. 39, no. 4, pp. 709–722, 2007.

[30] S. A. Spiller, G. J. Fitzsimons, J. G. Lynch Jr., and G. H. McClelland, "Spotlights, floodlights,andthe magic number zero: simple effects tests in moderated regression," *Journal of Marketing Research*, vol. 50, no. 2, pp. 277–288, 2013.

[31] K. L. Fiori, J. Smith, and T. C. Antonucci, "Social network types among older adults: a multidimensional approach," *The Journals of Gerontology, Series B: Psychological Sciences and Social Sciences*, vol. 62, no. 6, pp. P322–P330, 2007.

[32] R. M. Baron and D. A. Kenny, "The moderator-mediator variable distinction in social psychological research. Conceptual, strategic, and statistical considerations," *Journal of Personality and Social Psychology*, vol. 51, no. 6, pp. 1173–1182, 1986.

[33] C. G. Dumitrache, L. Rubio, and R. Rubio-Herrera, "Perceived health status and life satisfaction in old age, and the moderating role of social support," *Aging & Mental Health*, 2016.

[34] R. C. Moore, L. T. Eyler, B. T. Mausbach et al., "Complex interplay between health and successful aging: role of perceived stress, resilience, and social support," *The American Journal of Geriatric Psychiatry*, vol. 23, no. 6, pp. 622–632, 2015.

[35] Institute of Medicine, *Retooling for an Aging America: Building the healthcare Workforce*, Institute of Medicine, Washington, DC, USA, 2008.

[36] A. L. Rollins and D. Frantz, "Peer specialists in collaborative care for older adults with depression," *Psychiatric Services*, vol. 66, no. 9, pp. 1000–1001, 2015.

[37] N. G. Choi, M. T. Hegel, C. N. Marti, M. L. Marinucci, L. Sirrianni, and M. L. Bruce, "Telehealth problem-solving therapy for depressed low-income homebound older adults," *The American Journal of Geriatric Psychiatry*, vol. 22, no. 3, pp. 263–271, 2014.

[38] H. B. Jimison, K. A. Klein, and J. L. Marcoe, "A socialization intervention in remote health coaching for older adults in the home," in *Proceedings of the 35th Annual International Conference of the IEEE Engineering in Medicine and Biology Society (EMBC '13)*, pp. 7025–7028, Osaka, Japan, July 2013.

Permissions

All chapters in this book were first published in JAR, by Hindawi Publishing Corporation; hereby published with permission under the Creative Commons Attribution License or equivalent. Every chapter published in this book has been scrutinized by our experts. Their significance has been extensively debated. The topics covered herein carry significant findings which will fuel the growth of the discipline. They may even be implemented as practical applications or may be referred to as a beginning point for another development.

The contributors of this book come from diverse backgrounds, making this book a truly international effort. This book will bring forth new frontiers with its revolutionizing research information and detailed analysis of the nascent developments around the world.

We would like to thank all the contributing authors for lending their expertise to make the book truly unique. They have played a crucial role in the development of this book. Without their invaluable contributions this book wouldn't have been possible. They have made vital efforts to compile up to date information on the varied aspects of this subject to make this book a valuable addition to the collection of many professionals and students.

This book was conceptualized with the vision of imparting up-to-date information and advanced data in this field. To ensure the same, a matchless editorial board was set up. Every individual on the board went through rigorous rounds of assessment to prove their worth. After which they invested a large part of their time researching and compiling the most relevant data for our readers.

The editorial board has been involved in producing this book since its inception. They have spent rigorous hours researching and exploring the diverse topics which have resulted in the successful publishing of this book. They have passed on their knowledge of decades through this book. To expedite this challenging task, the publisher supported the team at every step. A small team of assistant editors was also appointed to further simplify the editing procedure and attain best results for the readers.

Apart from the editorial board, the designing team has also invested a significant amount of their time in understanding the subject and creating the most relevant covers. They scrutinized every image to scout for the most suitable representation of the subject and create an appropriate cover for the book.

The publishing team has been an ardent support to the editorial, designing and production team. Their endless efforts to recruit the best for this project, has resulted in the accomplishment of this book. They are a veteran in the field of academics and their pool of knowledge is as vast as their experience in printing. Their expertise and guidance has proved useful at every step. Their uncompromising quality standards have made this book an exceptional effort. Their encouragement from time to time has been an inspiration for everyone.

The publisher and the editorial board hope that this book will prove to be a valuable piece of knowledge for researchers, students, practitioners and scholars across the globe.

List of Contributors

J. van Hoof, R. A. Overdiep, M. E. Nieboer and E. S. Aarts
Fontys University of Applied Sciences, Fontys EGT-Centre for Healthcare and Technology, Dominee Theodor Fliednerstraat 2, 5631 BN Eindhoven, Netherlands
Fontys University of Applied Sciences, Institute of Allied Health Professions, Dominee Theodor Fliednerstraat 2, 5631 BN Eindhoven, Netherlands

E. J. M. Wouters, C. Vissers-Luijcks, C. S. van der Voort and M. J. G. A. Moonen
Fontys University of Applied Sciences, Institute of Allied Health Professions, Dominee Theodor Fliednerstraat 2, 5631 BN Eindhoven, Netherlands

M. H. Wetzels
Department of Industrial Design, Eindhoven University of Technology, Den Dolech 2, 5612 AZ Eindhoven, Netherlands

P. J. L. M. van Gorkom, A. M. C. Dooremalen and C. J. M. L. van Dijck-Heinen
Fontys University of Applied Sciences, Fontys EGT-Centre for Healthcare and Technology, Dominee Theodor Fliednerstraat 2, 5631 BN Eindhoven, Netherlands
Fontys School of People and Health Studies, Fontys University of Applied Sciences, Dominee Theodor Fliednerstraat 2, 5631 BN Eindhoven, Netherlands

A. M. E. Eyck
Fontys University of Applied Sciences, Fontys EGT-Centre for Healthcare and Technology, Dominee Theodor Fliednerstraat 2, 5631 BN Eindhoven, Netherlands
Fontys University of Applied Sciences, Institute of Information and Communication Technology, Rachelsmolen 1, 5612 MA Eindhoven, Netherlands

L. M. Zwerts-Verhelst
Fontys University of Applied Sciences, Fontys EGT-Centre for Healthcare and Technology, Dominee Theodor Fliednerstraat 2, 5631 BN Eindhoven, Netherlands
Fontys University of Applied Sciences, Institute of Human Resource Management and Psychology, Emmasingel 28, 5611 AZ Eindhoven, Netherlands

H. A. van de Vrande
Fontys University of Applied Sciences, Institute of Engineering, Rachelsmolen 1, 5612 MA Eindhoven, Netherlands

Megan E. O'Connell and Margaret Crossley
Department of Psychology, Room 183 Arts Building, 9 Campus Drive, University of Saskatchewan, SK, Canada S7N 5A5

Vanina Dal Bello-Haas
School of Rehabilitation Science, McMaster University, Hamilton, ON, Canada L8S 1C7

Debra Morgan
Canadian Centre for Health and Safety in Agriculture, University of Saskatchewan, SK, Canada S7N 5E5

Rebecca J. Green-LaPierre and N. Theresa Glanville
Department of Applied Human Nutrition, Mount Saint Vincent University, Halifax, NS, Canada B3M 2J6

Patricia L. Williams
Department of Applied Human Nutrition, Mount Saint Vincent University, Halifax, NS, Canada B3M 2J6
Atlantic Health Promotion Research Centre, Dalhousie University, Halifax, NS, Canada B3H 3J5

Deborah Norris
Department of Family Studies and Gerontology, Mount Saint Vincent University, Halifax, NS, Canada B3M 2J6

Heather C. Hunter and Cynthia G. Watt
Participatory Food Costing Project, Mount Saint Vincent University, Halifax, NS, Canada B3M 2J6

Teslime Ayaz
Department of Internal Medicine, Faculty of Medicine, Recep Tayyip Erdogan University, Rize 53100, Turkey

Serap Baydur Sahin
Department of Endocrinology, Faculty of Medicine, Recep Tayyip Erdogan University, Rize 53100, Turkey

Osman Zikrullah Sahin
Department of Nephrology, Faculty of Medicine, Recep Tayyip Erdogan University, Rize 53100, Turkey

Ozlem Bilir
Department of Emergency, Faculty of Medicine, Recep Tayyip Erdogan University, Rize 53100, Turkey

Halil RakJcJ
Department of Gastroenterology, Faculty of Medicine, Recep Tayyip Erdogan University, Rize 53100, Turkey

Raymond L. Ownby
Department of Psychiatry and Behavioral Medicine, Nova Southeastern University, Fort Lauderdale, FL 33318, USA

Drenna Waldrop-Valverde
Emory University, Atlanta, GA 30322, USA

Kelly Carr, Patricia L. Weir and Nadia R. Azar
Department of Kinesiology, University of Windsor, 401 Sunset Avenue, Windsor, ON, Canada N9B 3P4

Dory Azar
Dory Azar Architect, 870 Revland Drive, Tecumseh, ON, Canada N8N 5B2

Ellinor Edfors and Albert Westergren
The PRO-CARE Group, School of Health and Society, Kristianstad University, 291 88 Kristianstad, Sweden

Julie Norstrand
Boston College Graduate School of Social Work, McGuinn Hall, Chestnut Hill, MA 02467, USA

Keith T. Chan
School of Social Welfare, University at Albany, State University of New York, 135 Western Avenue, Richardson 277, Albany, NY 12222, USA

A. Nayena Blankson
Department of Psychology, Spelman College, 350 Spelman Lane S.W, Atlanta, GA 30314, USA

John J. McArdle
Department of Psychology, University of Southern California, 711 Seeley G. Mudd Building, Los Angeles, CA 90089, USA

Patrício Soares Costa, Nadine Correia Santos and Nuno Sousa
Life and Health Sciences Research Institute (ICVS), School of Health Sciences, University of Minho, 4710-057 Braga, Portugal
ICVS/3B's, PT Government Associate Laboratory, Guimarães, 4710-057 Braga, Portugal

Pedro Cunha and Jorge Cotter
Life and Health Sciences Research Institute (ICVS), School of Health Sciences, University of Minho, 4710-057 Braga, Portugal
ICVS/3B's, PT Government Associate Laboratory, Guimarães, 4710-057 Braga, Portugal
Centro Hospital Alto Ave, EPE, 4810-055 Guimarães, Portugal

Martin Sénéchal
Children's Hospital Research Institute of Manitoba, Winnipeg, MB, Canada R3E 3P4
Department of Pediatrics and Child Health, Faculty of Medicine, University of Manitoba, Winnipeg, MB, Canada R3E 3P4

Jana Slaght
Faculty of Kinesiology and Recreation Management, University of Manitoba, Winnipeg, MB, Canada R3T 2N2

Danielle R. Bouchard
Faculty of Kinesiology and Recreation Management, University of Manitoba, Winnipeg, MB, Canada R3T 2N2
Health, Leisure, and Human Performance Research Institute, Winnipeg, MB, Canada R3T 2N2

Carla J. Thompson and Nancy L. Bridier
University of West Florida, Pensacola, FL 32514, USA
Research and Advanced Studies, University of West Florida, 11000 University Parkway, Building 78, Office 121, Pensacola, FL 32514, USA

Elizabeth Procter-Gray, Jie Cheng, Kevin Kane and Wenjun Li
Health Statistics and Geography Lab, Division of Preventive and Behavioral Medicine, University of Massachusetts Medical School, 55 Lake Avenue North, Worcester, MA 01655, USA

Suzanne G. Leveille
College of Nursing and Health Sciences, University of Massachusetts Boston, 100 Morrissey Boulevard, Boston, MA 02125-3393, USA

Marian T. Hannan
Institute for Aging Research, Hebrew Senior Life/ Harvard Medical School and Beth Israel Deaconess Medical Center, 1200 Centre Street, Boston, MA 02131-1097, USA

S. A. Maris, D. Quintanilla, F. Xu and M. J. Delmonico
Department of Kinesiology, University of Rhode Island, Kingston, RI 02881, USA

A. Taetzsch and I. Lofgren
Department of Nutrition and Food Sciences, University of Rhode Island, Kingston, RI 02881, USA

A. Picard, J. Letendre and L. Mahler
Department of Communicative Disorders, University of Rhode Island, Kingston, RI 02881, USA

Shannon M. Sisco and Michael Marsiske
Department of Clinical and Health Psychology, University of Florida, Gainesville, FL 32610, USA

Sophie von Stumm
Department of Psychology, University of Edinburgh, 7 George Square, EH8 9JZ Edinburgh, UK

Md. Nuruzzaman Haque
Department of Population Science and Human Resource Development, University of Rajshahi, Rajshahi 6205, Bangladesh

Cecilia Fagerström
Blekinge Center of Competence, Karlskrona, Sweden
Department of Health and Caring Sciences, Linnaeus University, 391 82 Kalmar, Sweden

Lena Sandin Wranker
Department of Health Sciences, Division of Geriatric Medicine, Lund University, Lund, Sweden

Sathirakorn Pongpanich and Robert S. Chapman
College of Public Health Sciences, Chulalongkorn University, Pathumwan, Bangkok 10330, Thailand

Pattaraporn Khongboon
College of Public Health Sciences, Chulalongkorn University, Pathumwan, Bangkok 10330, Thailand
Prince Mahidol Award Foundation under the Royal Patronage, Faculty of Medicine, Siriraj Hospital, Bangkoknoi, Bangkok 10700, Thailand

Thiago Matheus da Silva Sousa, Tânia Maria Gaspar Novais and Paula de Lourdes Lauande Oliveira
Physical Education Department, Ceuma University, São Luis, MA, Brazil

Olivia de Moraes Ruberti, Bruno Rodrigues and Marco Carlos Uchida
Faculty of Physical Education, University of Campinas (UNICAMP), Campinas, SP, Brazil

Paulo Adriano Schwingel
Human Performance Research Laboratory, University of Pernambuco, Petrolina, PE, Brazil

Janaína Oliveira Bentivi Pulcherio
Health Science Graduate Programs, Federal University of Maranhão, São Luis, MA, Brazil

Gilberto Santos Morais Junior, Nathalia Oliveira Rodrigues, Adriane Dallanora Henriques and Otàvio Toledo Nóbrega
Universidade de Brasília, 70910-900 Brasília, DF, Brazil

Audrey Cecília Tonet-Furioso and Clayton Franco Moraes
Universidade de Brasília, 70910-900 Brasília, DF, Brazil
Universidade Católica de Brasília, 71966-700 ´Aguas Claras, DF, Brazil

Lucy Oliveira Gomes
Universidade Católica de Brasília, 71966-700 ´Aguas Claras, DF, Brazil

Ciro José Brito
Universidade Federal de Juiz de Fora, 36036-330 Juiz de Fora, MG, Brazil

Isabela Feitosa de Carvalho and Gianluca Loyolla Montanari Leme
Human Development and Technologies, UNESP, Rio Claro, SP, Brazil

Marcos Eduardo Scheicher
Human Development and Technologies, UNESP, Rio Claro, SP, Brazil
Physical Therapy, UNESP, Marília, SP, Brazil

Mathias Haeger and Otmar Bock
Institute of Physiology and Anatomy, German Sport University Cologne, Am Sport park Müngersdorf 6, 50933 Cologne, Germany

Daniel Memmert and Stefanie Hüttermann
Institute of Training and Computer Science in Sport, German Sport University Cologne, Am Sportpark Müngersdorf 6, 50933 Cologne, Germany

Richard C. Palmer, Anamica Batra, Chelsie Anderson, Timothy Page and Laura Seff
Robert Stempel College of Public Health and Social Work, 11200 SW8th Street, Miami, FL 33199,USA

Edgar Vieira
College of Nursing and Health Sciences, 11200 SW8th Street, Miami, FL 33199, USA

Christine McKibbin, Aaron Lee, Bernard A. Steinman, Catherine Carrico, Katelynn Bourassa and Andrea Slosser
University of Wyoming, 1000 E. University Avenue, Laramie, WY 82071, USA

Index

A
Active Ageing Index, 159, 162, 164-166
Activities Of Daily Living, 1-2, 15-16, 18, 23, 25, 33, 36, 51-52, 54-56, 58, 66, 68-69, 84, 126, 143, 148, 151, 160, 176, 185, 187
Aerobic Activities, 133
Alanine Aminotransferase, 39, 41-43
Alzheimer Disease, 15, 24-25
Anemia, 39-40, 134
Arthritis, 32, 59, 85, 131-132, 189, 199, 202
Aspartate Aminotransferase, 39, 41-42

B
Body Mass Index, 39, 66, 105, 111-112, 124, 126, 131, 133, 136, 196-197

C
C-reactive Protein, 39, 41-42, 196-197
Cardiovascular Disease, 28, 32, 39-40, 69, 133-134, 151
Chronic Degenerative Diseases, 190
Chronic Disease, 28, 51, 57, 101, 133, 180-183, 185, 187-188, 193, 221-222
Chronic Obstructive Pulmonary Disease, 41
Cognitive Dimensions, 69, 93, 95-96, 98-100
Cognitive Functioning, 51, 78-79, 81-82, 101, 103, 139, 157
Cognitive Plasticity, 147
Cognitive Skills, 78, 148, 214
Colorectal Cancer, 41
Comparative Fit Index, 80, 144, 162-164
Coronary Artery, 111, 189, 193, 196, 199-200
Coronary Bypass, 95
Crystallized Ability, 152-155
Cumulative Weight Exposure, 105, 107-108

D
Dementia, 2, 9, 11-12, 14-16, 18-19, 21-26, 41, 58, 103, 142, 169, 188
Depression, 15-16, 18, 22-24, 26, 30, 34, 41, 53, 59, 63, 82, 115, 117-120, 122, 141, 173-174, 185, 189, 229-230
Diabetes Mellitus, 38-40, 95, 103, 195, 197, 199
Diastolic Blood Pressure, 39, 189-190, 197
Dietary Screening Tool, 135-136
Disability Risk, 176-177, 181, 184

E
Engagement Hypothesis, 152
Episodic Memory, 78-81, 143
Erythrocyte Sedimentation Rate, 39, 41-42

F
Fasting Blood Glucose, 189-190

G
Gait Speed, 124, 126, 130, 134, 137, 201-206
Glycated Hemoglobin, 196-197

H
High-density Lipoprotein, 39, 41-42, 190, 197
Hopkins Verbal Learning Test, 143, 150
Human Development Index, 164
Hypernatremia, 38, 40-43
Hypertriglyceridemia, 38, 40-43
Hypoalbuminemia, 38, 40-43
Hypopotassemia, 38, 40-43

I
Intellectual Investment, 153, 157
Intima-media Thickness, 195-199
Investment Trait Scale, 152

L
Left Carotid Artery, 195, 197
Leg Extensor Torque, 135
Lewy Body Disease, 16
Life-span Perspective Approach, 113
Low-density Lipoprotein, 39, 42, 189-190, 197
Lower Limb Exoskeleton, 85

M
Mean Platelet Volume, 39, 41
Metabolic Complication Risk, 95
Metabolic Disorders, 197
Metabolic Syndrome, 39, 44, 101, 103
Mild Cognitive Impairment, 15-16, 25-26, 103, 157
Mini Nutritional Assessment, 59, 66, 174
Mini-mental State Exam, 79, 81, 131
Myocardial Infarction, 36, 41, 62, 95, 196

N
Neuropsychiatric Inventory, 18, 25

P
Physical Component Summary Score, 225-226
Posterior Cingulate, 16
Posttraumatic Stress Disorder, 114

Q

Quality Of Life, 1-2, 6, 13, 31, 36, 52-53, 57, 59, 65-67, 90, 139, 159, 167-168, 173-175, 188, 221, 223

R

Recreational Walking, 123-127, 130-131

Resistance Training, 133-134, 137, 139, 189-194

Robotic Exoskeleton, 85, 90-91

S

Sarcopenia, 57, 66, 133, 193

Short Physical Performance Battery, 124, 126, 131, 134

Single-nucleotide Polymorphism, 196

Somatosensory, 201

Subpatellar Bandage, 201-205

Systemic Arterial Hypertension, 195, 197

Systolic Blood Pressure, 142, 189-190, 197

T

Thyroid Stimulating Hormone, 40-43

Triglycerides, 189-190, 196-197

U

Utilitarian Walking, 123-127, 130-132

V

Verbal Fluency, 45-46, 95, 142, 147, 154

Visuomotor Guidance System, 85

www.ingramcontent.com/pod-product-compliance
Lightning Source LLC
LaVergne TN
LVHW081037210926
848485LV00004B/1041